The Ethics Police?

Other books by Robert Klitzman

A Year-long Night: Tales of a Medical Internship
In a House of Dreams and Glass: Becoming a Psychiatrist
Being Positive: The Lives of Men and Women with HIV
The Trembling Mountain: A Personal Account of Kuru, Cannibals and
Mad Cow Disease
Mortal Secrets: Truth and Lies in the Age of AIDS (With Ronald Bayer)
When Doctors Become Patients
Am I My Genes?: Confronting Fate and Family Secrets in the Age
of Genetic Testing

The Ethics Police?

The Struggle to Make Human Research Safe

ROBERT L. KLITZMAN, M.D.

OXFORD
UNIVERSITY PRESS

OXFORD
UNIVERSITY PRESS

Oxford University Press is a department of the University of
Oxford. It furthers the University's objective of excellence in research,
scholarship, and education by publishing worldwide.

Oxford   New York
Auckland   Cape Town   Dar es Salaam   Hong Kong   Karachi
Kuala Lumpur   Madrid   Melbourne   Mexico City   Nairobi
New Delhi   Shanghai   Taipei   Toronto

With offices in
Argentina   Austria   Brazil   Chile   Czech Republic   France   Greece
Guatemala   Hungary   Italy   Japan   Poland   Portugal   Singapore
South Korea   Switzerland   Thailand   Turkey   Ukraine   Vietnam

Oxford is a registered trademark of Oxford University Press
in the UK and certain other countries.

Published in the United States of America by
Oxford University Press
198 Madison Avenue, New York, NY 10016

Library of Congress Cataloging-in-Publication Data
Klitzman, Robert, author.
The ethics police? : the struggle to make human research safe / Robert L. Klitzman.
    p. ; cm.
ISBN 978-0-19-936460-2
I. Title.
[DNLM: 1. Ethics Committees, Research—United States.   2. Government Regulation—
United States.   3. Ethics, Research—United States.   4. Human Experimentation—ethics—
United States.   W 20.55.E7]
R853.H8
174.2'8—dc23
2014021924

9 8 7 6 5 4 3 2
Printed in the United States of America
on acid-free paper

Three umpires were once talking amongst themselves.
"I calls 'em as they is," the first one said.
"No, I calls them as I sees 'em," the second one said.
"No," responded the third. "They ain't nothing till I calls 'em"
—Old joke

Whoever hath an *absolute Authority* to interpret any written, or spoken Law, it is *He*, who is truly the *Law-giver*, to all intents and Purposes; not the Person who first wrote, or spoke them.
—Bishop of Bangor, *preaching before the King of England on March 31, 1717*

But who will guard the guards?
—Juvenal

To the men and women who shared their views and experiences with me for this book, and to Rénee C. Fox for her extraordinary guidance and inspiration.

CONTENTS

INTRODUCTION

CHAPTER 1

Protecting the People We Experiment on

"The experiment worked," the doctor told me, "but the patient died." The patient was my father. At the age of 78, my father had been diagnosed with acute myelogenous leukemia—skyrocketing numbers of white blood cells. Three months earlier, this same doctor had told me that my father would probably live only three months—that no effective therapy existed for adults with his disease, and that most doctors would not offer any intervention. "We could try chemotherapy," the doctor offered, "but it would be a bit of an experiment."

"What are the odds it might work?" I asked.

"Without it, he will probably die within three months. With it, there's a 50 percent chance he could live an additional 3 to 18 months." The doctor's tone was upbeat. He seemed optimistic.

Medicine inherently involves trial and error. Hence, as a newly minted physician and researcher—although in other areas, not cancer—I valued experiments in clinical care, whether for an individual patient or a large group. Doctors regularly publish the results of ever-evolving approaches to treating cancer and other diseases. Over the years, experimentation on human beings, whether formal or informal, has aided countless individuals, and advanced science. Such research has shed light on why we get sick, and helped us develop effective ways to treat everything from heart attacks to depression. Trial and error has yielded new drugs for bacterial pneumonia and HIV, and countless lives are now saved each year by reducing people's cholesterol and high blood pressure. New medical devices have replaced millions of broken hips, knees, and heart valves. Systematic studies to develop vaccines have shielded billions of people from lethal plagues. Science burgeons in ever-new areas, from stem cell research to treatments for the flu. We all are, have been, or will be patients—not to mention the friends and family members of patients—who benefit from these discoveries.

At the same time, every year many patients agree to treatments that may not work—that are, to varying degrees, experimental—for a wide array of diseases.

These efforts range from explicit research studies and clinical trials to risky interventions whose benefits, if any, are unknown or ambiguous. Some trials compare different common but competing therapies; others test new unproven approaches against standard interventions, placebos, or no treatment at all. Doctors may encourage patients and families to try these novel approaches when no proven cure is available; unfortunately, these strategies often fail as well, giving the patient no clear benefit.

When his physician offered chemotherapy, my father was torn. Raised in the Great Depression, my dad was a hard realist. He already felt terrible from the leukemia. But he wasn't ready to give up all hope. My mother thought that the chemotherapy's side effects, on top of his suffering from the cancer, made it too risky.

"What do you think?" he asked me one night by his bedside. He turned to me and looked at me intently, his eyes wide, concentrating on my response as he had only a few other times in my life.

The prospect of my father's death horrified me. I had also just finished my medical training, and was imbued with a sense of the possibilities that medical research offered. "I think you should try it," I said, surprised at how firm my voice sounded. The next day, he agreed—partly, I sensed, because of my answer.

For the next few weeks, he was extremely uncomfortable, with unremitting nausea and malaise. He lost weight, felt weaker, and looked worse. The physician who had suggested the treatment began visiting the room far less frequently.

Three months after he started the drugs, my father's blood count did, in fact, return to normal, but he died almost immediately. The side effects of his treatment had killed him.

The manner of my father's death and my part in it have haunted me ever since. I knew he could die, but I still felt shocked and let down by the fact that science had failed to prolong his life any longer than if he had declined the experimental drugs. Instead, the treatment had arguably made him suffer more, not less. I wondered whether my mother's wish to let him die in peace had been right—whether I had been biased, too "pro-science." Had my father valued my opinion too much? I kept wondering if I or the doctor should have acted differently, if the doctor had presented the chance of success too optimistically, and overly downplayed the risks, and if he should have guided us more thoughtfully through these decisions. My father may have sacrificed the comfort of his final weeks to help other patients in the future. If he had known that, would he have said yes? What unproven treatments *should* we offer patients, and how?

My father's treatment had been an informal experiment—an offer by a physician that we had decided to accept—which happens routinely. As a medical intern, I had worked in a cancer ward where large numbers of patients were on experimental drugs—some, but not all in formal clinical trials. Many of the patients in these trials died as well. They had been told that the odds of success were not high, but they were desperate. Hopefully, all of these deaths furthered scientific knowledge in some way—if only to demonstrate that certain approaches that seemed promising were ineffective.

My father's death made me far more sensitive to the plight of patients and family members confronting fatal illnesses, and the anguish of the decisions they face. I now understood more fully the criticisms that researchers take advantage of the patient's vulnerability pushing risky interventions, rather than encouraging the dying to focus on the quality of the time they have left. At the same time, as a doctor, I knew that the only way to improve treatment of leukemia and other devastating diseases was by experimenting on humans. Indeed, since my father's death, in 1994, subsequent studies have led to the development of a promising new experimental treatment for leukemia involving bone marrow transplants. This approach might have helped him, had it been available. But it was not.

Ethics and Science: Striking a Balance

We are living in a Golden Age of science. In the second half of the 20th century and the start of the 21st, researchers have unraveled the genetic code for all life, glimpsed the inner workings of the human mind as never before, discovered new particles inside of atoms that constitute all matter, and landed spacecrafts on the moon, Mars and comets. Many of the achievements that have advanced biomedicine have also, by necessity, involved human subjects, posing myriad cultural, ethical, and legal questions. These trade-offs are so intricate that every year scandals erupt, unforeseen by those involved. It is tempting to ignore the challenges they pose for the same reason—they represent profound puzzles about science, morals, ethics, greed, knowledge, globalization, and justice—but we must not do so.

Though integral to scientific research, trial and error has failed countless individual patients along the way before benefiting the common good. Ever since Mary Shelley wrote *Frankenstein* in 1818 and doctors began stealing corpses from cemeteries to study the human anatomy, the "mad scientist" who experiments on humans to satisfy his own intellectual curiosity or desire for power or wealth has lurked as a sinister figure in the collective imagination. Rebecca Skloot's 2010 book *The Immortal Life of Henrietta Lacks*, which explores the ethics of using human tissue samples for medical research without the donors' knowledge or consent, was on the *New York Times* best seller list for over a year, and has been translated into more than 25 languages. More recently, Facebook entered 700,000 users into an experiment without their knowledge, manipulating their news feeds—by reducing the number of posts with either positive or negative emotional content that they automatically saw from their friends. In July 2014 of the *Proceedings of the National*

Academy of Sciences, a prestigious scientific journal, published the results showing that the company had thereby been able to alter these users' moods but no informed consent had been obtained. Only after the experiment did Facebook add to its user agreement that it may use data for research. A public outcry erupted.

In July 2014, two Americans acquired Ebola as part of a growing epidemic in Sub-Saharan Africa. They received a new experimental drug that had never before been tried on humans, and over subsequent days, seemed to improve. A world-wide debate ensued as to whether this new drug should now be produced and distributed far more widely, without waiting first for additional tests to examine its potential risks and benefits—whether in this public health emergency, the usual standards for protecting research subjects should be abandoned, and if so, which patients should receive the experimental medication first. New possible treatments and vaccines being developed against Ebola, as of this writing, pose questions: how much evidence of effectiveness or safety should be required before these products are given to ever increasing numbers of individuals.

Most people take for granted that some mechanism exists to balance these often competing scientific and humanist agendas—that some set of laws or group of watchdogs is in place to ensure that scientists who experiment on humans do so in ethical and appropriate ways. Most of us have little or no understanding of what that mechanism is, however, and never will unless we come to feel that it has betrayed us—if even then.

In fact, such safeguards do exist, in the form of Research Ethics Committees (RECs) or, as they are known in the United States, Institutional Review Boards (IRBs). These committees regularly review and approve countless experiments involving human beings in this country.

In recent years, however, these committees have become increasingly contro-versial. Whereas the general public only hears or complains about this system of oversight when an ethical breach comes to light—when a healthy patient dies in a supposedly "low-risk" clinical study, or a researcher is caught falsifying data—researchers regularly criticize IRBs. Investigators frequently argue that these committees are now stymieing rather than supporting scientific progress. Indeed, almost every researcher I know has complained at some point, often vociferously, about an IRB having unnecessarily blocked or delayed his or her research.

The Growing Hostility toward IRBs

These complaints have been mounting, in part because over the past 40 years, since the development of the regulations began, science has burgeoned and evolved, becoming ever more complex. The past four decades have witnessed an extraordi-nary, unheralded explosion of medical research. Every year, the US now spends over $100 billion on biomedical studies—around 30 percent by government (mostly the National Institutes of Health, or NIH), 65 percent by industry, and 5 percent by others.[1] Between 1994 and 2003 alone, the amount tripled.[2] The NIH budget grew from $3.4 million in 1946 to $1.8 billion in 1974 (the year of the National Research Act) to $30 billion in 2009.[3] Since the law that prompted the creation of IRBs was written, the amount of NIH research has increased about 15-fold.

Researchers seek to explore the effects of increasing numbers of genetic and other biological and psychological factors on disease and human behavior, and therefore need to include ever-larger numbers of patients and consequently institutions. Studies of new treatments now often require thousands of subjects, and are therefore conducted at dozens of institutions simultaneously.[4] IRBs at 40 institutions may thus need to approve a single study, and vary in their deliberations, decisions,[5,6] and applications of standards.[7,8] Among placebo-controlled trials, the average number of sites per study has increased 20-fold—from 2 in the 1990s to 40 in the 2000s.[9] One committee might approve a project quickly, while another IRB might send the researcher pages of questions and require multiple changes; such requests for modifications can not only delay the study but also alter its design in ways that make the comparison of data between sites difficult.[10] Studies have shown that IRBs vary in their policies,[11] and can range dramatically in how long they take to approve the same study—from a few days to over a year.[12] Of 21 hospitals participating in one minimal risk study, the amount of time to receive IRB approval ranged from 12 to 960 days, with none of these institutions changing the basic study.[13] In other cases, IRBs at different institutions have altered the same study in different ways that have made the comparison of the results between the sites difficult, thus impeding the science.[10,14] In a study of 37 IRBs reviewing an identical protocol, 16 required no changes, while 21 required alterations, and 4 IRBs' hurdles seemed so insurmountable that the investigators at these institutions decided not to conduct the study at all.[15] IRBs can also require researchers to spend weeks if not months filling out extensive forms that divert limited resources from conducting experiments. For one study reviewed by 52 IRBs, each committee made an average of five changes—76 percent of which involved only differences in institutional language. No committees made substantial changes to the research. But the cost of the 52 separate reviews was over $100,000.[16]

I, too, have felt frustrated. A few years before my father's death, I had wanted to conduct a simple, anonymous survey of patients at my hospital, and had submitted the necessary forms to the IRB to receive approval to do so. I had a 12-month, state-funded fellowship, and therefore had only limited time to conduct the study. Yet, after three months, the committee had still not gotten back to me. The paperwork had taken me over a month to complete. I had phoned the committee *three* times to get an answer. "The reviewer misplaced your paperwork," a secretary finally told me. "You'll have to resubmit everything."

I had lost over four months, and was furious, but received no apology. I resubmitted the paperwork, and a month later received a memo asking for clarification of a few points. I responded the next day, and then waited two more months to receive approval to begin to interview participants. The committee had not asked for any changes in the study, but I had lost almost *eight* months of the 12-month fellowship. The committee also provided no evidence that they recognized the cost of their error to me, the research, or my fledgling career.

Many researchers and critics argue that IRBs now often go too far—that the pendulum has swung too much, and that IRBs frequently delay, alter, or block studies unnecessarily, and have too much power. These observers aver that IRBs have both too much authority and too little expertise to make decisions well. Evidence suggests that many IRBs review too much, too quickly, with too few experts; conduct minimal continuing review of approved research; and provide little training for members and investigators; and that too little attention is paid to evaluating these committees or their effectiveness.[17,18,19,20,21,22,23,24]

Many scholars assert that these committees have become more stringent in ways that do not increase participant protection and in fact detract from the scientific and hence social benefits of research—that these boards *now over*-regulate science. Designed to fight the power of pharmaceutical companies and greedy scientists, these boards, many observers say, now have too much power themselves.

Studies indicate that scientists support the importance of protecting human subjects but feel that IRBs have increasingly focused on small bureaucratic details that detract from the practice of science—and thus from the potential social benefits of the research.[25] Many observers contend that these local committees, established to protect patients, are instead now too often concerned about protecting *institutions* against potential lawsuits from patients. IRBs may engage in "tunnel vision," focusing on editing consent forms rather than on larger ethical issues.[26] Though intended to be instruments of good, these committees have now gone too far, critics argue—blocking important studies and scientific progress.

In some respects, local IRBs have absolute authority: no external appeals process exists. If a committee refuses to let a researcher conduct a study or a particular aspect of it, he or she can ask the same board to reconsider; if the board remains steadfast, however, the researcher must comply—even if the IRB lacks the sufficient necessary scientific expertise to evaluate the study in question.

Critics contend, too, that the current system spends too much time on low-risk studies; and that over the years, physical injury and death have only very rarely occurred in research. Every year, hundreds of thousands of individuals enter clinical trials and do fine and frequently benefit. Each year, in routine clinical care outside of research, medical errors injure and kill hundreds of thousands of patients[27]—doubtless far more than do unethical studies. It is also extremely difficult to judge how effective IRBs are. Ezekiel Emanuel, a bioethicist and oncologist, argues that IRB review cannot realistically prevent the kinds of harms that have occurred in the few well-publicized cases of serious injury.[28]

Granted, if the informed consent or privacy protections are not wholly suffi-cient, so-called dignitary harms may occur, even if the participant suffers no adverse consequences.[25] But critics insist that to prevent such possible non-physical harms, IRBs are diverting too many resources from research itself, hampering science. IRBs cost researchers and institutions significant time and resources,[29] and block certain research without sufficient ethical rationale.[30] Moreover, many research-ers in essence censor their own research by simply deciding not to pursue certain studies if they suspect that their IRBs will disapprove of or significantly alter the project, or require lengthy paperwork.[30]

Consequently, a few legal scholars have claimed that IRBs are in fact uncon-stitutional, impeding free intellectual inquiry and speech.[31] Historically, thinkers from Socrates to Galileo to Darwin have encountered staunch social and insti-tutional opposition, and attempts at censorship. Critics assert that IRBs are now doing the same. Scientists have argued that IRBs prevent them from investigating the issues that they want.

These committees have been chastised, too, for unnecessarily antagonizing researchers who, in response, may then seek to "bend the rules." Complaints about IRBs have become ever more widespread.[28,29,32,33,34,35] Clearly, some over-sight is needed, but many observers see the *status quo* as broken,[36] engaged in over-enforcement, and they recommend regulatory "de-escalation."[37]

If the majority of critics are concerned that current government regulations, designed to protect patients, are impeding science, a significant minority argues that current regulations are also keeping valuable new drugs from those who des-perately need them. Starting with AIDS activists in the late 1980s, patient-advo-cacy groups began to push the Food and Drug Administration (FDA) and the NIH to eliminate many of the bureaucratic hurdles to testing and releasing new medications. Many patient organizations continue to argue for more research on particularly lethal or debilitating diseases, contending that government regula-tions are impeding the development, approval, and availability of new therapies that could save thousands of lives.

But if, as various critics suggest, the current system should be altered and updated to protect subjects more effectively while still advancing science, how exactly should that be done? What changes should be made?

IRBs as a Subject of Study

From the beginning of my medical training, I felt that medical expertise and compassion were essential and complementary aspects of good doctoring, but were not always simultaneously present. As a physician and a son, I had wit-nessed patients dying of cancer because effective treatments didn't exist. Yes I had also observed doctors who were eager to put patients into experiments to try new chemicals that did not seem to offer much more than standard medications, but might benefit a drug company. When the results were later analyzed, my initial wariness often proved well founded.

I also knew first-hand that both doctors and researchers face stresses that can affect their care of patients, and I had witnessed occasional acts of appalling callousness by colleagues and supervisors. On my first day as a medical intern, for instance, my supervising resident gave me a list of the patients I would be treating, and I walked off to begin my rounds. I remember my first patient vividly: the morning sun poured through the window, illuminating the pink grapefruit she sat eating with a shiny metal spoon, as we discussed her cancer. Several minutes later, the supervisor asked me for an update in the hallway and I told him about our conversation.

"Don't waste your time with the dead!" he retorted.

"What do you mean?" I asked, perplexed.

"She's dead. Don't waste your time with her."

He meant that she had cancer spread all over her body, and had signed a Do Not Resuscitate (DNR) order—if her heart or lungs stopped, we would not try to revive her. In his mind, therefore, we could therefore simply ignore her. I felt as if my own heart had stopped.

I soon became interested in medical ethics, and over my subsequent years of training began to study how doctors and patients confront complex dilemmas. For decades, though, I wasn't sure how IRBs fit into the picture. I didn't know how to integrate my mixed feelings about them as a researcher, a doctor, and a son—were they good or bad? Did they do too much or too little? Certainly, I recognized the reasons for their existence; and IRB members and administrators I met over the years all seemed well intentioned. Yet these boards frustrated and angered almost all researchers—including me. How did a process that outsiders hated so much seem to make sense to those inside it? Clearly, a few researchers have behaved unethically, and patients fear research risks and being taken advantage of. But why did many well-respected, seemingly rational scientists so vehemently dislike IRBs?

As a psychiatrist, I was trained to examine how people thought about their lives, actions, and decisions—how they sought to act rationally but did not always succeed. I saw how patients, their loved ones, and their physicians come to view disease, treatment, and the ethical dilemmas they face, and seek to explain and cope with disease. I had also conducted research in medical anthropology and sociology, which made me interested in how organizations operate and can take on lives of their own.

As a doctor, family member, social scientist, and ordinary citizen, I have wondered more and more about the ethics of research on people, and hence about our nation's IRBs—who sits on them, and how they see themselves and weigh their own roles and responsibilities against those of researchers and the rights of subjects. How do or can they effectively sort through all these conflicts and make good decisions?

I searched the academic literature and was astonished to find that few studies of these committees had been published; moreover, these articles were almost all based on simple short questionnaires,[38,39] examining only small, particular aspects of these boards. No studies had probed how IRBs actually made decisions or viewed, or responded to, the full range of these problems or researchers' complaints. Conducting science is ostensibly objective, whereas defining, interpreting, and balancing ethical notions involves inherent ambiguities; despite this obvious fact, how ethical principles get interpreted and applied differently by different people has received little empirical investigation—observing or interviewing people to find out what they actually do.

We are also at a critical juncture—not only in the history of science, but also in the evolution of the university. We like to think that science takes place in a pure world, following pure ideals. And to a significant extent, it does. But increasingly scientists also work in a world of financial strains and constraints, as universities, academic departments, and professors slash budgets; tenure disappears; the NIH's budget flattens; and pharmaceutical companies face falling profits and layoffs.

It seemed to be a crucial moment to delve more deeply into the question of how, exactly, America's IRBs work. Hence, I decided to embark on a journey— interviewing IRB leaders, members, staff, and researchers about these realms to see whether the current system can be improved, and if so, how. What I learned consistently surprised me.

Science versus Human Guinea Pigs

Research on human beings is relatively new. Some historians credit James Lind with having conducted one of the first formal experiments on live humans when, in 1747, he equipped a group of British seamen with lemons and oranges, and then compared them to other seamen. By documenting how many cases of scurvy resulted in each group, he demonstrated both a cause and a cure for the deadly disease.[40,41]

Still, formal human experiments remained relatively rare until the 20th century. The horrors of the Nazi experiments illustrated the tensions between science and human welfare in particularly stark and grotesque terms. Hitler's doctors exposed prisoners to mustard gas, radiation, malaria, and bacteria, and then tried various experimental treatments. These physicians also took advantage of their captive victims to test the limits of physical endurance: for instance, these doctors forced inmates to remain in the snow to see how long it took for them to freeze to death. They also removed limbs to try to reconnect them, but the attempted reattachments all failed.

After the war, in response to these horrors, the Nuremberg Tribunal established principles of research, mandating that all study participants give informed consent.[42] In the following decade, however, even the US government failed to follow these guidelines, secretly infecting prisoners in Guatemala with syphilis to study the natural course of the disease.[43] Throughout the 1950s the US military also experimented on its own soldiers, exposing them without their knowledge to various biological and chemical warfare agents. In the early 1960s, researchers at New York's Willowbrook State School infected intellectually disabled children with hepatitis by feeding the children stool extracts from ill patients.[44]

Outside the US, the Nazi atrocities led the World Medical Association to develop the Declaration of Helsinki in 1964, to address the ethics of medical research.[45] Revised nine times since then, most recently in October 2013, this document now consists of a series of 35 paragraphs, articulating broad principles. It is not, however, legally binding, and translating these broad principles into specific regulations has been an ongoing challenge.

In 1966, in the *New England Journal of Medicine*, Henry Beecher, a Harvard anesthesiologist,[46,47] enumerated 22 cases of egregious ethical violations in research studies that had been published in leading medical journals—experiments conducted without informed consent that potentially harmed subjects without offering them any benefit.[48] The level of public outrage ignited by his article spurred the US Public Health Service (PHS) to require that institutions receiving federal research funds set up research review committees. These committees—early proto-forms of IRBs—reviewed all research funded by this agency to assure "an independent determination of the rights and welfare" of subjects, and to assess "the risks and potential medical benefits of the study."[49] But these guidelines remained vague and ill-defined, and did not mention many other aspects of research studies, such as which subjects should be included. Problems also arose regarding experiments that were not funded by this agency, and/or that researchers assumed were "minimal risk."

In 1963, for instance, Stanley Milgram, a Yale University psychology professor, asked participants to turn knobs on a "shock generator" to deliver electrical charges to a person hidden from view who was, Milgram explained, engaging in a memory test. Each time the examinee gave a wrong answer, Milgram asked the participant to administer a stronger shock. Even after the knob position had reached "XXX—extremely dangerous," and the examinee had screamed out in agony, Milgram told the subjects that the experiment required that they continue to deliver the shocks. Two-thirds of them did so—even after the examinee suddenly fell silent.[50] No shocks were, in fact, delivered: Milgram was using deceit to discover how long his *real* subjects would follow orders. Yet many of them were left traumatized by how far they'd been willing to go rather than question authority.

Similarly, in 1971, Stanford University Professor Philip Zimbardo randomly asked about two dozen college men to act as guards and others as prisoners in a mock prison. The Psychology Department and the University Committee of Human Ethics approved the Zimbardo Stanford Prison Experiment study and the University's legal counsel wrote the informed consent which stated that there would be an invasion of privacy, loss of some civil liberties and harassment.[51] But the "guards" soon began to abuse the "prisoners" verbally and physically; nevertheless, Zimbardo and 50 other observers let the experiment continue. Only after six days, when one observer—a graduate student whom Zimbardo was dating— complained about the severe abuse, did he end the experiment.[51]

In both cases, Milgram and Zimbardo had judged their experiments to be of minimal risk—since they did not expect the studies to cause any physical harm. Yet considerable psychological distress ensued.

Then, in 1974, a journalistic exposé revealed the now-notorious Tuskegee syphilis study, Through the early 1970s, the US government had continued to fund this investigation of infected poor African American men in rural Alabama, without offering penicillin when it became available as effective treatment.[52]

This scandal prompted Congress to pass the National Research Act in 1974, establishing IRBs as they exist today.[53] Specifically, the Act first established the National Commission for the Protection of Human Subjects of Biomedical and Behavioral Research in order to determine "the boundaries between biomedical and behavioral research and the accepted and routine practice of medicine." The Commission was to develop guidelines to address what the appropriate balance was between risk and benefit, and how that balance would be assessed; who could be selected for a particular experiment; and how the investigators should ensure that subjects gave their informed consent to be a part of it. Eventually, in 1978, the Commission produced The Belmont Report, which articulated three core principles: respect for persons, beneficence, and justice.[54] The Act also led to more precise federal regulations, creating local IRBs to review all federally funded research on humans. These regulations—the Code of Regulations (45 CFR 46)—were approved by 17 separate federal agencies that conduct research, from the NIH to the Departments of Justice, Education, and Defense, and hence are known as "The Common Rule."[55] IRBs are mandated to ensure that "Risks to subjects are reasonable in relation to anticipated benefits, if any, to subjects, and the importance of the knowledge that may reasonably be expected to result."[55] Many other countries have developed their own laws concerning IRBs as well.

IRBs Today

The US now has over 4,000 IRBs, and hundreds more have been established in 113 other countries.[56] Every institution that conducts research—universities, medical schools, hospitals, clinics, and freestanding institutions—has at least one IRB, or arranges to use one at another institution. Every year, these committees examine tens of billions of dollars' worth of research—all studies of people involving cancer, heart attacks, strokes, AIDS, diabetes, Alzheimer's, autism, depression, and obesity. They assess, too, all research on humans investigating the mind, brain, and behavior—how we think, learn, remember, forget, eat, sleep, dream, speak, lie, get sick, have sex, grieve, pray, and die.

In this country, the common rule dictates that IRBs must have at least 5 members, including at least one scientific member, one non-scientific (so-called "lay") member, and one member who is not affiliated with the IRB's institution. On average, these boards include about 14 members, but they can have as many as 40.[57,58] IRBs usually have a chair who oversees the process and is compensated about 20% of his or her salary for IRB work. These committees also have administrators—typically the only ones paid full-time for their work with these committees. Boards customarily meet once a month to decide whether research studies submitted for review ("protocols") by researchers (or "Principal Investigators"—PIs) are ethical enough to proceed or need alterations. Most boards review hundreds of studies a year, and many large medical centers have 5 or 6 of these committees.

To ease burdens on both committees and researchers, administrators or chairs can expedite studies that are "minimal risk" or only "a minor increase over minimal risk." In an expedited review, only a chair (or administrator on his or her behalf) reviews the protocol. Ideally, whereas a full committee review often takes months, an expedited review can take far less time. The regulations define minimal risk as not involving more than that "ordinarily encountered in daily life or during the performance of routine physical or psychological examinations or tests."[55] For riskier studies, one or two primary reviewers generally read the protocol in depth and present it to the committee as a whole, which then discusses it. Other studies are also exempt from IRB review—if they meet certain criteria, such as not involving human subjects. The US regulations stipulate that human subjects are involved if researchers either directly interact with them or collect identifying information about them.[55] Thus, giving a drug or questionnaire to a person is considered research, whereas reviewing the medical records of deceased patients in order to collect their diagnoses and lists of the drugs they took—if those data include no identifying information—would be exempt. The regulations also declare exempt certain kinds of research that involve "normal educational" tests[55] in particular settings, such as schools. Still, committees generally want to make these determinations themselves, not rely on the researchers to do so. Even for exempt studies, boards generally require that the scientist submit the protocol, or a description of it, for the chair or administrator to assess.[55]

IRBs must approve each study initially, and then review and reapprove it yearly.[55] If a subject unexpectedly dies or gets very sick because of the study itself—an "adverse outcome"—the researcher must report the event to the IRB, which then has to decide whether to stop the research and/or inform federal agencies and past or future participants what has happened.[55]

Although originally mandated to review only federally funded research, most of these committees now review *all* research on humans conducted at an institution. External grant agencies such as the NIH and private pharmaceutical and medical-device companies assess protocols to decide which to fund, but the burden of examining and vetting the *ethical* issues involved ultimately still falls on the IRB. The vast majority of IRBs are at institutions that conduct research, especially universities and hospitals. Recently however, private, for-profit IRBs have also sprung up, which review studies for pharmaceutical companies or others for a fee.

Ideally, appropriate IRB review can safeguard subjects, assuring they are adequately protected, uncoerced, and protected from unnecessary harms—all of which is essential for furthering science. As pharmaceutical companies fund larger proportions of research, IRBs can also help serve as bulwarks against any potential industry abuse.

IRB Failures to Protect Subjects

Most research proceeds without major problems, but despite IRBs, ethical violations have continued. Starting in the late 1990s, due to egregious practices, the US Office for Protection from Research Risks (OPRR) shut down all research at several institutions, such as the West Los Angeles (LA) Veterans Administration (VA) Hospital, the country's largest VA health care facility, in March 1999,[59] Duke University in May 1999,[60] and Virginia Commonwealth University in 2000.[61] For instance, at the LA VA, a patient refused twice to participate in a study that would prolong his surgery. The researcher decided to proceed anyway, and continued the patient's 105-minute surgery an extra 45 minutes, using an electrical probe in the patient's heart to collect data. Another researcher at the institution enrolled at patient with severe delusions who hid bullets in his hospital room. The researcher gave this man a drug to make his heart race, and kept him in the operating room longer with an electrical probe in his heart as well. The doctor claims that the patient gave his verbal consent, but no written consent was documented, as is required.[59] These shutdowns sent shock waves throughout the country and many

IRBs became stricter. In response, many researchers then began chastising IRBs for being too strict and blocking important studies.

Problems have nonetheless persisted, and several critics now lambast these committees for being too lax, not reviewing studies as closely and well as they should. Scandals have occurred in which committees have approved certain studies that later prove problematic.

In 1999, even after the LA VA and Duke scandals, Jesse Gelsinger, an 18-year-old-healthy volunteer, died in a University of Pennsylvania IRB-approved study designed to see if a new gene therapy, contained in a virus, was safe. The researcher, who was a leading figure in this new, much-hyped field, had suspected problems with the laboratory-altered virus but continued to inject it into subjects anyway, including Jesse. The scientist turned out to own part of the company making the therapy, and stood to gain millions if it worked.[62]

Other IRB-approved studies later triggered lawsuits and harsh condemnation from outsiders, including journalists and judges, who argued that IRBs were too beholden to their colleagues conducting research and their institutions. In 1993, researchers at the Kennedy Krieger Institute, which is affiliated with Johns Hopkins, undertook a study of the possible toxic effects on children of different levels of removal of lead paint in homes. Exposure to dust from lead paint, which was widely used in homes before 1977,[63] causes severe neurological and developmental problems in children.[64] In the US in the mid-1980s, approximately 675,000 children less than 5 years old suffered from high concentrations of lead in their blood that could cause such problems.[65] Yet eliminating lead paint from old homes was expensive—between $3,000 and $10,000 per home in the late 80s and early 90s.[66] In poor inner cities, landlords balked. Here, the researchers investigated whether less expensive, *partial* removal, rather than total removal, would also be effective.

The investigators moved families with young children into one of five sets of apartments—those with full lead removal, those newly built without any lead paint, and those with one of three levels of only partial lead removal. The experiment found that partial removal worked, but blood lead levels rose in two children. One child was in a partially abated apartment. According to the researchers, the other child's apartment was fully abated.[67] These families sued on the grounds that they were not sufficiently informed of the risks. The Circuit Court of Baltimore dismissed the case, but the plaintiffs appealed to the Maryland Court of Appeals, which ruled in their favor, and compared the study to research conducted at Nazi concentration camps and Tuskegee. The court's majority opinion stated that this study "... presents similar problems as those in the Tuskegee Syphilis Study... [in] research subjects being intentionally exposed to infectious or poisonous substances in the name of scientific research."[68] Moreover, the subjects were vulnerable—relatively poor African American children.[69] Other observers, however, including one of the judges who wrote a minority opinion for the court, felt that these comparisons were too extreme.[70] The case was remanded to the Circuit Court for the City of Baltimore and ultimately dismissed.[71]

Nevertheless, debates still rage as to whether the researchers should have placed families *only* in houses with no lead, rather than those in which the metal had been partially but not fully removed. The researchers argued that for inner-city landlords, full lead removal was not a realistic goal. Opponents contended that the researchers were thereby endangering these children's lives. The investigators responded that the youngsters in partially abated homes were less exposed than if they had remained in their former, fully leaded apartments; the researchers had hoped that partial lead-removal would eliminate health risks. Critics have argued that these investigators should have guessed that even small levels of the metal could nonetheless be dangerous,[72] but other commentators have pointed out that the two plaintiffs with elevated lead levels may not have been exposed at their own homes but elsewhere (e.g., at the homes of friends and relatives, or at daycare).[67]

The study raises profound questions of exactly how much responsibility researchers and IRBs have for promoting health equity as much as possible when it does not otherwise exist; whether researchers should be permitted to compare current suboptimal practices (patients living in apartments with only partial lead removal) with more robust interventions (i.e., eliminating all lead); and whether scientists should ever be allowed to endanger healthy children without disease—how much evidence is needed to determine that an intervention is safe enough.

Given these and other ongoing controversies, many IRBs have become even more stringent, but violations have nonetheless persisted, in which investigators appear to have been deficient. In 2010, Arizona State University settled a lawsuit with the Native American Havasupai tribe of Arizona.[73] The university's researchers had wanted to investigate the tribe's rates of schizophrenia—which were higher than those in the general population—and diabetes, about which the Havasupai were concerned. But these scientists feared that the tribe would object to the study of schizophrenia. Hence, these scientists told the tribe that the study was only about diabetes. The university's IRB knew the researchers' plan to study rates of schizophrenia but approved the plan, including the consent form, which did not mention any psychiatric diagnoses. In 1990, 200 members of the group gave blood samples. But in 2004, they learned that the researchers had published papers about the tribe's high levels of schizophrenia and alcoholism, as well as genetic evidence that the group had come from Asia, whereas the Havasupai believed that they originated in the Grand Canyon, where they now lived, and which they hence claimed to own. The legal settlement required that the university return the blood samples to the tribe, which then destroyed them. Had the researchers instead inter-acted with the tribe with more respect, they could perhaps have advanced science in many ways and even gained, rather than impaired, the tribe's trust, facilitating an ongoing relationship to improve the group's health.

Ongoing pharmaceutical company scandals, involving drugs such as Avandia and Neurontin, raise added concerns about the roles of industry in academic and other research. Corporations marketing Vioxx,[74] OxyContin,[75,76] and ciga-rettes[77,78] have hidden scientific findings that threatened to undermine sales.

In the recent era of multinational pharmaceutical companies, cutbacks in government funding for research, and rising academic pressures to "publish or perish," the goals of advancing science and protecting people are increasingly at odds. Scientists seek truth; corporations, profit. But pharmaceutical, biotech, and health care companies comprise over one-fifth of the US economy, fueling con-flicts of interest (COIs) for researchers, torn between their need to make money for themselves, their institutions, and their funders and their desire to uphold the ideals of scientific purity. As the pharmaceutical and biotech industries grow, ten-sions have heightened. Ever since the Bayh-Dole Act of 1980,[79] allowing universi-ties to patent discoveries made using federal grants, major academic institutions aggressively seek patents, earning hundreds of millions of dollars but heightening ethical strains. As the pipeline of new drugs is drying up, some analysts predict that pharmaceutical companies may search even more desperately, incentiviz-ing scientists to study so-called "me, too" drugs, and paying physicians to push patients unnecessarily into using experimental products.

Increasingly, US-funded researchers are also conducting studies in the devel-oping world, either because of particular epidemics there worthy of study (e.g., malaria and HIV) or due to the less stringent regulations and cost of the research. However, private industry, not government, now funds most clinical trials[80] and conducts most of this research in the developing world,[81] heightening the odds of abuse.

Government Responses

In 1998, in acknowledgment of these varied problems, the Office of the Inspector General (OIG) recommended recasting IRB requirements, granting these com-mittees greater flexibility, holding them more accountable for results, and ensur-ing that investigators and board members are adequately trained and insulated from conflicts.[18,19,20,21] Yet few structural changes have occurred since that report, and numerous problems persist. In 2002, the Institute of Medicine (IOM) called for increased assessments of research protections and oversight[82] and rec-ommended several approaches, including identifying and disseminating best practices, enhancing Quality Assurance/Quality Improvement, examining the type and number of FDA and OHRP audits of IRBs, and enhancing accountability and transparency. The report also suggested differentiating IRBs from other institutional compliance, risk management, and COI offices, and having institutions provide adequate resources for these activities. *Yet the authors of this report felt "repeatedly confounded by the lack of data regarding the scope and scale of current protection"—underscoring the need for more research on IRBs*—and the impact of this report has been limited.[83]

Increasingly, some observers have thus called for essentially revamping the entire system, discarding IRBs, and instead letting research participants sue if they are harmed. Yet this model, used in medical malpractice, may be very inefficient. Others have suggested only slight alterations,[28] or leaving the current regulations unchanged. Standard questions have been proposed to reduce IRB variability, but have not been widely used.[3284] Although some opponents suggest eliminating or greatly reducing the roles of these boards, what the alternatives might actually look like, or how well they would function, is unknown.

Increasingly, these debates have also been rigidly polarized—pro or con, black or white—the system is either crucial or should be scrapped. Researchers and IRBs each argue that the other side needs to change.

In July 2011, the US Department of Health and Human Services under President Barack Obama issued an Advanced Notice of Proposed Rule-Making (ANPRM), proposing several dramatic shifts in IRB regulations.[2885] The Obama Administration's proposals focused on only three areas: making minimal-risk research automatically exempt from IRB review; using central IRBs (or CIRBs) more in multi-site studies; and questioning how to improve research involving storage and use of biological specimens. The administration also included a list of 74 questions, asking how IRBs in fact work, and might best be changed. The document highlights how vast areas of the current system remain uncharted and unknown.

Yet this lengthy document, too, has generated debates. For instance, under these proposals, researchers would decide for themselves whether their study is "minimal risk" and therefore exempt from IRB review. Investigators would simply then register their study with their IRB, complete a simple (approximately one-page) form, and immediately begin conducting the research. But under this arrangement, investigators conducting research similar to the Milgram and Zimbardo prison studies could simply claim that their projects were of minimal risk, and then proceed to conduct them—with no one reviewing these decisions. If, as also proposed, IRBs become more centralized, local committees may still regularly modify or veto the central IRBs' decisions, thereby diminishing key potential benefits of centralization and possibly creating more—not less—paperwork. The document presented more questions than answers regarding storing biological specimens, too.

The Administration invited public comments to this report through October 2011; yet as of this writing, the fate of these proposals remains utterly uncertain. This document, and the Obama Administration's involvement, resulted in large part from the fact that Ezekiel Emanuel was involved (at the time, his brother, Rahm Emanuel, currently the mayor of Chicago, was the President's chief of staff). But he has since left the federal government to become vice provost for global initiatives and professor at the University of Pennsylvania. Whether any of the changes suggested will be instituted—and if so, when, how, and with what results—is unclear. In the end, the Administration's efforts may alter the status quo little, if at all. Moreover, other aspects of these committees, on which the Administration has not even commented, need attention as well.

Strikingly, as the document discussed, relatively little data about IRBs are available, and the underlying causes of their difficulties have received scant attention: many key questions remain unaddressed. It is still unclear, for instance, *why* IRBs vary so much, and inappropriately block, delay, or approve certain studies; how they themselves view these debates; and how much inconsistency between them, if any, is acceptable.

Hence, regardless of the fate of this recent proposal, critical tensions and questions will no doubt persist, given our ongoing advances in science and widely differing views of ethics. We need IRBs, but have they become too stringent, or too lax? As a society, we face fundamental dilemmas as to how to proceed: how to balance the social benefits of research against the potential risks to subjects, how much to trust *vs.* monitor researchers, and how to avoid either over- or under-regulating science. Debates mount and yet, astonishingly, these controversies rage in a relative absence of data.

Similar debates boil in other countries as well, though many other nations, in Western Europe and elsewhere, rely much more on national committees, which thus have much more influence. In addition, the US faces these issues more acutely since it conducts far more research than does any other country.

I therefore decided that to understand these vital issues I first needed to examine these committees themselves—to explore how they view and confront these complex problems, how they make the crucial decisions that shape science, medicine, and biology—and hence all of our lives—and whether the various problems mentioned above can be ameliorated and, if so, how.

Past Studies of IRBs

It is striking that only a few past studies of how IRBs make decisions have been conducted. In 1969–70, before IRBs as they exist today were created, Bradford Gray, a Yale sociologist, investigated one of the "clinical research committees" that then existed. He examined 54 projects submitted to the committee, read the records, and interviewed 15 of the researchers and subjects in five of these projects. He found that the committee may be biased in favor of research, and that the informed consent forms sometimes contained vagaries—that subjects may feel they understand studies when they in fact do not.[86]

It is remarkable that the question of how IRBs themselves actually work, make decisions, and view and understand these quandaries has received relatively little attention. Only a few studies of IRBs have been published, and these have focused on procedural and logistical issues. In addition, almost all of this published research has been quantitative, based on very short surveys using multiple-choice questions. These studies have not generally used more descriptive, qualitative methods to explore the language and concepts the committees themselves use to understand and describe these areas. Moreover, these past studies have usually each looked at only one or another of these multifaceted issues, ignoring the whole.

Nonetheless, even these few published studies focusing on the logistics of IRBs—quantitative assessments of size, types of members, workload,[87] gender, ethnicity, and aspects of training[88]—have highlighted several problems. IRBs vary in size and the number of studies they review each year. Overall, they confront heavy workloads, competing priorities, and difficulties in criticizing colleagues' studies, and understanding complex science. Eager to recruit subjects, researchers can sometimes overlook deficiencies in the informed consent. Many institutions and IRB members also have financial ties to a study; in one survey, 36% of IRB members had one or more such industry connections,[89] though this study didn't address how these individuals understood and justified this. These studies have also suggested limitations in the training of IRBs. In another survey of IRB administrators, 75% felt that 80% of committee members did not have "ethical expertise." IRB members use criteria such as "scientific merit" in their evaluations, but how they judge these criteria, or what they consider acceptable or not, is unknown.[90]

These limited findings are provocative, and suggest areas where further study is needed. Nonetheless, the quantitative studies have not examined the *contents* of committee decisions or disagreements; the reasons variations occur; committees' responses to researchers' complaints; or a host of other crucial issues. Forty-five years have passed since Bradford Gray's qualitative research exploring the inner workings of committees, and he examined only one board. Many questions arise as to how these issues have evolved, and how they differ across institutions.

Recently, two qualitative studies of IRB members have been published. The sociologist Chuck Lidz and his colleagues[91] approached several IRBs and managed to observe a few committees—many said no. These researchers found that community members on these committees spoke less than the other members and were more likely to discuss confidentiality issues.[92] One or two members usually serve as the primary reviewers for any protocol.

Among other members at meetings, community members, when they did speak, discussed consent forms more than did other members. In 2012, Laura Stark, an anthropologist now at Vanderbilt University, observed three IRBs for her doctoral dissertation. In her subsequent book, she noted several valuable points: that members drew on personal as well as professional experience, and on local precedents; and that IRBs used the fact that they would need to write a concrete memo to investigators as a way to focus committee discussions, motivate the group to reach a decision, and hide the identities of individual reviewers.[93]

Still, a great many essential questions remain concerning how IRBs in fact operate, make decisions about specific protocols, and view and fill their roles. Manuals on how to run an IRB have been published, but no study has systematically examined how these boards themselves grapple with the content of dilemmas they confront, and the full range of uncertainties, pressures, conflicts involved (e.g., how attitudes and contexts shape their decisions). The perspectives of IRBs themselves are essential—to grasp what problems these committees face from their own points of view, and how they perceive possible solutions. Whatever criticisms IRBs provoke, reforms cannot be designed or implemented effectively without fuller comprehension of the perspectives of the individuals serving on these boards. Although many critics deride IRBs as powerful, unresponsive bureaucrats, the degree to which IRB members are even aware of and try to address these problems has not, for instance, been explored. Given this lack of knowledge, the sociologist Raymond De Vries recently concluded, "The next step in IRB research must include ethnographic studies...that document how members of IRBs interact and make decisions."[94]

Methods

One of my professors, the late anthropologist Clifford Geertz, argued that to comprehend any social situation we should try to obtain a "thick description" of the lives and decisions of the individuals being studied—not by imposing external preconceptions or theoretical structures on them, but by trying to grasp their own views in their own words.[95] This approach ideally illuminates not only what these individuals are doing but also what they *think* they are doing, and how they understand their activities and the challenges they face.

For over 30 years, I have interacted with IRBs: submitting protocols, communicating with staff, and speaking at and observing various IRB meetings. To comprehend the inner workings of IRBs as best as possible, I decided to interview individual IRB leaders in depth about their experiences to explore these issues. Unfortunately, many IRBs have refused to allow researchers to observe and study them, requiring these scientists to obtain consent not only from all IRB members and staff, but also from the investigators of the protocols being discussed, and the funders of those protocols—an essentially impossible task.

To understand these committees more fully, I first held focus groups with IRB members and researchers, and subsequently conducted in-depth interviews with 46 chairs, IRB members, and staff from a total of 34 IRBs. I have described the methods far more fully in Appendix A.

As shown in Table 1.1, these 46 interviewees included 28 chairs/co-chairs, 10 administrators (including 2 directors of compliance offices), 1 IRB director, and 7 members. Some have occupied more than one of these roles, changing over time. In all, 58.7% were male, and 93.5% were Caucasian, reflecting the larger imbalances on these committees more broadly.

I also surveyed 76 chairs and administrators of IRBs in the US and 37 from South African (SA) Research Ethics Committees (or RECs), as they are called in many other countries. I focused on their attitudes concerning reviews of HIV vaccine trials. I found that in both countries these individuals were split on key ethical issues, and agreed they needed more training. Yet REC members in South Africa were much more likely to call for major changes in studies and to think that study participants in the developing world did not understand risks and benefits.[92] I also interviewed 17 REC chairs, members and administrators from 7 RECs in South Africa, and recently 12 REC members from other developing countries in Africa, Asia and Latin America, and found that these individuals turn out to confront many similar challenges to their counterparts on US IRBs.[96] These interviews have informed my thinking here as well.

The questions (as seen in Appendix B) explored these individuals' experiences and views of research ethics and integrity, and related areas—specifically, what challenges IRBs faced concerning the ethics of research and related areas, how they addressed these challenges, and why. I used follow-up questions to grasp these issues as fully as possible. In the course of our conversations, these men and women reflected on a wide range of issues concerning their roles and work.

I am deeply grateful and indebted to these interviewees for their willingness to share their views and experiences—for their openness and candor. They discussed how they think, feel, and make and view decisions that affect us all. Their opinions may not always be wholly objective or include the "full reality." In a few instances, it also became clear that some interviewees even misunderstood the regulations. Still, their errors are revealing, indicating areas where larger confusions persist.

To protect confidentiality, I refer to associate, vice, co-, and former chairs simply as "chairs." For the same reason, I do not provide identifying characteristics about these interviewees. Yet I do not want them to be utterly faceless, or have

Table 1.1. **Characteristics of the Sample**

	Total	*% (N=46)*
Type of IRB Staff		
Chairs/Co-Chairs	28	60.9%
Directors	1	2.2%
Administrators	10	21.7%
Members	7	15.2%
Gender		
Male	27	58.7%
Female	19	41.3%
*Institutional Rank in NIH funding**		
1–50	13	28.3%
51–100	13	28.3%
101–150	7	15.2%
151–200	1	2.2%
201–250	12	26.1%
State vs. Private		
State	19	41.3%
Private	27	58.7%
Region		
Northeast	21	45.7%
Midwest	6	13.0%
West	13	28.3%
South	6	13.0%
Total # of Institutions Represented	**34**	

*Due to rounding, percentages exceed 100.

them all blur together. I have therefore tried to provide some sense of them as people by giving each a pseudonym and identifying their position—as seen on Table 1.2—and then later by mentioning a few general, non-identifying characteristics about them.

not appear as whole people. This book gives a more complete sense of each interviewee and his or her thoughts. The index lists the pages on which each speaker appears, allowing readers to trace how each person perceived not only one topic but many.

To understand how the system can be improved, a fuller and more nuanced understanding of the world of research ethics is essential—how these committees view and try to fulfill their mandate, how they make decisions, and why. This book reveals what I learned, probing this relatively little-known world. These men and women profoundly altered my views. Much of what I found has not been described before. Much of the literature and most of the debates about IRBs center on whether these committees are good or bad, and whether they should be kept, eliminated, or changed. Many IRB critics argue, for example, that all social-science and minimal-risk studies should simply be exempt from review. This book provides new data, examines issues that have not been probed, and offers new suggestions and perceptions.

I came to appreciate far more the struggles and obstacles these men and women face, and why the current system has frustrated other researchers and me. I saw how the crucial questions are not whether IRBs are good or bad, but what their roles should be, how and why these committees differ, who should be a member, whether these boards should be altered, and if so, how. I set out on this journey to enhance and/or reform the status quo, but soon confronted underlying issues about IRBs themselves—how they operate at both the macro and the micro level—who their members are, and how they make decisions, interact with, and are affected by larger social forces, including federal agencies, industry, institutions, and researchers. We first need to understand and diagnose these committees before we can fix them.

In brief, as shown in Figure 1.1 and elaborated through the chapters that follow, these individuals shed unique light on how the current system functions and can possibly be improved, providing rare glimpses into the conflicts they face. Within intricate social, political, historical, and scientific worlds, they wrestle with a series of dilemmas. They face complexities defining science, assessing and weighing possible future risks and benefits of studies, deciding what exactly subjects should be told, how much to trust *vs.* monitor scientists, and how to balance advancing science against allowing institutions, researchers, and others to make money and foster reputations and careers. In an age in which, on any given day, many of us online simply scroll down and click "I accept"—scrolling, but not reading or understanding—these committees wrestle with quandaries of not only how much scientists should tell subjects while avoiding information overload, but also how to protect the privacy of individuals who give sensitive personal information—whether to a researcher, a doctor or a web site.

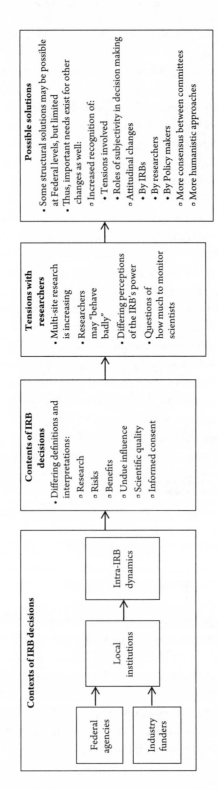

Figure 1.1 Overview of Issues Concerning IRBs.

Perhaps most of all, these interviews taught me about how we view and interpret ethics in our lives at this particular cultural moment—how we view moral principles in everyday life, and how complex social systems can affect us and our definitions and applications of these precepts. Ever more frequently, our increasingly globalized world witnesses warring moral beliefs. While some critics decry a widespread decay of morals in the US, others fear that moral discourse exercises too much of a role in public and political life.

In working on this book, I came to understand how far ethical perspectives can conflict, and how we can potentially bridge these tensions. Some philosophers believe that in any debate, a single, best-reasoned ethical argument always exists. But I saw how people at times interpret and apply ethical terms in equally reasonable, though different ways. *I often saw how ethical principles did not collide as much as differing interpretations of these principles did.* This distinction can potentially help clarify many misunderstandings and debates.

I came to see, too, that the work of IRBs is in fact closer to the humanities and social issues than to the hard sciences—filled with complex questions of meaning and interpretation, shadowed by uncertainties, and confronted within particular social contexts. A few years ago, in Greece, I visited the largest intact ancient theater in the world in Epidaurus, once the center of the cult of Asclepius, the demi-god of healing and medicine. This famed theatre was in fact part of a compound that included a temple and a hospital. From the Ancient Greece of Hippocrates through the late 19th century, medicine combined science with humanistic concerns about the patient. Yet ever since the late 19th century, academic medical centers have sought to follow a far stricter, scientific model, and cultivated a positivist sense that an absolute answer exists for any problem. This notion extends, I would argue, to attitudes about IRBs as well. Of course, scientists themselves are not always objective either, and may be affected by various preconceived notions, but arguably they see themselves acting objectively, nonetheless. These interviews, however, showed me how much *we need a different model—a more humanistic approach that recognizes and incorporates far more the complex psychological, social, and cultural dimensions of these decisions.*

"Power corrupts," Lord Acton famously quipped,[97] but does it do so here? And if so, how and why? For centuries, power has intrigued thinkers from Aristotle and Machiavelli to George Orwell, Franz Kafka, and Michel Foucault. Orwell, for instance, explored the rhetoric of power—how authority may downplay or deny its power, recasting its might in language of seeming beneficence.[98] Kafka, too, described the disturbing tendency of institutions of authority to be anonymous and unresponsive.[99,100] Echoes of these tendencies at times surface here, albeit in muted ways.

Psychologically, decisions about risks and benefits have increasingly been demonstrated to be subjective. Daniel Kahneman received the 2002 Nobel Prize for showing how individuals perceive risks and benefits not objectively but by using "biases and heuristics,"[101] and overvaluing possible risks more than benefits. I soon found that such phenomena operate on IRBs as well.

"We try not to be the 'Ethics Police,'" one of my first interviewees told me. Researchers commonly use this nickname in referring to these boards. The title of this book includes this phrase—not as a label, but instead as a question that I seek to explore and answer. While investigators frequently see IRBs as possessing great power, these committees themselves tend to disagree. Why do these two views conflict so radically? What does this contrast tell us? Do these committees or researchers at times fall short, and if so, how, and what should be done?

But this is not an "anti-IRB" book. These committees do extremely valuable work and, in some form, they are here to stay. Key questions arise, however, as to whether the current system can be improved, and if so, how.

Within the relatively small world of IRBs and trained social scientists, a few individuals may feel that these interviewees' comments are not totally surprising—that IRB variation is not very startling. Yet the extent, scope, reasons, and many of the implications, have been very little explored or documented, at best. More important, IRBs themselves generally defend these variations, failing to see these differences as a problem. They tend to ignore or dismiss the frequency, breadth, nature, and extent of these differences, and often do not recognize or appreciate either the causes or the consequences. These deficiencies are significant, because such discrepancies and the lack of publicly documented decisions and precedents by IRBs trigger major battles, frustrations, and costs for researchers. Lack of consistency undermines the authority and legitimacy of local reviews. Hence, understanding these phenomena is vital.

In addition, this book is intended not just—or even primarily—for IRB members and scientists, but much more widely for doctors and other health care professionals, policy makers, patients and their family members and friends—in short, for all of us—as this little-known world directly or indirectly affects us all.

In recounting the battles between IRBs and researchers, it would be simpler if each group consisted entirely of either "good guys" or "bad guys"—a perspective taken by much prior scholarship. Some IRB members may feel that certain suggestions in this book's conclusion are too radical, whereas some researchers may think that this book is far too sympathetic to these committees and does not go far enough. But the realities proved far more nuanced than critics have admitted. The often competing goals of advancing scientific benefits while reducing risks as much as possible can only be reconciled if we better understand the causes of conflicts that arise.

The widespread public sense that these committees are removed from most of our lives is a dangerous illusion; instead, they serve as crucial prisms through which many of the vital struggles of our time—between science and ethics, individual freedom and government control, industry greed and individual patients' rights—are refracted. Ultimately, whether at the hospital bedside or the prescription counter, the decisions of these men and women impact us all.

PART

II

WHO IRBs ARE

CHAPTER 2

"Inside the Black Box"

BECOMING AND BEING IRB MEMBERS

"I was volunteered," one IRB member told me. "My chairman said that the department needed to assign someone to the IRB. I was now 'it.' But I was surprised—I had no training in ethics." Repeatedly, I heard such stories. Increasingly, I saw how these committees are in the end merely a collection of individuals on whom many pressures fall. They are the keystone—the fulcrum—balancing opposing forces of scientist, university and drug company desires *vs.* subjects' rights and government regulations. Who then are these individuals, and how did they end up in these positions?

Surprisingly little has been published about why individuals join these committees—whether as members, chairs, or staff—and how they got these jobs. Yet understanding who is making these decisions is crucial to better understanding how IRBs function. The regulations stipulate that committees must "be sufficiently qualified through the experience and expertise of its members, and the diversity of the members, including consideration of race, gender, and cultural backgrounds and sensitivity to such issues as community attitudes." Boards must include 5 members, including "at least one member whose primary concerns are in nonscientific areas," and "at least one member who is not otherwise affiliated with the institution and who is not part of the immediate family of a person who is affiliated with the institution."[1] For research on prisoners, IRBs also need an advocate for this population.

A few surveys have examined logistical and sociodemographic aspects of IRBs.[2,3] In a 1998 national study conducted by the NIH, 95% of chairs were white and 77% were male, reflecting patterns of authority within medical centers as a whole.[4] Of members, 92% were white, 58% were male, reflecting patterns of authority within medical centers as a whole.[4] This report found that 72% of committee members had "doctoral degrees," but it did not examine whether these were MDs and PhDs, or whether the degrees were in any way related to members' attitudes. Once appointed, members have been found to stay an average of 4 to 7 years.[4] A few institutions have begun instituting term limits (e.g., 3 years), but doing so is by no means the norm.

Given the importance of the work they do, and the potentially grave consequences of IRB lapses and oversights, the lack of preparedness for the work is especially striking. Both general members and chairs have been found to have little if any formal training in ethics. One study found that more than 95% had not received any special education regarding their IRB work.[4] Of members, 77% had learned what was expected of them through "an oral briefing,"[4] but it is unclear what these "briefings" consisted of—how long they were, and what information they included. When I surveyed IRB members in South Africa, I found that 40% were "self-taught" in ethics.[5]

IRBs have a "check the box mentality," one researcher and former IRB member recently told me. "They think that reviewing a study is a matter of simply checking the box—a principle is either there or not. They don't think much about it. If the researcher disagrees with the interpretation and application of a regulation: that's tough. The staff do not think that the researchers, in seeing the regulation differently, may have a legitimate point."

Indeed, the bioethicist John Lantos has described IRB members as "well-meaning amateurs"[6] who usually lack training for these tasks.

Who Becomes an IRB Member?

"My department head needed to fill a hole, and wanted a voice on the IRB," Anthony, a researcher and chair, reported. "[He] said, 'Would you be willing to do this?' I said fine...I didn't see it as a career aspiration to be going down this road. I still don't." Many committees face particular challenges recruiting and integrating members, especially so-called community members (note: I use this term below, as IRBs regularly do so). These individuals' professional and personal backgrounds are important to grasp, as these can profoundly affect committee decisions.

Members and chairs may be chosen for a range of reasons, and vary from having had strong to slight to no prior interest in ethics. Generally, one cannot choose to join an IRB, but is put up for the position by a department chair, administrator, or IRB chair; and one may or may not then have the clout to decline. At times, individuals may have a *modicum* of interest in research ethics, but no formal training. Interests may grow over time, but even then not be part of an explicit career plan. Still, over several years—especially for chairs—ethics can become an important part of one's career.

Experience is also valued. Often an individual who has served on one institution's IRB will be asked to do so at a new institution, as well. At institutions where relatively little research was performed, members or chairs may be chosen simply because they have conducted studies. These faculty become IRB members and/or chairs because they have worked in research broadly, even if not in ethics per se.

Others joined because they wanted to learn more about studies at their institution—out of either intellectual curiosity or hopes of getting involved. "I was a statistician, and started on the IRB because my interest was research," said Warren, an IRB member. "I saw this as a way to familiarize myself with a hospital on a research level." Being a member can strengthen one's network within a medical center, which can help one in other ways professionally. He continued:

> *It's a medical education.*... researchers get to know me.... So it's been professionally helpful. I enjoy the social recognition... [It] has led to my being used as a statistician or consultant on projects.

Committees may recruit individuals as members for other complex political and institutional reasons as well. The inclusion of chairs and members who are also researchers can help in gaining investigators' cooperation; it also may make it easier for IRBs to withstand external pressures to approve certain protocols. As Nancy, a researcher and chair, said:

> We think it's pretty important that the IRB chair be a practicing researcher, and we want lots of researchers on the IRB who...have the respect of their colleagues and are pretty distinguished, so that they can't be intimidated by any department heads or vice presidents.

Having too many non-researchers as members or chairs can pose multiple challenges in reviewing studies. As Christopher, an IRB chair, said, "A non-researcher is then trying to make decisions about specific qualifications of the faculty." Some such members may not be qualified to judge the scientific value of a particular study; others may be biased against scientific research generally—excessively unsympathetic to experiments involving human subjects across the board.

In cases like this, if ongoing, IRB chairs or institutional leaders may appoint new committee members to try to make the board more research-friendly. Greg, a social scientist and former chair, reported,

> Some researchers were having the hardest time getting their protocols through. I didn't replace members, but added a few members. I inherited a committee that was great, but didn't have a lot of research background.... Only one or two members were researchers. I added a number of actual researchers, and they have added a lot...

Yet other IRB chairs may be less proactive in changing their board, or feel unable to do so. Altering the status quo can be hard. Christopher said, "We *should* get new chairs who do research. But that's not going to happen any time soon."

At the same time, having chairs or members who are *too* pro-research could interfere with IRBs fulfilling their mandate to protect subjects. Balancing the various characteristics of members can prove important in ensuring that IRBs are neither overly harsh nor overly lax. Nancy added,

> Some people just love to argue, nitpick, and be critical. You can't have people like that. But you don't want people who are just going to put in their time and leave and not read protocols carefully!

When such a balance is established, it needs to be carefully maintained, but committee turnover can make this difficult—especially on boards that have brief and fixed terms of service. "Once you get good members, a lot of IRBs rotate them off after two years—like it was an onerous duty," Nancy continued. "I'm not sure that's good." Term limits, as established by several committees, thus have important pros and cons.

"BEING VOLUNTEERED"

I found that some members get appointed without any particular interest or background in ethics. Membership may serve as a routine committee assignment, and seem utterly random—because everyone in an academic department is assigned to a committee. IRB director Liza, for instance, tells department chairs that they *must* supply a member in order to have their protocols reviewed ("If I...am having a problem with getting an immunologist on my IRB, I just go to the department chair and say, 'No member: no review.'"). This quid pro quo may guarantee that Liza has a particular academic discipline represented, but it doesn't yield particularly experienced faculty members. "They usually bring in the most junior person who hasn't yet been assigned a committee," she confessed.

Given the time commitment that IRBs require from members—several hours a month, uncompensated, reading and reviewing complex protocols—many faculty resist joining these committees. Senior investigators, busy writing grants and conducting studies, may decide not to be board members because it takes time away from research. As a result, faculty members on IRBs may not be the researchers with major ongoing research projects, but rather be either younger or fully or semi-retired. Junior faculty may even "be volunteered," and have less power and authority in their departments. Hence, IRBs can end up with a disproportionate number of junior faculty—and some senior members—who have scant ethics education or experience.

Ideally, the head of a researcher's department would read a protocol for possible problems before the researcher submits it to the IRB; in practice, many departments are lax about this. In response to this problem, an IRB may actively appoint investigators to join the committee who have resisted IRB regulations in the past, or who are members of a department that has regularly done so. IRBs may see such recruitment as a form of intervention. Helene, an IRB administrator, said,

> Some departments think, "We'll do it the way we want…We won't spend much time on IRB submissions. Let the IRB critique it, and tell us what we need to do." In retaliation, we appoint a member from that department on our IRB. It has worked very well. We get this person in here, and this person comes to appreciate the IRB.

"We humorously call it 'his sentence,'" Olivia, an IRB chair, said about one such appointee—suggesting not only education, but punishment. "I feel bad for this investigator," she continued, "because he just kept telling me, 'I had no idea.' Nobody had trained him about informed consent." And yet such strategies can be effective. Olivia added,

> He joined our committee, and everything changed. He is now totally *sold* on what has to happen. He's training his fellows, and not doing anything without sending it to us first.

"See One, Do One?": Orientations for New Members

Committees differ widely in whether they provide any orientation for new members, and if so, what. Many boards provide little formal training. Sometimes only after an IRB has faced a scandal—and as a result received more resources from its governing institution—does it provide a fuller orientation.

In medical school and internship, as other trainees and I learned new procedures—from inserting catheters into patients to extracting arterial and venous blood or spinal fluid—a common adage was "see one, do one, teach one." Similarly, a few boards simply give new members a manual and say to read it and "just do what everyone else is doing." Orientations can potentially provide more specific procedural context and mechanisms, and training in applying principles and regulations. IRB member Andrea suggested:

> Having a better orientation that didn't just focus on "see one, do one" could be more helpful…It's been almost entirely word of mouth…My training consisted entirely of coming and watching the meeting.

After watching how protocols were reviewed, she was thus expected to review and present studies herself.

Other IRBs may provide some orientation, which members found helpful but still generally insufficient. Interviewees felt that not all members were equally knowledgeable on key topics, and that they and many others could benefit from additional training. One IRB provided a one-hour meeting with the chair to review the committee's overall purpose, and issues to look for in reviewing protocols. Yet more "concrete" approaches of how to review studies (e.g., a checklist rather than just a general discussion) can also help. As Patrick, a physician and committee member, said,

> As an orientation, we had to sit in on at least three sessions as an observer...I also had a one-hour meeting with the chairman...But that was the extent of it. More would've been good—a little more detailed. For every protocol review, they give us a sheet: "This is what you have to do." But that sheet is fairly new. I was expecting the chair to be a little bit more concrete: "This is how you go about it; this is what you need to be aware of. These are our expectations...picking up things that fall through the cracks, or red flags." I wish somebody would've been more specific.

Training must thus balance abstract principles with concrete interpretations and applications of these. Patrick felt that the chair should have:

> realized the struggles that *you* might have the first couple times—as opposed to somebody who's been doing it for 30 years, forgetting what it's like to be a "newbie"...

Like Patrick, Andrea, a nurse and IRB member, had to attend three sessions before she could vote. When she was then given a consent form to review, however, she had no idea how to go about it. These forms are critical to ensure that patients give informed consent—that they understand the relevant details about the study in which they are considering participation. As such, these forms are supposed to be written at no more than an eighth-grade reading level, but studies show that most are far too complicated, lengthy, and inscrutable. Andrea recalled her own experience reviewing a consent form:

> They...told me a person would help me with it. That was it. One man on the committee for 15 years is down the hall from my office. I go and say, "I don't get it...where am I supposed to find this...?" He would just explain it.

New members may thus have to rely on *informal* interactions that they themselves initiate to do their job properly. The full knowledge needed could take a few years to acquire. Additional initial and ongoing training of chairs and members could potentially assist IRBs, and need not require exorbitant resources. IRB member Frank suggested "a more systematic checklist, or how-to guide, or sit-down with the chair."

For assessing informed consent forms, some IRBs have instituted checklists for each reviewer. Such lists can help, but can also become cumbersome and bureaucratic. "Reviewer forms are 12 pages for every consent form," Christopher explained, "with 65 items to check off!" Checklists can potentially help to a degree to make sure key areas are considered, but do not address how principles and regulations are interpreted and applied. Still, briefer, more basic checklists can potentially be developed to aid protocol reviews.

Physician members tend to feel comfortable relatively quickly. Yet even they still take time to fully learn key details. Members also learn much "on the job"— an education that can take several years. As IRB chair Nathan explained,

> I was on the committee for 8 years before I actually understood what was behind the whole organization: how the policies were set up, how the interpretations of what we should ask people to do were established.

Some other members, however, face more challenges. Even after a few years of membership, individuals may remain uncertain about several types of IRB issues. Andrea initially felt intimidated and somewhat lost due to lack of training. She now finds her role comfortable and rewarding, but is still unaware of many aspects of committee procedures, and uncertain about the board's full scope:

> I don't have a good understanding of the whole process…the roles of the various people involved. How does the consent even get generated?…I'm never sure whether I have all the information I need, because I'm not positive what it should include. Do I have *all* of the adverse reports [i.e., researchers send IRBs reports of all serious unanticipated adverse events that arise in a study—such as whether a patient in a drug study experiences severe unexpected side effects]? That makes me feel insecure. I never had a sense of the scope of the responsibilities of the IRB, how it relates to the federal government…who's supposed to sit on the IRB, what it's supposed to do…In the beginning, I didn't understand that if there are protocol violations, they come to us. It would have helped me from the beginning if someone had said, "These are the areas where the IRB has purview and responsibility."

Over time, through experience, members acquire not only factual background and knowledge, but confidence and skills. Their acclimation is not only cognitive but emotional, as well. Gradually, members can reduce their apprehension and hone their judgment as they learn more fully what is *vs.* is not important, partly through feedback from others; these processes are highly dynamic. As Andrea, the nurse and IRB member, added,

> Initially, I was terrified. I used to think I had to mention every last thing. I was concerned I was being too nitpicky, mentioning things I should've just ignored, or worried that what I had to say was going to sound lame. Now, I don't feel that way...If the researchers don't underline this here, it's not the end of the world...I've become more comfortable asking questions.

At first, Andrea was afraid of saying too much *and* saying anything at all; of not fulfilling her ethical responsibility ("I had to mention every last thing") *and* unnecessarily obstructing research ("mentioning things I should've just ignored"). Over time, she adapted to the ecology of her IRB and now feels more comfortable. Of course, given both the individual and the nature of the group, these ecologies are not consistent; even IRBs that run well may differ greatly. As a nurse, her experiences differ from those of many physicians, and thus of many members of these committees. Still, her feelings are not unique, and hence are important to grasp.

New members are therefore often reticent, although other factors such as personality and professional discipline can also come into play. Andrea said of her IRB:

> New people never say anything. It takes them months. They don't know what's going on, and are just overwhelmed, because they see us come in with these stacks, and all these little stickies to mark our places. It's just very daunting. Some people are more comfortable than others.

Yet over time, members generally become more comfortable, and realize what they can uniquely contribute. As a nurse, Andrea said "I found I probably have a *better* understanding of what patients and families would care about." The positive feedback from other members can also mitigate feelings of being inadequate or dismissed. "People have said, 'I never would have thought of that,'" Andrea added "or 'I wouldn't have picked that up.' That makes me feel that what I do here is important."

Personal Rewards

Generally, interviewees come to like working on the IRB, becoming genuinely engaged and finding the work satisfying.

IRB personnel tend to have high levels of commitment. Most members and staff appear to have a strong sense of the moral importance of the job, and work additional unpaid hours—at home and on weekends—to review protocols as best as they can. This ethos can become mutually reinforcing. As Jeremy, an IRB chair, said:

> Members are so committed, and hold themselves to standards in terms of doing the right thing, carefully reading, analyzing, taking it all seriously, trying to protect subjects. It's very inspiring, and it makes me want to do a better job.

IRB members see themselves as grounded in *ideals*, "picking up this IRB torch." They are aware of historic research scandals such as Nazi experiments and Tuskegee, and see themselves as upholding the good, "fighting" "bad science."

At the same time, many members may also identify strongly with the science they are overseeing. In discussing studies conducted at their institutions, many IRB chairs and members refer to the "research we are doing here," their choice of pronoun reflecting pride and a sense of collaboration. Yet this feeling of collaboration is not always shared by all researchers, and can suggest potential COIs as well.

Members may gain other personal, professional, and intellectual satisfaction and advantages from the work as well. "I really enjoy it, actually," Patrick said, "It's interesting to know what's going on in research arenas I'm not too familiar with." Members not only uphold ethical standards, but learn about exciting cutting edge science.

Some members, such as Warren, enjoy the work so much that they remain on IRBs for over 40 years (underscoring how much IRBs are seen differently across institutions). Extended terms (e.g., 20 years) allow some members to become very experienced "pros," which has advantages. But arguably, younger members could provide fresh perspectives and question incorrect assumptions. Ideally, committees should seek and maintain a balance between new and more seasoned members.

Compensation

Generally, chairs, administrators, and sometimes community members get compensated, whereas ordinary members do not. A few members cite indirect, non-monetary "perks." Maggie, a community member and office manager for a small research company, said, "The community members are not paid. We're volunteers; glad to do it for lunch." Warren, an IRB member for over 40 years, said,

> Retired people like me, no longer paid, have worked for years on the IRB, and enjoy the perks—a free lunch. That's been very persuasive: a nice free lunch, coffee mugs from time to time, free parking, and recognition

for participation. Little things like that make a bit of difference in your commitment and interest in the board.

In Warren's answer there is also the suggestion that it isn't simply the perks in themselves but what the perks symbolize—*recognition for participating* when he is not financially compensated for doing so—that strengthens his long-term commitment to his IRB.

Faculty members work many hours for committees and at times have to face research colleagues' hostility toward the IRB. Compensation can stymie these possible erosions of member and staff enthusiasm and morale. Staff may work many extra hours, and end up demoralized. Scott, a director, said,

> A few years back, there was no pay for members. Now, we compensate them. They spend quite a bit of time, and put themselves at risk—in positions that may not be favorable to some of their colleagues.

For many, however, the funding still wasn't seen as fully covering the effort. "On an hourly rate [the institution] is getting a bargain," Anthony, a chair, said.

Members of IRBs that did compensate relatively well thought that other institutions should do the same. Jeremy argued that members *should* be paid, given their competing demands:

> Members were doing this work before they were compensated, and took it just as seriously. But now they are being compensated. It's not a ton; and they're spending a lot of time. Institutions should all compensate, if they can. As a clinician, I'm not making a ton of money. Every year I'm scrambling. So, I could not be on the IRB, if I wasn't compensated.

Jeremy also thought that lack of compensation might diminish the quality of the reviews:

> Maybe a lot of people are doing the exact same job as they would if they were getting compensated. But how much time can you devote to carefully reading a protocol, when nobody's carving out protected time for that?

Scott felt that paying members would also further motivate them to interact with researchers more, facilitating the review process.

Becoming a Chair

Individuals become IRB chairs in several ways, but customarily begin as regular members, and occasionally as administrators. The candidate generally has some say, but at other times medical center deans or directors may simply state their interest in making the appointment. While some of the chairs I interviewed had had a strong interest in ethics prior to their IRB service, others developed an interest in the area only after joining the committee. Often, a chair was appointed simply because he or she was the longest-serving member of the IRB. As Jack, who is at a rural institution, said, "I don't have a professional background in ethics. I've just been here long enough that when the chair left I was the most experienced person."

Others were surprised to be asked to chair. "Out of the blue I got a phone call," Nathan said, "wondering if I'd become the chair. I said, 'You've got to be joking!' I was interested, but didn't know exactly what it entailed."

Not all members want this position, in part because they are wary of the large time commitment, or of bureaucracy more generally. "I'm not that sort of bureaucrat," Eric explained, "I'm much more the person who thinks up ideas." Others are grateful for the salary support, since they have had difficulty procuring research grants to cover their salary and as regular members received no compensation. Their motives may thus not be solely the protection of subjects. "I'm not much of a researcher," Christopher said, "so I was happy to have something like this that reduced my research obligation."

Often, chairs did not have prior training in ethics or know the federal Common Rule well. Such chairs frequently "run things by" their paid administrative staff, who are more intimately familiar with the regulations. Several chairs told me that they wanted to know the regulations better. After 18 months, Pam remained unsure about the essential elements of informed consent, and wanted to develop more of an ingrained sense of the basis for decisions.

> I've only been here a year and a half, and am coming up to speed…just knowing my way through all the regulations would be helpful—to…have a good gut feeling for what's good, and what's not. Are there eight elements in informed consent, and are they all here?

Like regular IRB members, chairs, too, commonly learn on the job, and detailed and nuanced understandings can take time to acquire fully. As Nathan added,

> I was on the committee for 8 years before I actually understood what was behind the whole organization: how the policies were set up, how the interpretations of what we should do were established.

Over time, for various institutional, professional, and/or personal reasons, chairs may rotate. Institutional leaders may switch IRB chairs to make an IRB more accommodating to research. As Maggie related, "The chair had a number of conflicts with researchers, who started saying, 'Can't we get a new chair? Isn't there a term limit?'" Scandals and audits can also trigger leadership changes.

Over time, many of the IRB members I interviewed had switched roles. Some administrators also later became members or chairs. Maggie explained that 10 years earlier she had been the IRB administrator:

> Then I left the organization and was unemployed for a period, and then was asked to chair. I chaired the IRB for two or three years and then, after my tenure as chair ended, I stayed on as a community member.

Chairs and members may also come and go depending on their other teaching, clinical, and administrative responsibilities. Judy, a chair, explained:

> When I first came on, I did two terms of two years each. Then I had a lot of teaching responsibilities . . . and had a pretty heavy clinical schedule. So I went off the committee, and then was asked to come back to chair it.

Several former chairs I interviewed stayed on their committees afterwards as regular members. Since the training takes so long, there is an incentive to keeping people who are both experienced and good on the committees. Generally, if such members want to stay, committees are glad to have them.

What Are Good Chairs?

Being a "good chair" can require sophisticated interpersonal skills. Members may disagree with each other and/or the chair about a protocol, and negotiating these differences can be challenging. Most boards seek consensus, but that is not always easy. A board leader's arrogance or openness can raise or lower IRB staff morale. As Jeremy explained,

> The most challenging thing about being a leader is *mediating differences* of opinion. Usually, we come to a pretty easy consensus. But some cases elicit strong opinions on either side: not approving, or requiring something. That's always challenging—having the skill to further explore members' thinking and reasoning.

Chairs often need to redirect discussions. Maggie described her efforts to herd wayward members:

> The most difficult part of being a chair is when you get a rogue committee member. One member tends to go off on tangents. That's the most difficult: trying to keep him on task, and bringing him back.

Maggie and others described how chairs sometimes have to "cut members off and say, 'we're not going down that path.'"

Committee leaders also serve as the public face of the IRB, and are therefore responsible for conveying an IRBs' concerns to researchers; so they must also learn to interact as diplomatically as possible with investigators. Jeremy added,

> It's a challenge writing the letters to investigators, communicating clearly and precisely our concerns, and what researchers; need to do about it. I'm getting better at that. But *there's a learning curve* [emphasis added].

Some discomfort is usually inevitable. "It's difficult fielding the disgruntled PI calls and e-mails," Jeremy elaborated. "Somebody's unhappy because I've delayed approval, and they disagree."

DIFFERENCES IN INDIVIDUAL TRAINING
AND EXPERIENCE

Although everyone on an IRB is considering the same protocol, chairs' and members' professional training, experience, and attitudes can shape their decisions, too. These individuals can fall across a spectrum in the degrees to which they are pro- or anti-research. Jeremy said,

> There is a continuum of IRB chairs. There are fierce advocates for investigators, who tend to err on the side of not impeding progress of research. Others are non-interventionists: *let's not doing anything* [emphasis added]. Other people are more inclined to favor requiring something *more*, recognizing that it is going to be a burden, but trying to protect subjects optimally.

These differences in background and views may prompt individuals to weigh the relative costs to researchers differently. Jeremy continued:

> Whether the IRB leadership are PIs, and what their temperaments are, can make a difference. On our IRB, most members are investigators, which helps. We're sympathetic to PIs' concerns, and the challenges of trying to get research approved.

In contrast, many members on other IRBs, and administrative staff more generally, may have no experience doing research, and consequently may not always fully grasp the costs of requesting protocol changes.

Chairs who are also investigators may encourage committee members to support studies. Jack, the rural chair, for instance, reminds his IRB that current oncology treatment is poor, and that they should therefore encourage research as much as possible. "We have a pretty low threshold to say, 'This scientific question needs to be answered. So, let's do it.' I suspect that other IRBs have many more issues." He thinks that committees elsewhere would not like studies of treatments that have relatively high risks and unclear benefits. But he encourages his committee to view such experiments in the context of the limited efficacy of current treatments. Other committees may not do so, and instead focus on the risk-benefit ratio in itself—not as compared with other existing treatments.

He tries to emphasize the need for research, though how much committees can do so is unclear. "Sometimes that's the trump card: there's no good definitive treatment," Jack continued. "It's a matter of *very subtle shades* of gray as to where those lines need to get drawn."

Based on their experience, clinicians may also be more comfortable than non-clinicians with the risks involved in treatments that can be invasive. A study may, for instance, involve injecting a powerful experimental drug directly into the patient's muscle, blood, or spinal fluid. Physicians, experienced with these procedures, may see this as routine and relatively low risk, while others may feel much more uneasy. Whether IRB personnel have had *clinical training*, and if so, what kind, can affect their views. "It's very difficult to be detached," Cynthia, an administrator, said. "Most of our clinicians are more detached than I am. It just makes me hold my breath."

"Community Members"

The views of non-scientists and of individuals outside academic medical centers are important to provide wider perspectives. But many IRBs have difficulty finding appropriate such people to keep and remain on the committee. The regulations were intended for these outsiders both to reflect the concerns of potential subjects and broader communities and to counter possible financial and non-financial conflicts of interest. Yet, the government does not address *who* exactly these nonscientific and unaffiliated members should be, how they should be chosen, and what precise roles and functions they should fill. Many boards therefore struggle with uncertainties about these categories.

Given difficulties finding appropriate individuals, the NIH Office of Human Subjects Research, OHRP's precursor, decided that a single person could fit both these roles.[7] Yet does such a determination meet the intent of the regulations? A non-scientific member who works in the university is most likely affiliated with the institution, not unaffiliated, with strong ties and allegiance to it. Only one person, then, may be outside the ecology of the IRB as described above, and therefore may feel much more an outsider and potentially unsupported, alienated and uncertain.

Only a handful of prior studies have examined issues concerning so-called community members. Dismayingly, prior research about these members has usually lumped these two groups together, as if there were no significant differences between them. One study found that 16 "nonaffiliated/nonscientific" IRB members from 11 institutions were unclear about whom they represented, and felt they would like more respect from the rest of the IRB.[8] Another one of the only studies on these two groups, also failed to differentiate between these, and found that in aggregate they saw themselves as playing a variety of roles, and valuing several traits as ideals (e.g., "assertiveness" and "communication").[9] Robert Allison and colleagues[10] also combined the two groups as "non-scientists" in examining how these individuals viewed their specific functions; they found that this group was more likely than scientists to think that their major role was to review informed consent documents. In one question, however, Allison[10] compared affiliated *vs.* nonaffiliated nonscientific members, and found that nonaffiliated members were more likely, as a trend, to see themselves as laypersons.

In another study, Sohini Sengupta and Bernie Lo[11] found that, of 32 nonaffiliated and nonscientist members from 11 IRBs, who had been on IRBs for an average of 8.4 years, 71.9% held advanced degrees, 88% had occasionally felt intimated and disrespected by the scientists on the IRB, and 78% wanted more education. In this study as well, nonaffiliated and non-scientific members were combined together, rather than differentiated. But an outside researcher and an outside clergyman will bring different perspectives. Here, the regulations had intended that IRBs include both—not just one—of these perspectives. Moreover, the individuals who participated in this survey are extremely well educated, suggesting that they may not be representative of all non-scientific, nonaffiliated members. Nonetheless, even *they* still felt intimidated and disrespected. Anecdotally, many community members are nurses and social workers—"clinicians," even if not scientists *per se*. These "affiliated" clinicians may then vary markedly from unaffiliated non-clinicians, due to training. Nurses and social workers from the institution are not as external as they probably should be and are not always very far from the world of science. Along with individuals unaffiliated with the institution, they may have indeed conducted research now or in the past, and hence, arguably, may not be "non-scientists."

Another study surveyed 284 IRB members, and for "IRB role" listed 105 as physicians, 28 as nurses, and 59 as "unaffiliated member." These researchers found that unaffiliated members were less likely than physicians and nurses to see, as personally important to them protecting confidentiality and privacy and ensuring IRB oversight of a study after it had been approved.[12] It is unclear if these nurses were considered by their IRBs to be "non-scientific." Nonetheless, this study suggests that unaffiliated members perceive certain issues differently than the rest of their committees.

The interviews I conducted revealed how IRBs face several challenges in obtaining, training, and maintaining independent (community or "lay") representation; deciding who these members are, or should be, and whether they do or should represent anyone; and if so, whom. Non-scientific members, by definition, have no scientific background, but frequently therefore have difficulty understanding key aspects of protocols. "Unaffiliated" members, too, may lack scientific training, and then feel "unempowered" to contribute much. Committees vary substantially in how much they encourage these members to participate, how, and with what success.

Because these members potentially have critical roles, regularly pose dilemmas for IRBs, and have received scant attention, I have decided to explore their roles here in greater detail.

Many boards appear unclear who these members should be. Indeed, these individuals are generally referred to as "community" rather than "unaffiliated," "lay," or "non-scientific" members. Though I interviewed only a few community members, almost all of the other interviewees commented on challenges involved in finding, retaining, and appropriately using these members. In fact, on IRBs of 30 or 40 members, only one is a community member—making their numbers relatively small, though their role as stipulated in the regulations is essential. IRBs often seemed to find community members not in any systematic way, but indirectly and at times haphazardly through informal networking and word-of-mouth.

These individuals may be from the community, yet not necessarily representative of the community *per se*. As Martin, a researcher and chair, said,

> They tend to be well-educated people, generally retired—lawyers, social workers, some in health. They generally have an interest in the welfare of human research subjects. They often come from a background where they were involved in providing a service, or involved in care.

Gray areas obviously exist regarding the degrees to which community members are, and should be, unaffiliated or nonscientific. These roles can be fuzzy. Maggie, the former IRB administrator and chair, said, "After my tenure, I stayed on as a community member while working as the office manager for a smaller research company whose protocols are reviewed by that IRB." Maggie is no longer affiliated with the institution, but was in the past; moreover, some might see her present affiliation with a research company as presenting another possible COI. Employees at a research organization, even if they are not scientists by training, may still not fully contribute perspectives of a nonscientist to an IRB, and presumably would be relatively pro research.

Many IRBs then wrestle with whether these members should be more representative of communities from which research subjects are, in fact, recruited, or whether these members are valuable simply for providing some outside perspective. Jeff, the social scientist and former chair, would like more guidance in this area:

> We have not had people like leaders of local churches, nongovernmental organizations or other social service agencies—something with a strong minority membership... One long-term community member is a medical malpractice attorney. He's been a great member, and contributed important things. But I don't think that's the idea of what a community member really is or brings. Another community member is a retired director of research at a few local institutions. During retirement, he's been on our IRB and another institution's IRB. He contributes a lot, and brings a nice cross-fertilization from the other institution. But he's not what you think of as a community member.

Indeed, this last member that Jeff describes may have a pro-researcher bias. At times, IRBs wonder whether these individuals can merely reflect the interests of vulnerable populations, rather than necessarily being members of these groups themselves. Such individuals, in part due to their training—some are even scientists—may understand studies and the ethical complexities involved, but not reflect the views of vulnerable communities. Jeff's misgivings reflect his awareness of this discrepancy. Many IRB members assume that the "spirit" of the regulations was to include members who can present attitudes of patient communities. Thus, while the regulations stipulate only that these two members be, respectively, nonaffiliated and nonscientific, interviewees often think that these individuals should ideally somehow represent research populations.

Still, not all IRBs are certain that committees need such direct or broad representation. Instead, these members might presumably understand the study subjects' viewpoints. Several interviewees felt that their IRB had valuable community members—for example, lawyers or nurses who help clarify and improve consent forms—even though they do not necessarily "represent" the community per se. As Christopher explained,

> They may not be *representative* of the community as a whole, but we've had a law professor for a number of years... He's interested in people's ability to understand consent forms and he's been a very strong advocate of making things clear. That's very nice. We have a woman with a Master's in Counseling. She's also a very good layperson.

A therapist with a master's in counseling, which may have required a thesis that involved conducting research, may not, however, constitute a "non-scientist," and certainly poses a question as to the definition of this term—whether some-one who conducted research at some point in the past, but not at present, fits this category. Christopher also described having had several clergy members on his IRB—which many might feel came closer to representing a wider swath of the community. In fact, however, he valued them for their *pro-science* bent.

> We've had some reverends, which has been very good because they've been able to talk about these studies at their churches on Sunday: "They're doing good stuff if you've got diabetes or hypertension." So they've been able to help promote the *science*, too, and actually help recruit subjects.

Yet such assistance with recruitment and promotion of research is *not* the regulations' intent, and can potentially raise problems, including COIs.

Generally, IRBs seemed to feel that that broader representation is more important when the research is explicitly about a vulnerable community (e.g., low-income minority populations). Almost all patients may have trouble suffi-ciently understanding consent forms, and non-scientific members can presum-ably help committees here, too.

A "community member" may also seem to represent a particular commu-nity, but not in fact do so very well. Membership in a community does not nec-essarily guarantee ability or interest in representing that group's perspectives or best interests. One IRB trusted a Native American representative who turned out not to know much about that culture. Charlotte, the administrator, said,

> We learned that just because someone says they're an Indian...doesn't mean they know anything about doing research in Indian country. We made some assumptions in the expertise we called in...

She added about potential community members that simply being from a par-ticular group does not make one a good community member on a hurly-burly IRB. "Some individuals just have clunky ways of being in the world," Charlotte continued, "and rub other people wrong." Other individuals may know about a particular community but not be eager or especially able to facilitate relationships or interactions between that community and researchers.

Communities may also be divided, and finding an appropriate single rep-resentative may be difficult. Often, the IRB has to rely on researchers having chosen the right community gatekeeper. But an inappropriate community rep-resentative may be involved. Charlotte described this problem as it applies to researchers' efforts to forge useful connections within the community:

[You] go in a community, and find a leader or a gatekeeper, and they invite you into the community, and then [you] find out that you're talking to *the wrong person*. You've gotten a bad reputation because you've aligned yourself with the wrong person. So investigators need to have and understand that level of smarts.

But these goals can be hard, and some IRBs struggle to assess the representativeness of potential community members. However, how to do so, and how to know whether an individual is representative *enough* is difficult. "If you're not dealing with an Indian tribe that is organized and has a government or structure," Charlotte added, "the IRB has to trust the investigator."

Arguably, though, even a small amount of potential representativeness may be helpful. Andrea, the nurse and IRB member, bemoaned that her committee had no African American or Latino regular or community members. "I think there is one person of color on the other committee. There's no minority person at all on my section. Everybody's Caucasian."

WHAT DO COMMUNITY MEMBERS DO?

Committees vary widely, too, in the roles and functions they have these members fill—from only reading consent forms to being primary or secondary reviewers of entire protocols. Some IRBs have non-scientific members evaluate just consent forms—not the rest of the study—though they still vote with the rest of the committee. Andrea said,

> The doctors review the protocols, and other folks do consents. At first, I didn't realize that's what was going on...Nobody ever told me that that's what they do, but that's what they do. I get a copy of a protocol, but my assignment is just the consent...I don't review the protocol itself.

Because the regulations are so minimal (only 17 pages long), committees vary considerably in these details.

IRBs who do not have these members serving as main reviewers may still try to give these individuals' opinions special consideration. Some chairs try to call on community members regularly or periodically for input. Yet, even within the same institution, IRBs can differ in these practices. Christopher said,

> We tend to give extra weight to the community members' opinion in terms of "Do we table this protocol?" or "Is this a minor revision?" If the consent form isn't clear, it'll get tabled...Some other committees don't

empower their community members as much. Our committee members are happier.

This committee is very interested in community representation because their institution is located in an area with a large minority population. Christopher and several of its members are physicians who treat these groups clinically. They feel a special connection with, and responsibility to protect the rights of, this population, and thus take these concerns seriously.

On many IRBs, community members may play a particularly unique and important role by reviewing consent forms, in part because physician members recognize that they themselves have difficulty reading these documents as a layperson would. As Christopher added,

> A doc reads a consent form and it's straightforward. He knows what all the words mean. It's very hard for us to put ourselves in the shoes of someone with a sixth grade education, trying to make sense of what they're being asked to do. We say, "OK, we can't read that as a layperson; so let's hear what our laypeople have to say."

Several IRBs have found that schoolteachers and clergy may be good community members. As Greg, a social scientist and former chair, said about teachers, "They tend to want to be involved in something like this. We have a lot of students from our education program, which is a good pool to draw from."

RELATIONSHIPS WITH REST OF IRB

IRBs generally appreciated and valued their community members, and were often aware of wide social, economic, and educational gaps between themselves (as mostly physicians) and some of these other members (e.g., school teachers). The social context of the rest of the IRB can play a critical role in helping to integrate new members—or failing to do so. Community members face difficulties, since other committee members tend to have far more education, especially about science. Andrea said,

> I've often wondered what they think, and how comfortable they are saying something. They are in this committee with doctors who have grants and all this kind of stuff. It must be intimidating for them, as well. Some of them just sit there and look scared all the time.

Committees vary in how much they encourage these individuals, who may feel intimidated, though uncomfortable articulating their predicament. As most

IRB members are white male physicians, new appointees who are not can feel anxious, overwhelmed, and uncertain about what points to raise. As Andrea explained,

> I'm a nurse, so I'm used to not being in charge of situations where there's also a doctor and other high-level people. That was intimidating at first. One physician on the committee tends to be dismissive. That's still intimidating.

Even Liza, a long-time IRB administrator, said, "I'm not a scientist or physician, so sometimes I think my questions are stupid." She did not feel "looked down on" or purposefully disrespected, but was nevertheless aware of—and sometimes constrained by—her perspective of the gulf between herself and the room of white men in white coats.

A few very well-funded institutions, with hundreds of IRB members, have a full-time staff member to orient and train members—particularly community ones. Many others, however, provide little or no orientation or ongoing logistical on hands-on educational support. Not surprisingly, many committees end up having difficulties finding and retaining effective community members. As Warren said,

> Community members are hard to keep motivated. Most are overwhelmed with the conversation...Medical people use many acronyms. So unless the community member is a former nurse or a doctor—hardly a community member—[they]'re not going to be able to follow that very well. Community members from minority communities are probably totally at sea.

Self-selection may ensue. Christopher said, "Not every community member has been great. We've had a few disasters, though they don't last very long."

IRB Staff

Administrators play critical roles in running IRBs, but range widely in background. Many have had little if any prior ethics training. In one survey, of the total number of hours spent on IRB work, most (58%) are from IRB administrators and administrative staff. Of administrators, 85% were female, 89% were White, 7% were Black, 3% were Hispanic, and 1% were other. Their highest levels of education were high school (19%), bachelor's (28%), master's (18%) and other (35%).[4] A smaller number were lawyers and PhDs. Administrators generally do not vote, but attend meetings, take minutes, and compose memos to researchers, summarizing reviewers' concerns.

They work with impressive dedication, feeling they are part of an important moral cause. As Jaime, an administrator, said,

> Most people who stay in this arena believe they're doing something bigger than just pushing paper. They're part of the human-subject-protection philosophy…helping ensure that research subjects are protected, informed—the principles of the Belmont Report.

Effective administrators tend to be very detail oriented. Chairs themselves, for instance, do not always perform all the bureaucratic steps that must be followed—writing the minutes of meetings and memos to investigators—and staff then do so. Often, administrators handle all correspondence with researchers, and expedited reviews for minimal risk research, assessing whether these investigators have responded appropriately to the committees' concerns. Generally, IRB chairs and co-chairs will review and sign these memos, but staff does the major work involved. As mentioned earlier, chairs may not fully know all the regulations and administrative requirements. "The administrative side is quite complicated," Dwayne, a rural researcher and chair, said. "I really only know the basics." Jack, the rural physician and chair, concurred, "I have to rely on our staff who knows these things very well." He depends on them to comprehend what he calls "the hard bottom line of the regulations." They inform him, "You can do this in this circumstance," or where the rules are "gray"—for example, all the situations in which research is exempt from IRB, or informed consent, can be waived.

Ideally, therefore, the administrators must keep up with all the relevant legal and regulatory developments, and this task can be challenging. Maggie said,

> IRB administrators have to have their finger on the pulse of all of the trends in IRBs and research. Networking with other IRB administrators is fabulous. Researchers and IRB members go to [these staff].

Some administrators seemingly "fall into" the job, and may not be trained in the complete set of skills and background needed. Some begin in the office as secretaries and then take on more responsibilities. As Elaine, an administrator, said,

> It's certainly not what I set out to do in life. I stumbled upon my last job, and moved here, and that's what was open…I'm not practicing what I went to school for.

At a few institutions, a savvy and smart administrator essentially runs the office, functioning as a *de facto* director and chair, and having the most expertise. Many staff, however, focus on smaller parts of the picture: sending and tracking memos to researchers and protocols to reviewers, and keeping track of due dates for annual renewals of all studies and progress report data. As Katherine, an administrator, said,

> Since I stepped into a system already in place, I haven't really had a chance to think about certain issues. We have our nine meetings a year, deadlines, processes, and things that have to get done. It works pretty efficiently. I don't really see how we could do things differently.

In 1999, PRIM&R set up a system to establish Certified IRB Professionals (CIPs).[13] Applicants agree that they will follow good practices and take an exam to show that they know the facts of what the Belmont Report and the Common Rule say. There is a great deal of talk now about IRB administrators becoming "professionalized," but what this means exaclty, and how much it will reduce discrepancies between IRBs is unclear. Frequently, IRBs require complex conceptual assessments. Liza, a director of compliance, said,

> Now, there's certification of IRB professionals, professionalization. It *can't just be a clerical person.* You need to have someone trained and thinking, who can interpret, and be flexible. The chairs are busy.

Yet given this range in their training and skills, and in others' views of them, administrators generally face obstacles. They may fear jeopardizing their position if they are too outspoken in formal or informal meetings with physicians, investigators, members, and chairs. They may have far less education than the doctors with whom they work—who are chairs, members, and researchers—and yet they are commonly "the face of the IRB," in being the only IRB-affiliated person with whom researchers interact. Often, they are the ones who tell researchers what the latter can and cannot do. In IRB meetings, administrators frequently point out when the regulations do or do not support chairs and members' opinions (e.g., when the regulations justify waiving of consent). Yet this difference in knowledge *vs.* hierarchy can prove touchy. As Elaine said,

> If I speak up, I'm not going to have a job...It can really vary depending on the institution and the chairs. At the beginning, I tried to say if I disagreed with the chair's expedited review [i.e., determination that a study doesn't have to come before the full committee]. Then, I didn't. You don't want to fight with certain people. If I think the committee is doing

something wrong, or I don't understand, I will try to voice an opinion. But putting things in writing can destroy you. You have to protect yourself, because everyone wants to blame someone else. You have to hold up to your ethics and morals. I don't know who's qualified to do it. No one has gone to school in all these areas.

In certain ways, these members can bring valuable perspectives akin to those of "community members"; yet some feel they must be careful in offering strong opinions about protocols, since they are relatively low in the institutional hierarchy of academic medical centers. Surprisingly, however, scant other research has been done on administrators' experiences, views, and attitudes. To help IRBs run as efficiently as possible, far more studies are needed to understand more fully how administrators interact with members and chairs and see their roles, how much power and discretion they have, and of what exactly their training consists—how much background in ethics *per se*.

Intra-IRB Dynamics

As a whole, IRBs seek to work by consensus, discussing issues and having members who wish to express an opinion about a certain study do so. "Any other concerns?" a chair might say. A member might respond, "Is the sample size big enough? Shouldn't the consent form also mention risk to privacy and confidentiality as a possible risk of the study?" Another member might wholly allay the concern. Otherwise, concerns and questions are listed on a memo to the researcher. "Okay, so we'll have the investigator respond to the following issues," the chair may conclude. If a debate has ensued and continues, the chair might take a vote. On most issues, IRBs reach agreement fairly readily. Discussions and clarifications facilitate concurrence. Yet for a significant number of other studies, achieving uniformity can be hard. Personalities and other factors can shape opinions and decisions. Pam, an administrator, observed,

> You have 15 personalities in a room: 15 ideas about whether something meets our definition of an adverse event, or is a mistake. We read the definition and look at the events, and go back and forth about whether it meets the definition. We may or may not talk about similar past things that have happened, to set a precedent. But everything's unique. We try to come to the conclusion the actually meets the definition.

Many IRBs tend to follow their "gut feelings" at any one point in time. As with any group of diverse individuals, personal feelings can mold decisions. As Vicki, the chair, said,

> There's always a lot of idiosyncrasies amongst the members, which has its upsides and downsides. This is in any group—particularly with highly motivated and professional people. Frequently, something is brought to the fore that people hadn't thought of. Somebody mentions it, and everybody says, "You're right!" On the other hand, somebody can be flogging a dead horse.

Interpersonal dynamics can be hard to negotiate. At times, particular members may articulate strong attitudes that can be hard to redirect. For instance, attorneys on the IRB can press legal rather than ethical concerns. As Vicki described,

> We have lawyers, and they drive the board and researchers nuts. One isn't bad, but another will not make a decision to save his soul. All he does is raise roadblocks. He doesn't say, "No," but won't say "Yes." He's difficult. Sometimes I can go around him. If I talk to him directly, we can generally come to a conclusion. Or, we say, "Things don't have to be unanimous," although typically they are, or close to it. We always vote. Finally, I'll say, "I think it's time to stop. Can I get a motion?" Suddenly you get this dead silence. He knows he doesn't know the science, and we have a very bright lawyer with some science training. So if she is in the room, he will defer to her. The best thing is to try and get them together.

Adroit chairs will thus try to arrange discussions outside of full board meetings with one or more members. Within the local dynamics and politics of boards, such informal discussions and negotiations can be critical. Savvy IRB leaders can seek interpersonal interventions. Vicki, for instance, assists researchers in trying to navigate responses from the male lawyer she mentions:

> When investigators need his OK that something is legal, he basically won't give them an answer that is doable in this lifetime. Usually, they come back to me. I'll say, "We'll do it *this* way."

At meetings, members may try to parade their special knowledge, creating additional tensions. "There's occasional showboating," Olivia said. "People showing how much they know. But mostly, depending on the chair, it can go well." Meeting tone can thus vary considerably, depending on size and other characteristics. In influencing both the form and content of meetings, chairs can play decisive roles.

At times, some chairs thought IRBs can be "dysfunctional." "Having a good, well-functioning versus dysfunctional IRB can be a challenge," Greg said. In these interviews, social scientists such as Greg tended to appear more attuned than physicians or administrators to these larger social dynamics and processes.

LACK OF INSTITUTIONAL MEMORY

Ideally, an IRB will respond to certain questions regarding studies in a consistent way over time, using the same logic, rather than being wholly fickle or idiosyncratic. No two protocols are exactly the same; they differ from each other in various major and minor ways. Yet if IRBs draw on their own past decisions as the rationale for similar ones moving forward, the committee doesn't have to formulate, argue, and negotiate difficult issues from scratch with every protocol; and determinations on subtle points may subsequently be less difficult. In reality, though, IRBs frequently have little or no formalized institutional memory, or mechanisms to build or enhance it; and they thus end up being less efficient and consistent over time. Often, in fact, there seems to be little incentive to follow established precedents and avoid discrepancies. Frank said,

> IRBs have a certain institutional memory, but it's not standardized. Someone will object to a protocol that asks for a biopsy after treatment. Someone else will say, "Yeah, but I remember a couple of years ago, we allowed that to go through!" One way to standardize it would be more written checklists. But even that wouldn't guarantee it.

An IRB would also have to remember and know to look for past decisions, which can be arduous. As Anthony said,

> We talk about how to ensure that our institutional memory and consistency are appropriate. We don't do a great job. We have some mechanisms in place, subject to human error: simply having long-standing members of the committee, which is not perfect. We're still relying on our own *individual* memory.

Yet categorizing all past decisions and periodically searching through them for precedents would take large amounts of staff time. He continued,

Often, we say: instead of relying just on our memory, we're going to go back to those files, and establish some sense of coherence. But given our massive amount of paper, the burden on our staff is pretty high. If staff can't answer it by the end of the committee meeting, it can take hours to days to dig that up.

Yet increasingly, study protocols and committee responses are becoming electronic, which may potentially help improve institutional memory; still the transition to electronic systems is generally not easy or complete, and would presumably involve only post-electronic decisions, not earlier ones. Anthony felt it is "going to take an enormous amount of time." Yet, he is concerned here with improving uniformity only within a single IRB, not across multiple ones. Still, search engines can make looking for potentially relevant cases among recent cases much easier than in the past, and web sites with password-protected areas limited to IRBs could allow for interchange of relevant cases and decisions to foster collaboration and consistency within and between committees.

ONGOING EDUCATION

Future education of IRB chairs, members, and administrators can help. CIPs, who are mostly administrators, must fulfill continuing education requirements every year. Several efforts to enhance education and build consensus on and between committees can be beneficial. PRIM&R holds large national conferences that hundreds of individuals—mostly IRB administrators—attend every year. Sessions cover topics such as "IRBs 101," informed consent forms, protecting data, biobanking, research on the Internet, improving IRB procedures, and handling alleged researcher misconduct. But federal policy does not require IRB chairs, administrators, or members to have any initial or ongoing training in ethics or the regulations, and most chairs and members have little if any of either. Other national conferences may provide education on other aspects of bioethics, at times related to research on humans. Such national conferences can aid to a certain degree, but are expensive to attend. Hence, not all chairs, staff, and members go. A few institutions pay for members to travel to trainings. But far more commonly, institutions lack the extra funds. As Scott explained,

A problem is not having the resources to send our reviewers to more conferences. It's a lot of money: $1,000–$2,000 a pop. With 30 members, you need a lot of funds. But they come back with information, and can serve as ambassadors to their respective academic departments, spreading the knowledge.

Recent budget constraints exacerbate these limitations.

Surprisingly, several chairs and administrators here have *never* attended national IRB meetings. "They don't go to out-of-state trainings," Dana, an IRB chair, said, "and may not even be aware of these."

Some IRBs are completely isolated from others, and may avoid a national meeting not only due to the expense, but because they believe that they already possess sufficient knowledge. As Dana added, "It's far, and they think they know it all."

Nonetheless, these large professional meetings can allow for discussion about valuable approaches to common problems. "One *should* go," Dana continued. "Sharing information would help."

However, given the different possible interpretations of regulations, national conferences do not always provide clear answers or consensus on disputed cases, and speakers at large meetings may offer their own view, rather than the fullest and most correct answer. "PRIM&R drives me crazy," Joe, a chair, said. "Speakers may or may not be right, depending on the topic. Yet people then walk away thinking that's the answer."

Again, research ethics is closer to the so-called "soft" social sciences and humanities than to the hard sciences. As we will see, more awareness of needs for rigor, coordination, and use of precedents are thus vital.

Conclusions

In sum, these interviews, the first to explore several key aspects of the inner dynamics of IRBs—how and why IRB members and chairs are chosen, oriented, trained, and interact—reveal several complexities. These individuals undergo socialization processes—formal and informal, cognitive and emotional, and personal and professional. "Socialization"—the processes by which individuals learn to adopt a particular social role—has been described among physicians and other groups.[14,15,16,17] These processes vary in effectiveness, and create tensions, but can be unexamined by the individuals and organizations involved. Research in other realms suggests that people enter organizations with differing personalities, expectations, and knowledge,[18,19] and these processes of initiation can be more or less successful. When these mechanisms fail to allow for relatively smooth transitions, individuals leave, resulting in high turnover.[18]

IRB member and chair selection and training are often informal, unsystematic, and haphazard. Members and chairs may be chosen for complex political or institutional reasons; they range widely in whether they have had formal ethics education or orientation, and if so, what, how much, and when. Few if any faculty may have had more than a few hours of online research ethics learning, although some chairs have had a long-standing interest in the area. Most learn "on the job." Yet what, how much, and how rapidly they absorb what they need to know can vary. Surprisingly, many members, chairs, and administrators have never attended a national ethics meeting.

Given criticisms of these committees as inefficient and inconsistent, as mentioned in Chapter 1,[20,21,22] these issues are particularly important. In considering changes in IRBs, these wide variations in ethics education, experiences, and motivations for joining committees pose concerns. No policies or guidelines provide any details concerning how to choose members—other than specifying that expertise, and an unaffiliated and non-scientific member, are needed—nor what kinds of training and background they should have. The government, through NIH and the National Science Foundation (NSF), mandates minimal ethics training for *researchers,* but not for any IRB personnel. Initial and ongoing training requirements for IRBs, chairs, and members should be established, too.

Some chairs feel that they do not require much additional training, since their staff members know the regulations well. But as we will see in the next few chapters, committees struggle with several specific questions and challenges, for which knowing the specifics of the regulations, and how to apply them in different situations, would help, since several recent controversies have involved specific interpretations. At times, IRBs at prominent institutions have misinterpreted the regulations. Hence, though committee administrators play crucial roles, often knowing more about regulations and procedures than do members and frequently chairs, they themselves may not all have sufficient training to address the complicated and nuanced dilemmas in interpretation and application of the regulations that may be involved. Enhancing the education of members, chairs, and staff is thus crucial.

More study of community members is also needed. "Non-scientific" and "non-affiliated" members may feel intimidated; it is important to glean how often, among whom, and to what degree that is the case. Yet these areas may be difficult to investigate, as members who feel apprehensive about their roles may hesitate to discuss these sensitive topics.

Still, many of these problems can be ameliorated. Minimal standards for initial and continuing education are needed. A critic may aver that institutions lack resources for such training, but each year IRBs review billions of dollars of research. The NIH gives out $24 billion in research grants per year.[23] Potentially, a small proportion could be used to ensure that these committees have sufficient training. Such an investment could yield valuable returns.

Particularly as many biomedical and social scientists criticize these boards, these committees need to demonstrate that their power is justified, if that is the case. Possession and demonstration of sufficient education can help. Additional training can be developed and instituted, perhaps with IRBs sharing materials they put together. Since not all personnel can travel to national conferences, interactive webinars can be further established. In other realms,[24] formal mentoring and role models have helped. Such formal mentoring on IRBs—whereby a long-standing member is explicitly assigned to mentor each new member—may be valuable. "Best practices" should be developed to include such mentoring and what areas it should cover.

Efforts have also been made to improve the education of IRB members, but the focus and success of such attempts remain unknown. In general, how ethics can best be taught in the "real world" remains uncertain.[25] After all, not only knowledge, but also attitudes, beliefs, and social settings can shape human decisions.[26] IRBs should draw on certain ethical principles—autonomy, beneficence, non-maleficence, and justice—but education needs to focus not simply on general principles per se, but pragmatic considerations of how to apply these notions and make decisions in varying, evolving contexts. Increasingly, IRB administrators are becoming CIPs and PRIM&R emphasizes that IRB staff sees themselves as "professionals." Becoming a CIP requires taking an exam; yet this certification remains optional. Moreover, the test does not assess how administrators interpret ethical principles that committees define and apply differently. In addition, IRB chairs and members ordinarily do not take such an exam. How much initial and ongoing ethics training and background, in what specific areas, they do and should have is not wholly clear.

These phenomena have several implications for future research: to explore more fully exactly how much and what type of initial and ongoing training chairs, members, and staff do and should have, of what it consists, and what specific gaps persist. Several members felt that to become fully knowledgeable and comfortable on the IRB took a few years, raising questions of what is learned over that time "on the job," and what exactly heightened their confidence and comfort. These processes of *socialization* over time—how individuals enter these committees and come to stay, thrive, or become demoralized and leave, and how these processes may affect IRB functioning and decisions—needs further investigation.

Quandaries emerge, too, as to whether so-called community members do or should represent anyone, and if so, whom, and how well, and how to assess that. Current guidelines define these members by what they are not—non-scientists and nonaffiliated. But what they *are* is unclear. Confusion exists even concerning their name—whether they are "nonaffiliated" or community or "lay" members—underscoring the ambiguities surrounding who they are supposed to be. The degree to which committees are disturbed by this apparent lack of representativeness varies, as do the ways they interpret the regulations. Other means of identifying these and other potential members can also help; IRBs often struggle with finding, choosing, and using non-scientific and nonaffiliated members.

The fact that these members are generally found in unsystematic ways, through happenstance, may seem inevitable, but can certainly be improved. Community members may have friends who work in the institution, and thus be indirectly affiliated, which could cause COIs. The lack of attention or guidance concerning these issues is disturbing.

Getting "community" members to stay on an IRB poses challenges, too. The sample in one prior study[11] stayed an average of 8.4 years, which may not be representative of those who ever join the IRB, since this research may have included nonscientific *affiliated* members (e.g., hospital social workers). Many nonaffiliated members may leave earlier, feeling ill-prepared or overwhelmed.

This raises another deficit in the prior research. While prior studies have tended to analyze "nonaffiliated" and "non-scientific" members together (except in one question in the study by Robert Allison and colleagues),[8,9,10,11,12] these two types of members can dramatically differ. Combining them does not appear to reflect the "lived realities" of their experiences. Instead, these categories constitute two very different groups, with different functions, backgrounds, roles, attitudes, and approaches concerning reviews. Affiliated *vs.* nonaffiliated nonscientists can also differ since the former but not the latter may have COIs, working for the institution.

Future research and discussion should thus separate these groups, given their very different characteristics and roles, and should investigate more fully who these members in fact are, as well as how different IRBs find these members, how long these individuals stay on IRBs, and how often one individual jointly fills both roles.

Similarly, the OHRP should reconsider the decision that a single individual can simultaneously serve both roles. Given recent scandals involving financial and non-financial COIs[27,28]and tensions with communities (e.g., in the case of the Havasupai),[29] IRBs should include *both* nonaffiliated *and* non-scientist members to avoid both types of problems. Guidelines are needed regarding whether these members do or should represent others, and if so, who and to what degree; whether such representativeness should be assessed, and if so how; and whether these individuals should no longer be called community members. Arguably, IRBs should also include *more than* one member in each category. Since feeling fully a part of an IRB can be difficult even for "insiders" within its ecology, increasing the number of "outsiders"—of both nonscientific and unaffiliated members—could also help these community members feel more empowered and visible.

Approaches that have worked more or less well in recruiting, maintaining, and helping these members could also be presented and shared. Educational chat rooms and modules could be developed, since these and other members often cannot afford to travel to conferences.

As we will see, *who* is on these committees, and how they interact is critical to understand *what* these boards decide. Many of the decisions of who should be on an IRB within an institution are based on different kinds of knowledge about the candidates. With outsiders, there is no easy way of wholly predicting their fit—psychologically, intellectually, emotionally. They may slow the process for researchers. Of course, they are required for precisely this reason—because they are not part of the institution. But questions then arise of how smoothly IRBs should run. As Henry Beecher argued in his 1966 article, enumerating unethical research practices in studies published in major journals, these committees are essential, to serve as a check on researchers.[30] Hence, non-scientists and outsiders are especially important. Yet the fact that these members are intimidated poses concerns. As we will see, such intimidation can become too much. Again, proper balance is key.

WHAT IRBs DO

The Contents of IRB Decisions

CHAPTER 3

Weighing Risks and Benefits, and Undue Inducement

Weighing risks and benefits can seem straightforward, but is at times extremely complex.

In June 2013, one of the most divisive recent debates in bioethics erupted concerning the risks and benefits of a study that examined how much oxygen to give premature infants. Every year, approximately 500,000 babies are born prematurely, and 5,000 of them die.[1,2] The vast majority of premature and low-birth-weight infants require supplemental oxygen.[3] Pediatricians in Neonatal Intensive Care Units (NICUs) have, however, faced a dilemma. If they give too much oxygen, babies are more likely to survive, but also to develop vision problems and become blind. If the doctors give too little oxygen, more babies die, but the survivors are more likely to be able to see. Thus, doctors give a wide range of oxygen levels, hoping to avoid either too much or too little. But within this wide spectrum, doctors vary. Some choose 89 percent oxygen saturation, while others give closer to 95 percent. Until 2004, no study had been conducted to determine definitely which was, in fact, better.

Hence, from 2004 to 2009, 23 institutions, including Yale, Stanford, and Duke, conducted the Surfactant, Positive Pressure, and Oxygenation Randomized Trial (SUPPORT) study. IRBs at all 23 institutions approved the study. When the mothers were in labor, researchers randomly assigned the future infants, before they were born, to one of two levels of oxygen saturation: 85–89 percent or 91–95 percent. In May 2010, the results were published,[4] showing that the higher amount was more likely to avoid death, but also to cause blindness. At the higher level, 16.2 percent died before leaving the hospital and 17.9 percent developed eye disease. At the lower level, more died (19.9 percent), but fewer (8.5 percent) developed eye disease.

Two years later, in 2011, the Office for Human Research Protections (OHRP) received a complaint about the study and, in response, sent a letter to the investigators. The agency wrote that the informed consent forms had been inadequate, and asked the institutions to take corrective action.[5] Public Citizen, the consumer advocacy group founded by Ralph Nader, vociferously attacked the study and argued that OHRP had "failed to demand adequate corrective actions."[6] A *New York Times* editorial, entitled "An Ethical Breakdown," concluded that the study's failure was "startling and deplorable."[7] A major battle erupted, with competing groups of 45 and 46 bioethicists each publishing opposing letters to the *New England Journal of Medicine* in June and July 2013. In December 2013, *The American Journal of Bioethics* devoted an entire issue to the controversy, publishing three major articles, and 17 responses from leading bioethicists—disagreeing significantly on which side was right and why.[8]

OHRP argued that the study's informed consent forms significantly overemphasized the benefits and downplayed the risks of the study, and failed to mention death as a possible outcome. The forms said, for example, that "subjects may have a possible decrease in chronic lung disease . . . and/or a decrease in the need for eye surgery"[9] But these documents did not mention the possibility that the subjects, conversely, may have an increased risk of lung disease or eye problems. OHRP also stated that the study was not minimal risk, as the researchers had contended, but rather involved substantial risks since many infants would receive oxygen levels that were different than those they would have otherwise gotten.

Some observers supported OHRP, concurring that the consent forms had significant deficiencies. But the study's defenders maintained that, in questioning this study, OHRP had "over-reached."[10] They argued that death was a possibility for these premature infants even if they were not in the study; and that these consent forms only needed to mention those aspects of the study that were *not* part of the care that participants would receive anyway.[11] Since the risk of death for these infants was not greater than it would have been outside the research, they said that the consent form did not need to mention this danger. Moreover, these study advocates averred that when doctors are divided about the use of two different treatments and both approaches are considered "standard of care," studies are needed to decide which is better. Such comparative effectiveness research (CER), as it is called, is vital to improving health care. These proponents argued that this study exemplified such research, and that to oppose it would impede further such investigations. In fact, Simon Whitney, a physician and lawyer at Baylor Medical School, had argued that for this study, informed consent could be waived altogether, since the research was minimal risk.[12] He pointed out that obtaining consent for this project cost $200,000, and took the study more than twice as long to enroll the needed number of subjects. In the meantime, without the results of the experiment, many infants would continue to die. Since doctors were divided, both levels of oxygen were acceptable. Randomizing infants to one of these two doses may change which one each patient would otherwise receive but, the study's supporters argued, does not in itself necessarily make that treatment better or worse.

Opponents countered that randomization itself *was* a risk. In the study, modified oxygen machines controlled and masked gas levels in ways that do not usually occur. Hence, physicians would not be able to monitor and adjust the infants' level over time as they otherwise would. Randomization, rather than the clinician's judgment about each individual patient, would determine the dose, which would be fixed through the course of the treatment.

In addition, a central tenet of research ethics is that subjects can be randomized to one of two interventions only if so-called clinical equipoise exists—that is, if scientists do not have reason to believe beforehand that one approach is better than the other. If the researchers think one treatment is superior, they should not knowingly be giving subjects the other, inferior treatment. Yet earlier research, on which the SUPPORT study was based, showed that 93 percent of NICUs used higher, rather than lower doses. Only 7 percent of NICUs had maximum targets of less than 92 percent, and 93 percent had targets of more than 92 percent. Moreover, *some* hospitals use a much narrower range of 88–92 percent. Hence, in assigning many infants to lower amounts of oxygen (85–89 percent), the study increased their risk of death.[13] Critics have thus argued that equipoise did *not* exist. Presumably, many parents would not want their premature baby randomized to receive a level that only 7 percent of centers provided (while 93 percent of centers gave more), knowing that the risk of death would probably increase. Granted, lower doses would presumably reduce the risk of blindness. But to many parents, these two risks would undoubtedly not be equivalent—they would understandably prefer to have a blind child than a dead one.

Ideally, if doctors are divided in their practices 50/50, randomizing patients to each treatment is fine; but if 93 percent of doctors prescribe a higher level, and only 7 percent aim at a lower amount, questions emerge about giving 50 percent of the ill subjects the less popular dose. The consent form stated that both levels were considered "acceptable." The parents were *not* told that 93 percent of doctors give the higher oxygen level. Half of the parents might not want their child to have only the lower level, if they knew that only 7 percent of doctors provided it. Critics argued that the study, as it was designed, did not have equipoise, and hence should not even have been conducted.

Debates continue as to whether randomization was a risk. John Lantos[14] argued that in earlier studies of oxygen saturation, infants in studies did better, regardless of which treatment they received, than did those outside the study. Nurses and doctors may be extra-motivated and devote special attention to patients in a study. Therefore, Lantos wrote, randomization should in fact be listed as a benefit of studies.[xiv] But as Public Citizen points out, infants in SUPPORT were healthier than those excluded by researchers from the study,[15] and hence did better—not because study subjects received extra attention in the study. Moreover, in many other studies, patients receiving a new treatment do *worse* than those receiving standard of care.

These debates thus open larger questions of when exactly equipoise exists—exactly *how* split doctors need to be about two competing treatments to conclude that *patients can be randomly assigned to each*. In these debates, each side seems to raise several valid points, but neither group is entirely right or wrong. Though study proponents argue that critiques of SUPPORT imperil all comparative effectiveness research, the question is not whether such research can be conducted, but *how*—exactly which treatments should be compared, and what subjects should be told about them.

At the same time, though OHRP asked the University of Alabama to take corrective action, it is not clear what action would be appropriate at this point.

In June 2013, however, under intense pressure from NIH and others, OHRP backed down. These debates continue, and parents whose infants died are suing the researchers, bolstered by OHRP's charge of unethical behavior

As I saw when my father wrestled with whether to undergo chemotherapy with its terrible side effects and unclear benefits, weighing potential unknown risks and benefits can be extremely hard—especially when life and death are involved. Even in one family, individuals can differ widely about participating in research. IRBs, I soon found, often struggle and argue about these questions, too.

Since the federal regulations governing IRBs are relatively minimalist, individual committees have a great deal of leeway concerning these issues. Law, like ethics, is not a science, but is bound by many more rules and seeks to follow precedents very seriously. Attorneys and even judges can interpret laws in different ways, but appellate courts exist with the sole purpose of adjudicating and often overturn the rulings of lower judges. The Supreme Court serves as a final arbiter, though its nine justices are divided rather than unanimous in 70 percent of cases.[16] Moreover, even when the judges are unanimous, they may disagree widely on the legal reasoning behind their conclusions.[17] Interpreting and applying ambiguous language, these courts draw on published decisions, and document and disseminate their own interpretations, thereby establishing and building on widely published precedents. Judges regularly refer to this large body of case law. But for IRBs, no such mechanisms exist. Committees and researchers lack these tools. *Instead, in many ways, local IRBs serve as their own police, judge, jury and Supreme Court*. Institutions and OHRP can affect IRBs. Nevertheless, these committees maintain enormous autonomy.

Once a committee has determined how to interpret and apply the regulations for a particular study, it tends to see its decision as incontrovertible, rather than as subject to differing alternative interpretations. Even many philosophers have seen principles as either present or absent in an argument. While some philosophers feel that for any ethical problem or question, only one best answer exists, in practice wide disagreements persist about many areas in bioethics, even among experts. Every month, *The American Journal of Bioethics* publishes target articles followed by six to 12 commentaries that usually offer a range of contrasting, if not dramatically conflicting, views.

Balancing Risks *vs.* Benefits

When evaluating a study, one of the IRB's chief charges is to examine and weigh the potential risks to the patient versus the potential benefits—to the patient and to the expansion of scientific knowledge and society at large. IRBs often struggle with this balance. In general, researchers should follow the principle of clinical equipoise—a patient should be entered into a study comparing two therapeutic approaches only if the researcher is genuinely uncertain at the outset whether one of these treatments is better than the other.[18] However, applying this principle can be tricky.[19,20]

In general, people view probabilities subjectively, using biases and so-called heuristics—simplified ways of conceptualizing complex competing odds. As the Nobel Prize–winning psychologist Daniel Kahneman has argued, if a wild boar is suddenly running toward us, we instantly gauge whether it is better to run left, right or backward—climb the tree or run to the cave[21]—without precisely calculating and comparing the risks and benefits of each possible alternative. So, too, we tend to rely on gut feelings in assessing risks. Studies have shown that, psychologically, most people overrate rare but traumatic events, weighing responses to possible losses more than responses to potential future gains[21]—overvaluing risks and undervaluing benefits. So, too, in making risky medical decisions, patients and doctors frequently face uncertainties, and make and rely on rough assumptions.[22,23] Patients may also differ from providers in perceiving risks and benefits, based on their respective education and past experiences.[24,25,26,27] Perceptions of danger and risk can also involve subjective elements related to cultural rather than simply individual fears. In *The Immortal Life of Henrietta Lacks*, for example, Rebecca Skloot explains that many African American residents of Baltimore in the 1950s believed that members of their community were sometimes snatched off the streets at night and used in medical experiments,[28] reflecting histories of grossly unequal treatment during and after slavery.

How IRB chairs, members, and staff should respond to these complexities—how they are to weigh risks and benefits from the researcher's and patient's perspectives and also their own—remains unclear. Often IRBs must weigh many possible risks and benefits simultaneously. Committees must decide whether researchers should be allowed to test any two drugs against each other, if the products are ethically equivalent (i.e., that so-called clinical equipoise is present). A new drug might reduce a patient's symptoms more than the standard treatment, but cause worse side effects. Another drug might have fewer side effects, but be somewhat less effective. Yet the likelihoods of each of a study's possible future risks and benefits are frequently highly uncertain. The exact amounts of the possible differences—whether 10 percent more possible benefit is worth 20 percent more risk—can be crucial, but unpredictable and hard to weigh.

As we saw in the Kennedy Krieger study of lead levels in different homes (see Chapter 1), IRBs, courts, journalists, researchers, and subjects may perceive potential risks and benefits of a study differently. The court, and many journalists and observers, suggested that not only was the informed consent form deficient, but the study lacked equipoise—that the risks of only partially abated apartments were too great, and that the consent form inadequately described these.[29]

Yet, in making these assessments, individuals—whether IRB members, researchers, or subjects and their families—frequently rely on subjective "gut feelings" and highly personal assessments. As a nurse, Andrea was very aware of how idiosyncratically patients, families, and committees all perceive risks and benefits.

> It's very hard to weigh risks and benefits.... Everybody has to make calculations on their own. We thought a drug might help a sick patient, but a side effect was stroke. The likelihood was extremely small; but one patient turned it down because his mother had had a terrible stroke. He was a sick man—why would he turn down the possibility that this could help him for a 2 percent chance of a stroke? He wouldn't take that risk. All the IRB can do is try and make things as clear as we can. We have "likely," "less likely," and "rare but serious." I think "likely" is 20 percent, which in my mind is *not* likely. I would say "likely" is 50–60 percent—better than an even chance.

She felt strongly that IRBs need to ensure that consent forms conveyed these vagaries as best as possible. Yet *to describe risks not in percentages, but in descriptive language—as "likely" or "less likely"—is hard, and open to wide interpretation.*

DIFFERING DEFINITIONS AND THRESHOLDS OF RISK

"Truly Safe"? How Much Risk Is Okay?

When participants suffer or die in research studies, as did infants in the SUPPORT study, and Jessie Gelsinger in the gene transfer experiment, questions arise of whether these studies were too risky to have progressed as far as they had. IRBs therefore wrestle with exactly *how* safe a study is or should be. The difficulty of this question is compounded by the fact that the outcomes of experiments are by definition unknown, and risks can range from direct to indirect. Anxieties can thus shape IRB assessments of both the likelihood and seriousness of harm. Gauging potential benefits and harms is not a science, and is therefore shadowed by uncertainties. "When you don't know for sure what the risks and benefits will be, it's really hard, involving perceptions," Judy, a chair, explained. "You know what they *might* be, but you really don't know."

Consequently, I found, individuals and boards differ on the standard—whether a protocol needs to be *completely* safe to be approved, or whether the benefits only need to justify the risks. In fact, the regulations stipulate only the latter, not the former, and state that committees should reduce risks. Yet many IRBs feel they should "go beyond the regulations" and get rid of risks in some way. Olivia, the health care provider and chair, said,

> I worry: is the study *truly safe*? We do a lot of studies that are potentially high risk. We worry, but have to trust the investigator. That's why we look so carefully at the progress reports.

An IRB must rely on local researchers to do what they have claimed they are going to do, and to document what they have done. But establishing sufficient confidence can be hard. The IRB may not know of the researcher, or the PI may have a bad track record, or the risks can seem high. IRBs may be *overly* cautious, seeing their job as promoting subject protection, not science as well. Committees have ample reason to be vigilant, and no strong incentive to countervail this stance. Others feel that the cost of this vigilance to science is at times too high. Patrick, a physician and regular member, said,

> Being cautious is the IRB's job, but they may be *overly* cautious. For most IRBs, nothing good can come from approving a protocol. Every time you approve a protocol, there's a risk for bad things happening— including bad press.

Committees may thus avoid risk as much as possible, rather than lowering it to the point at which it is commensurate with the potential benefits.

IRB members and chairs who are not themselves investigators or clinicians may be especially wary of research. As an investigator who was new to his IRB, Patrick found this startling:

> Sometimes I get the impression that non-clinical IRB members and staff think that researchers are trying to harm people! Certainly, researchers

have a vested interest and are biased—that's why it's good to have the IRB. I think HHS [The U.S. Department of Health and Human Services] says, "The protection of research subjects is the IRB's primary purpose." But that, almost by definition then, presents a tension in getting the research done.

In fact, Patrick misquotes the current regulations, which stipulate instead that risks should be weighed against benefits. But his misunderstanding is revealing; since he is a researcher, this impression comes probably from his IRB. He continued, "You hear this mantra of, 'What is the safest thing?' We're always going to err on the side of safety. But in clinical medicine, there's a justified risk/benefit ratio."

CHALLENGES IN QUANTIFYING RISK

Assessing dangers can be hard because many patients are already sick, like my father, and desperate for any interventions. Many ill patients also have what are called *therapeutic misconceptions*—even though they are participating in a blinded randomized study, they believe that their white-coated doctor is nonetheless choosing a treatment that is best for them individually, when in fact they may be randomized to a placebo. Despite being told otherwise, many patients persist in this belief.[30]

Participants may not understand the limitations and restrictions of research—especially in early-phase studies that are designed only to assess the side effects of drugs or initial possible effectiveness on small numbers of patients before being tried on larger numbers, and that usually have little promise of providing clear benefits. Andrea said,

> In their heart of hearts, subjects believe they're going to be the lucky guy who might get cured with this unlicensed therapy. Patients may agree to pretty onerous things because they're *desperate*.

Patients may fail to grasp the complexities involved, and just want to enroll. As Andrea said about consent forms,

> I'll say to subjects, "You should take it home and read it." "No, I don't want to read it. I just want to sign it." Some people are quite militant. They don't want to hear about it. They're scared of dying, and the doctor said he thought they might be interested in this. So they believe that the doctor is recommending what's best for them, even though the doctor may have clearly said, "I don't know if this is going to work." Patients don't necessarily hear what you tell them.

Patients with no other treatment alternatives may enroll in so-called last resort studies that have high risks and very uncertain potential benefits, posing additional challenges. Unfortunately, both experimental *and* existing therapies may be high risk and offer little benefit. IRBs must then struggle with when and how much to be paternalistic—by attempting to protect the patient against his or her own desperation and potentially poor judgment, and when to let patients choose to enter such trials, despite the potential harms. As Cynthia, an administrator, said,

> One of the most difficult issues is: is it OK to let people enroll in last resort studies? What is our responsibility for people enrolling in a study in which the prospect of benefit is very slim—almost entirely risk? But the alternative is no treatment. The study can make their last days worse! One of the hardest things is to allow people to have self-determination, and just make sure that all the information has been presented—that they're not coerced.

But if some doctors may try to pressure their patients too much, others may be too vague: Cynthia added, "Some doctors just tell such patients, 'Yeah, we've got a research study.'"

SOCIAL RISKS

A researcher may want to study rates of psychiatric problems, drug use, criminal behavior or IQ tests among a particular group—whether the Havasupai, African Americans, or gay men. But the results of such a study, if it found higher rates of problems in these populations, could be used to discriminate further against these groups. IRBs then face questions of whether to allow, change, or disapprove such protocols.

According to federal regulations, IRBs should assess potential social *benefits* of research, but not such long-term social *risks*. The regulations stipulate that:

> The IRB should not consider possible long-range effects of applying knowledge gained in the research (for example, the possible effects of the research on public policy), as among those research risks that fall within the purview of its responsibility. [31]

For example, if a researcher wanted to study rates of HIV and drug use among inner-city teenage girls, in order to help design a preventive program, the IRB may be hesitant to approve the research, fearing that there is a risk that these girls will become stigmatized and that law enforcement officials may "crack down" on this population and arrest them. The regulations dictate that the IRB should not consider such a possibility in the risk–benefit assessment. Yet the Obama Administration's proposals on IRBs posed questions about this stipulation:

> Do IRBs correctly interpret this provision as meaning that … it is not part of their mandate to evaluate policy issues such as how groups of persons or institutions, for example, might object to conducting a study because the possible results of the study might be disagreeable to them?[31]

The pediatrician and ethicist Alan Fleischman and several colleagues have felt that local IRBs *do* nonetheless at times consider broad social risks, though the regulations tell these committees not to.[32] These authors considered four realms—behavioral genetics, adolescent behavior, harm reduction, and human genetic enhancement—and concluded that IRB considerations of these social risks "sometimes create significant delays in initiating or even prevent such research."[23] These scholars oppose IRBs' considerations of these issues, since "predicting negative effects of new knowledge on populations or social policy is highly speculative and essentially political."[32] Instead, they argue, national review bodies should address these issues. Yet it is unclear what would be involved in having such national committees performing this task. After all, national committees may not be better equipped than IRBs to resolve the dilemmas that arise.[33] Committees face these issues concerning not only the four specific realms these authors discussed,[32] but more broadly.[22]

Strikingly, no prior empirical studies have examined whether IRBs do in fact consider social risks, and if so, how. I found that these categories in the regulations—"social risk," "individual risk," and "justice"—seem to be more distinct in the abstract than in the messy real world, where they can blur and become vague.

I discovered that IRBs do in fact at times oppose studies that exacerbate existing inequalities in health services. Yet this exacerbation would seem to fit the current regulatory definition of what IRBs should *not* consider. Morally, however, such a consideration may be important, suggesting that the revision of the regulation should be contemplated. Obviously, though, the specifics of when exactly IRBs should consider such risks need to be carefully assessed and decided.

Investigators may not all recognize potential social harms, which can exist even in seemingly "minimal risk" research. These interviews showed me how IRBs struggle with how to define and balance social risks, and whether and how much to do so. In practice, this category often proves related to potentially amorphous issues of stigma, vulnerability, and social inequity. After all, risks to a group can affect individuals within the group. Hence, IRBs regularly consider possible long-range social risks. Committees consider social and psychological harms to a population (related, for instance, to stigma), and social vulnerabilities that affect groups as a whole (related to the benefits and burdens of research), but have to decide how much to do so. For example, as noted in Chapter 1, researchers had published data on high rates of schizophrenia among the Havasupai tribe. Such data about rates of mental illness in a population can increase the amount of stigma and discrimination that that group already faces. Certain cultural groups may perceive potential harms, even if the IRB might not do so. As Anthony, referring to the delicate issues surrounding human tissue samples, explained:

> Just because a sample has been de-identified from an individual stand-point doesn't mean it has been from a racial or ethnic group stand-point. There could be harm at *that* level. A group may have spiritual or worldview-related beliefs about that tissue that are much different than ours: we want bones of our ancestors returned to us, because they're not merely bones. From their perspective, it's very unpalatable that you have my blood or genes in a freezer somewhere.... So we have to expand our vision.

Consequently, while regulations explicitly state that IRBs specifically should *not* include long-term social harms as risks, some committees do so anyway, since social harms can include stigma and concerns about vulnerable populations, which the regulations do mandate IRBs to consider. Social harms can also endanger individuals who are members of the affected group.

These attitudes reflect in part the Havasupai recent lawsuit—of which many interviewees were aware, and which entailed social harm to the tribe.[34] Hence, IRBs may ignore this provision of the regulations *not* to consider "long-term" social risks, due to concerns and fears about perceptions of potential legal liability.

Risks to Vulnerable Groups

In 2004, Dan Markingson, a 26 year-old celebrity tour bus driver hoping to become an actor or screenwriter, developed schizophrenia with paranoid delusions and thoughts that he needed to murder his mother. Doctors committed him against his will to a psychiatric hospital affiliated with the University of Minnesota, and enrolled him in a study of new antipsychotic drugs. Two weeks later, they discharged him to a halfway house. His mother phoned his doctor, saying that he was getting worse, becoming suicidal, and that he did not understand the study (and should not be a participant in it). But the researchers continued. Five months later, he slit his throat and died.[35]

The FDA investigated Dan Markingson's death and did not find wrongdoing, but a bioethicist at the University, Carl Elliot, alleged otherwise: that the researchers should *not* have enrolled him in the study, and that the university was trying to protect the researchers. After Markingson's death, the Minnesota State Legislature enacted a law preventing involuntarily hospitalized psychiatric patients from participating in drug trials, unless the treating psychiatrist submits an affidavit citing the benefits to the patient; the treating psychiatrist also cannot be a researcher working on the drug trial.[36]

The reasoning behind this decision is that this population is particularly vulnerable. Patients who have been involuntarily hospitalized may not understand that they have a right to say no, or may not be mentally fit to make a reasoned decision. They also may feel coerced into participating—perhaps believing that they will never be allowed to leave if they don't follow their doctor's recommendations. At this point in time, however, Minnesota's law, enacted because of Dan, appears unique among the 50 states.

IRBs, however, frequently wrestle with questions of who is vulnerable, and whether researchers should recruit them into studies anyway. The regulations dictate that committees "should be particularly cognizant of the special problems of research involving vulnerable populations, such as children, prisoners, pregnant women, mentally disabled persons, or economically or educationally disadvantaged persons."[37] Vulnerable individuals, lacking power, may also fail either to understand that they can readily withdraw from a study at any point, or to feel empowered to do so. They may fear angering powerful researchers. IRBs thus seek to prevent researchers from exploiting vulnerable groups, such as the poor, semi-literate black men in rural Alabama examined in the Tuskegee syphilis study. Arguably, Dan Markingson, severely psychotic because of schizophrenia, should also not have been allowed to participate in research because he both may not have sufficiently understood the study, and was involuntarily hospitalized. His rights had already been taken away. He may have felt obliged to consent in order to get treated better.

The Belmont Report and the Common Rule each suggest several differing notions of the term *vulnerability*—as related to diminished capacity, possibility of undue influence, injustice (e.g., to being unfairly burdened by a study),[38,39] and "inequitable distribution of the burdens and benefits of research participation."[40] The Declaration of Helsinki states, too, that research on a vulnerable community is only justified if the group "stands to benefit from the results."[41] In all of these documents, vulnerability is a characteristic of *populations* (i.e., it is social, not individual, in scope).[22] According to the *Oxford English Dictionary, vulnerable* means "open to temptation, persuasion...liable or exposed to disease,"[42] suggesting that both individuals *and* groups may be inappropriately recruited into a protocol and also be harmed because of it. But how IRBs in fact approach these issues has not heretofore been examined.

The regulations require that the benefits and burden of the research be distributed fairly,[36] and thus that "selection of subjects is equitable." Hence, IRBs must weigh the risks to vulnerable subjects against both the social (i.e., scientific) benefits of including these individuals, and the inequality of excluding them. Here, committees grapple with several challenges: to construct safeguards to protect vulnerable subjects, and to gauge how effective these protections need to be. Balancing possible harm to vulnerable subjects against possible scientific benefits to society can be among the most difficult decisions an IRB faces, and committees vary in how they respond to this tension.

Even studies consisting merely of interviews might harm stigmatized groups in unforeseen ways. "We try to build safeguards," Phil, a social scientist and chair, said about research on HIV, drugs, and suicide, "but know that something can go wrong."

Removed as they are from the field, IRBs find such potential dangers hard to assess—whether these harms will occur, and if so, how commonly, to what degree, and with what effects, and how to weigh all these factors. Even after IRBs erect protections, they may still worry, given lingering uncertainties. As a researcher himself, Phil thought it was important that the research proceed, but other IRBs may disagree. Additional vulnerable groups might also warrant special protections. "Lots of other populations are special and vulnerable," Henry, a chair, said, citing "people who are economically disadvantaged, have low levels of health, or literacy, or are in poor countries."

The regulations do not specifically address, for instance, psychiatric patients. Dan Markingson was vulnerable, and his case highlights the challenges in researching patients with mental illness. IRB members may feel that mental health is relevant, but psychiatric disorders vary from mild to severe—from situational anxiety to severe depression and psychoses. The boundaries of a vulnerable group are also not necessarily demarcated. Not all individuals in a so-called vulnerable group may indeed be vulnerable. IRBs can differ in where they draw the line. Christopher, the physician and chair, said,

> If you're clearly psychotic, you're vulnerable. But if you have social anxiety disorder, I don't think you are, and the investigator doesn't need to have an independent psychiatrist interview each patient, and assess whether the person understands the consent and the study.

IRBs may thus struggle to decide on a case-by-case basis, defining, applying, and determining the boundaries of "vulnerability." "It's not cut and dry," Christopher concluded. "You need flexibility."

How Much Justice?

My father had insurance to pay for his care, but innumerable patients both in the United States and abroad lack such resources. Many broader questions therefore arise on IRBs concerning whether investigators and committees have responsibilities to address such ongoing health inequities when they intersect with ongoing research, and if so, how much. American bioethics has been criticized in general for overemphasizing individual autonomy at the expense of social justice and communitarian concerns.[43]

While Western European countries all guarantee certain minimum levels of insurance and care for all citizens, President Clinton's proposals to expand health care coverage and President Obama's Affordable Care Act have produced acrimonious battles. In the US, prevailing values have supported maximizing individual choices for those with health insurance (emphasizing individual autonomy), not guaranteeing that all patients receive coverage (which would maximize social justice). These tensions arise in research ethics as well. How much should these committees weigh not only individual, but broader *social* risks and benefits?

Martin, a researcher and chair, described, for instance, a study in which the pharmaceutical company:

> "will provide the drugs for free, but bill the insurance company for all the doctor's visits, the time in the hospital, the CT scans, and tests. Some private insurance companies will pay. Others won't—if it's an experimental treatment. But then, either the drug company has to pay, or the study won't get done. Issues then come up: what about *poor people* who don't have insurance? Here's a potential life-saving treatment that *only the rich* can get. The drug companies claim that they can't otherwise afford to conduct these studies. But many of our IRB members, especially our lay members, get upset about this."

Different opinions about these issues may therefore partly reflect members' own backgrounds and positions on the committee. Even with the Affordable Care Act, insurers may vary widely in whether they will cover such experimental treatments. Unfortunately, certain studies may necessitate lengthy hospital stays, for which insurance coverage is key. Hopefully, drug companies won't abuse these limitations, and seek to avoid paying for research-related expenses that they could potentially afford.

Generally, interviewees felt that they could *not* eliminate the larger health care inequities in the US and the developing world—these larger health policy issues simply lay beyond their scope. Nevertheless, IRBs may confront closely related questions—for example, whether to consider reduction or exacerbation of existing social inequities, respectively, as a social benefit or risk.

Committees thus face questions of how and to what degree to incorporate and weigh justice and injustice. When researchers want to exclude from a study patients without insurance, IRBs must decide how to respond. Including all populations equitably into a study can heighten logistical and financial costs. IRBs thus wrestle with how to balance advancing justice *vs.* facilitating research. In the US and abroad, subjects may lack health insurance, and IRBs must then decide *how much responsibility* funders and researchers have for treating medical problems that may occur during a study or afterwards as a result of the intervention. These boards encounter dilemmas in what standard to use—*how much* social justice to require, how to decide, and how much to incorporate broader justice and health inequity concerns into decisions.

Committees often try to address these ambiguities and tensions by seeking compromises. IRBs may debate, for instance, how small the criteria for exclusion can be—what to do with studies that require that participants have a high-speed Internet connection, since certain subjects may lack one. Committees may develop informal "rules," permitting exclusion of Internet-less subjects in a *pilot* study, but not in a full protocol. Charlotte explained,

> We decided our *rule of thumb* is: it's OK to exclude people for a six-month preliminary study. But for a Phase II program, a PI needs to get high-speed Internet to the participants—have them use the Internet at a clinic, or pay for it for them.

Yet even when such compromises are attempted, problems can ensue and objections can arise, based on other interpretations of the regulations. Charlotte recalled,

> A grant reviewer said, "You're still excluding a whole population of people!" The PI answered: "We're not going to be marketing this intervention to people who don't have the technology to support it. So it doesn't matter." But to exclude people flies in the face of justice!

IRBs must decide whether to compromise or make exceptions, depending on the type or extent of the study.

Committees may allow inequalities to continue partly because doing otherwise would significantly burden researchers. In predominantly white regions, for instance, IRBs face tensions concerning how ethnically diverse a sample needs to be. If the population near an institution is 98 percent white, an IRB could potentially urge or require the researcher to collaborate with researchers in other regions. But doing so imposes burdens that IRBs may not recognize. At other times, committees may allow low ethnic or racial diversity, given the obstacles to proceeding otherwise. Jack, the rural physician and chair, said:

> Occasionally, if the PI is trying to study some rare cancer, the committee says, "The tumor registry here sees one case per year. You need to find collaborators elsewhere." But it's usually due to rarity, not diversity.

IRBs may overlook justice concerns about sampling in part because the regulations do not *clarify to what extent* IRBs should ensure or further justice. However, IRBs may consider justice only after all else—particularly the individual risks and benefits—have been assessed. IRBs may thus be unsure how much additional justice, if any, to require.

A few interviewees wondered if protections against social harms to vulnerable groups may at times go too far, impeding potentially beneficial research. Given past lapses of research ethics, sensitivities arise in studying certain vulnerable populations such as Native Americans. As Elaine explained,

> It can take months to get tribal permission, even for a really low-risk study. So a lot fewer investigators are doing research targeting Native Americans because it'll take so long to get it approved.

Wide, ongoing health disparities therefore exacerbate these dilemmas. The regulations themselves do not directly address whether researchers, funders, and IRBs have responsibilities concerning these broader social injustices, and if so, who does so and how much.

For instance, the Kennedy Krieger lead paint study sparked controversies because researchers gave subjects amounts of an intervention that were lower than the quantities known to be effective. The researchers justified their decision by arguing that the subjects would be unable to access the full treatment otherwise, and that providing and studying the medical intervention (amount of lead paint removal) at a lower dose was thus necessary. These claims remain contentious, highlighting underlying quandaries about how much effort all of us, whether as researchers, IRBs, clinicians, or taxpayers, should devote to reducing global and domestic health inequities directly *vs.* advancing science or pursing other goals.

Yet, studies may exclude patients without insurance, forcing IRBs to decide whether to disapprove such plans. Committees face dilemmas about who should pay for certain parts of these protocols, and how to present any costs to potential participants. Full disclosure may be essential, but researchers and pharmaceutical companies may not want to scare off possible subjects. As Christopher said,

Our biggest disagreements are about who's responsible for paying for extra things. If you're in a National Cancer Institute [NCI] protocol, and get randomized to a surgical *versus* non-surgical intervention, in addition to chemo and radiation, and your insurance won't pay for the surgery because it's *experimental*, who pays for it? Should the NCI or the patient with terminal cancer pay? The researchers can tell patients, "It's going to cost $5,000. You can be in it or not." But when no one knows *how much* it will cost, there are issues. So IRBs differ. We try to come up with standard consent forms and templates, and have as much standardization as we can. But one IRB says patients should pay. Another IRB says that NCI should pay, or that it should be more explicit in the consent form: "You may be responsible for paying additional dollars. We don't know how much it is, but it could be up to $100,000." The consent forms now just say, "You will be responsible…" but not *how much* it could be. It used to say, "Please call your insurance company." But patients won't call. Some sponsors don't want patients calling up or having to pay, because subjects will drop out.

Committees confront quandaries, too, about not only direct, but *indirect* social benefits. In public health research, for example, IRBs may look for indirect benefits such as improving public health policy, since direct benefits to patients may be absent. Committees encounter questions as well of how to weigh free general medical services offered as part of a study. Laura, a lawyer and IRB administrator, described a study of tuberculosis (TB) prevalence in the developing world,

> The study results will go to the Ministry of Health and inform policy, affecting new programs that serve people. We make sure that circuit is in place, because you're often not going to have direct benefit. By being in the study, poor populations are likely to get better medical attention for other diseases than the one being studied. A secondary benefit is that they'll be treated for free for sexually transmitted diseases [STDs] that are diagnosed, even though the study is on TB.

DEFINING MINIMAL RISK

IRBs must decide which studies are minimal risk, since the regulations for such research are different and less onerous, but making these judgments can be hard. Researchers conducting the Stanford prison, and Milgram (and as we will see, restaurant [in Chapter 11], and "fake grad student" [in Chapter 5]) studies all thought that their experiments were minimal risk. An IRB reviewed only the last of these and concurred, concluding that the researchers didn't need informed consent. Yet in each of these four cases, controversy ensued.

IRBs can vary widely in deciding if a protocol is minimal risk. In 2002, David Wendler and colleagues at the NIH surveyed 188 IRB chairs about how, in pediatric research, they applied the categories of risk in the federal regulations—minimal risk, minor increase over minimal risk, and more than a minor increase over minimal risk. These investigators asked about performing 12 procedures on an 11-year-old, and found wide variations.

Among these chairs, 27 percent thought allergy skin testing—part of routine care, and thus arguably minimal risk—was more than a minor increase in minimal risk.[44] A single car trip is part of an ordinary activity of daily life, and would thus be minimal risk; it causes death in 1/100,000 cases. Hence, any activity with that degree of risk would be minimal risk. Yet 59 percent of chairs thought that a pharmacokinetic study that had a risk of death of 1/100,000 was the *maximal* level of risk. Older chairs were more likely to see several procedures as less risky.

IRBs can encounter difficulties gauging minimal risk in part because it is relative and involves predictions about the future. Researchers' own self-assessments can be biased. As Judy, the physician and chair, said,

> The anesthesia department thinks that any anesthesia protocol is minimal risk because they have such a low rate of complications—they lose only one patient in 100,000. But none of the rest of us think that to be anesthetized is minimal risk.

Since the requirements for minimal risk research are is less burdensome, researchers may push to squeeze their studies into this category, while IRBs are cautious. Administrators may come to resent such investigator desires. "Researchers think 'expedited' means in a hurry," Cynthia, an administrator, explained. But of course, it does. Yet IRBs often see this word narrowly in procedural terms—that it refers to a category of studies—and may lose sight of the fact that the category was designed to allow for quicker reviews.

The phrase "minor increase over minimal risk" can also be ambiguous, triggering other definitional debates. Judy questioned, for example, having children spend five more minutes in a catheterization lab if they did not directly benefit:

> If three more biopsies are taken in a colonoscopy, is that a minor increase in minimal risk; or is it not allowable? We discuss that a lot. If a kid is getting a cardiac catheterization because of underlying cardiac disease, and spends five extra minutes in the cath lab getting an injection—but would already be having a cardiac catheterization for an hour

and a half—is that a minor increase over minimal risk or allowable? The child is not normal. The risk is more than that of everyday life. It's really hard to know how to interpret that for sick children already undergoing that procedure. So we debate it. In the end, we decided that five extra minutes in the cath lab is OK.

Yet others might contest this conclusion. Judy feels more government input is needed concerning these definitions. "The guidelines should clarify what the criteria should be for full board review." She felt that threshold should be not more than minimal risk, "but *the risk over what risk is already happening*" [emphasis added].

Ambiguities also exist as to whether for minimal-risk studies IRBs need to review every alteration researchers make, no matter how small, after the committee has approved the project. The consensus among those I interviewed felt that IRBs do need to do so, despite consequent delays to research. Yet some chairs think this practice should be changed. In the meantime, IRBs generally say that all alterations require approval. Jeff, the social scientist and chair, said,

> If the PI is going to add one more highly standardized instrument that takes ten minutes, or realizes that a demographic is left off one of his questionnaires, does he need an amendment? In medical studies, every little change like that needs to be reviewed for safety of patients. But in a psychology study?

Certain changes in studies can pose other questions, such as definitions of when a study becomes "coercive." Jack, the rural physician and chair, said, "A sponsor just realized that it's a drag to have people sit in clinic just to hang out for blood draws, and wants to pay them $500 per day." In doubt, Jack asked the full committee.

> $500 is a lot of money. We have poor people here. That could be a little coercive. This study happens to be zero risk. But if this were a new chemotherapy study, or a Phase I study, and the risks were more severe, the money could be more coercive. I tend to feel a whole lot more comfortable if I have *all* the committee's thoughts.

These decisions may thus partly be matters of *comfort*—not wholly rational, but reflecting in part emotions, underscoring how moral decisions do not always result from entirely logical processes per se. "We have a pretty low threshold," Jack added, "for tossing things back to the full committee." As a minimal-risk study, the regulations permit him to make a decision about it quickly by himself without having to consult the entire board, which would then need to read and review the protocol, and may only meet once a month.

Given ambiguity, many "err" on the side of caution and try to be conservative. "If it's not clear," Greg, the social scientist and chair, said, "we make it expedited, rather than exempt." Such caution can, however, alienate researchers. It can also consume the IRB's own resources and time. Liza said, "IRBs just don't understand what they can expedite...to leave time for the important, challenging protocols."

Whose Daily Risk?

Since regulations define minimal risk as the risk ordinarily encountered in "daily life," questions surface of *whose* daily life. Normal, healthy volunteers, for example, face different risks than sick patients do. These questions arise in a variety of settings involving a range of potential dangers from relatively mild to more severe. Aaron, an IRB chair, cited the recommendation of the Secretary's Advisory Committee on Human Research Protections, which says,

> "It should be the everyday life of a *normal, average person*." But I'm in my 60s—if you throw *me* on a treadmill, and run me up to twice my heart rate, there's a risk. But not for a conditioned athlete. So to me, the everyday life of *a subject* makes sense.

Moreover, even "healthy" populations range in their daily risks. Homeless inner-city street youth, for instance, even if they are healthy and drug free, may face more dangers in their lives than do middle-class suburban adolescents of the same age. As Charlotte, an IRB administrator, added:

> An intervention with street youth may not be risky to them because they're already living on the street in a dangerous environment. But if you propose it with kids living at home, it would appear risky. We argue about it, but tend to choose the norm of the population the researcher's working with. IRBs could benefit by having this articulated.

RISKS TO RESEARCHERS

IRBs also wondered whether they should extend beyond the regulations in considering risks to *researchers*, and if so, when and how much. The regulations discuss IRB responsibilities to protect subjects, not researchers.[12] Yet though not technically within its purview, a committee may try, for example, to protect student or other investigators. An additional motivation in such cases may be that the IRB is also protecting the institution—in this case, its employees—from physical or other harm. Arguably, however, such concern may be beneficial. Committees struggle with how to weigh and address these risks. Elaine said,

> One study would be exempt because the researchers are interviewing convicted sex offenders, but not recording names. The topics weren't real sensitive. It actually went to the full board because the committee was concerned about the safety to *researchers*, going to subjects' homes. The IRB was less concerned about the subjects than about the researchers, and required at least a male and a female researcher to go together.

These problems can become especially vexing with studies in politically unstable countries. Scott, an IRB director, said,

> A researcher wanted to study the trauma associated with being refugees from a war-torn country. The rebels there have been accused of genocide, conducting border raids, placing the subjects, if not the researchers, at risk. Our researchers are great, but gung-ho, Indiana Jones types. So are we going to contribute to the potential for harm befalling our own researchers? We debated, and at first rejected it. Then, after we received certain assurances that minimized the risks, we approved it.

These considerations are not called for by the regulations, but suggest how much IRBs can see themselves as overseers of research, and protectors of colleagues and institutions more broadly—how much their roles as loyal employees can blur into and affect their roles following the specific regulations. In some ways, if they had the resources, they could and perhaps should take on broader roles in certain ways—though not necessarily primarily to help the institution *per se*. Here again, tensions emerge about which wider discussion and debate are needed—of whether IRBs should go beyond the regulations, and if so, when and how much.

Committees thus wrestle with whether, when, and how much to consider social risks, indirect social benefits, fair distribution of benefits and burdens of research, broader health inequities, and vulnerability of participants, *and* how to balance these against individual risks and benefits. IRBs also face underlying tensions concerning the degrees to which they *should* weigh these concerns, and the inherent ambiguities in interpreting the relevant terms.

These issues may be much harder to assess than individual risks and benefits, which can often be measured—a particular drug, for example, may have a 25 percent likelihood of eliminating symptoms or causing a side effect, whereas the likelihood of a study finding an effective new drug is harder to quantify. In response to the Obama Administration's questions about IRBs' interpreting regulations about social harms, IRBs appear to be taking these risks into account frequently, but wrestle with how to do so. While the Obama Administration's policymakers sought to see "social harms" and "justice" as clearly distinct, in practice these terms are closely intertwined. Stigma and widened social inequity are commonly related to social harms. At times, committees develop "rules of thumb," or compromise, or accept limitations in their ability to reduce broader health and social harms.

"Coercion," "Undue Influence," and the Question of Compensation

Dan Markingson's death revealed several problems. For instance, the researcher didn't inform the IRB of the mother's report of Dan's suicidality, which this investigator should have as an adverse event. The fact that doctors entered him into the study when he was involuntarily hospitalized also raises concern about possible coercion or undue influence.

In experiments performed by Nazis in death camps, by the US Army, and at Willowbrook,[45,46] scientists gave vulnerable subjects no choice. Federal regulations require that research minimize the "possibility of coercion or undue influence,"[12] but do not define these terms. Critics have argued that IRBs are *overly* concerned about the potential danger of undue influence, obsessing over whether small increments of money—paying a subject $50 rather than $25 for participating in a study—may unduly influence him/her. IRBs may prevent a researcher from paying, say, $50, yet lower compensation may decrease enrollment.

I once placed an ad for subjects in a magazine and accidentally left out the compensation ($30). I got no subjects. I then reran the ad with the payment and got several. Potential subjects are often busy, facing competing demands on their time. Payment can thus help incentivize participation. But money also has a range of symbolic meanings, raising sensitive concerns. I soon saw how IRBs wrestled with dilemmas of how much to pay subjects, how much is too much, and whether participants should participate only for the money or whether science should be "above" the taint of monetary concern. Some critics contend that IRBs spend too much time worrying about what relatively small amount of money to pay subjects. Yet IRB over-concern about possible undue influence can unreasonably hamper science.[47] How IRBs actually view and make decisions about these concepts, however, has not been explored. Money can distort research—for instance, at times when drug companies pay university researchers—but does money overly influence research subjects?

The Belmont Report states that coercion involves "an overt threat of harm...to obtain compliance, and offer of excessive, unwarranted, inappropriate reward"[36]—for instance, if a doctor were to tell a long-standing patient, "enter this research study or I will no longer treat you." A milder concern is potential "undue influence." More recently, OHRP has distinguished on its website that:

> "Coercion occurs when an overt or implicit threat of harm is intentionally presented by one person to another in order to obtain compliance.... Undue influence, by contrast, often occurs through an offer of an excessive or inappropriate reward or other overture in order to obtain compliance...undue influence also can be subtle....Because of their relative nature and lack of clear-cut standards on the boundaries of inappropriate and appropriate forms of influence, investigators and IRBs must be vigilant."[48]

Coercion occurs at times in clinical psychiatry, but overall is probably relatively rare in research.[47,49,50,51] IRBs frequently end up worrying, however, about the possibility of exerting undue influence by paying subjects too much.

Recently, the philosophers Alan Wertheimer and Frank Miller have argued that IRB members mistakenly see offers of payment as coercive.[51,52,53] Yet these authors conclude, "The question as to when the offer of financial payment actually constitutes an undue influence is a topic that merits separate analysis."[51]

How much exactly should subjects get paid to be in a study? IRBs often wrangle over this question. How much should researchers pay healthy subjects to be in risky, invasive research? Should a lawyer and a McDonald's cashier get paid the same amount? Neal Dickert and Christine Grady[54] have outlined several models for determining how much to pay participants. These scholars outline three possible models and advocate a "wage payment" model—providing a low, standardized wage that could be increased for uncomfortable or other onerous tasks. They present limitations of a "market model" (based on supply and demand, and potentially offering more payment for taking on more risk), or a "reimbursement model" (covering expenses, including costs from missed work).

But, what such a wage should be, how IRBs should determine it, and how much participants actually get paid are very unclear. Online recruitment sites usually offer compensation.[55] Most journal articles, however, do not mention whether or how much participants have been compensated in the studies they describe.[56] One study gave a quantitative survey to IRB members and found they vary widely in their views.[52] Many questions remain, though, about how IRBs themselves actually make these decisions concerning studies they review, and how they perceive and experience these issues.[54,55]

Table 3.1. **Ambiguities and Dilemmas Faced by IRBs Concerning Coercion and Undue Inducement**

IRBs Struggle with Dilemmas Concerning:

- *Content*
  - o How much to give subjects
    - ▪ Should subjects get paid differently based on their income?
    - ▪ Will selection bias result?
    - ▪ Is the provision of free care coercive?
    - ▪ What to give subjects (e.g., cash *vs.* vouchers)?
    - ▪ What types of studies
  - o Added challenges in several situations:
    - ▪ Research on children
    - ▪ Research on students
    - ▪ Research in the developing world
  - o Whom to compensate
  - o When to compensate subjects
  - o Whether, when, and how to inform potential participants about compensation
  - o How to define undue influence:
    - ▪ Based on "gut feelings" and "common sense"
    - ▪ Can be subjective

- *Process*
  - o IRBs can take time to make these decisions
  - o Decisions often reflect compromises
  - o Underlying tensions arise:
    - ▪ "Undue inducement" is inherently subjective and difficult to assess in others
    - ▪ Questions arise of whether subjects should "volunteer" *vs.* do it for the money
    - ▪ Lack of a consistent standard
      - ▪ Between IRBs
      - ▪ Even in one IRB over time

As summarized in Table 3.1, IRBs wrestle to define "undue influence," and often rely on "gut feelings." Yet IRBs vary—even single IRBs shift their views from one meeting to another—reflecting underlying quandaries of whether subjects should be motivated by altruism *vs.* money.

IRBs struggle with how much money is "too much," and how to decide. Determining at what point exactly an amount becomes an "undue inducement" is hard. As Elaine said,

> Researchers were approved to pay participants $225 in a longitudinal study with follow-up interviews. They wanted to increase it to $300 due to the length of time. The chair said, "*That's* coercive." There was a compromise of $250. I was once a Research Assistant on a study, and we weren't getting people. My boss said, "We're paying them $30. Let's change it to $50."

Elaine and others misuse the term *coercion*, employing it instead of *undue influence* when no threat is involved. IRBs often use this term as a catch-all phrase for incentives that may motivate participation that might not otherwise occur.

Countless employees take jobs they don't like because of money. But should the same incentives be allowed for research subjects? "Research just seems different," Elaine felt. "It's a voluntary thing, and you don't want people to be trying just to put up with something because they're going to get paid." Yet the reasons for these differences are not always clear. The belief that research should be "voluntary" appears to reflect the notion that science should be "pure"—that everyone engaged in it should be doing it solely for the advancement of scientific knowledge. But of course this is hardly the case. IRBs may fear "undue influence" because money may thus "taint" both researchers and subjects, though for different reasons. IRBs may extend the view that researchers need to be "pure" to participants as well, raising fears of overcompensation.

Yet compensation can in fact motivate subjects; and IRBs can debate these issues at length. As Henry, the chair, said,

> We spend an inordinate amount of time on compensation levels, and whether it is adequate, or too much and coercive. We don't apply a common standard across all studies—developing countries *versus* the US; and within the US, impoverished communities *vs.* volunteers through Craigslist.... Investigators may get quite different and inconsistent advice from the committee *depending on what it feels like that day*. I don't think there's any agreement in the field. You come up with different numbers—if you think it's just to pay for people's transport *vs.* opportunity costs of being away from work.

Questions also arise of whether payment to subjects should vary based on the amount they usually earn *vs.* a single amount, regardless of their income.

In the latter case, selection bias may occur, skewing the sample. As Henry continued,

> Should you compensate a radiologist much more than a laborer? Or should they get the same?...If you pay people differently, or the same, you're going to attract different groups of people, and that may cause adverse selection or targeting.

Many IRBs still determine acceptable amounts of compensation for each study on a case-by-case basis, but wide idiosyncrasies can result within and between committees.

CHALLENGES ASSESSING UNDUE INFLUENCE IN PARTICULAR SITUATIONS

Particular types of studies pose additional challenges. For instance, the provision of free care by researchers could unduly influence poor participants. But how to proceed otherwise is not always clear. As Christopher said,

> We have an 80 percent Medicaid population....Are people participating in studies because it gives them free medicine, not because there's any real benefit to it? [They] get a free appointment and physical. Otherwise, they won't get treated.

Yet Laura, in describing the TB study in the developing world that also provided better medical attention for other diseases, including free STD treatment, added, "It might be coercive. But do you then not do research?" She does not answer whether the research should then not be conducted. Yet I would argue that the research is vital to do, but requires very careful review.

Committees then encounter quandaries about whether and how to inform potential participants about compensation. Given the uncertainties involved, IRBs may shift their positions over time. As Dana said,

> We used to not allow [researchers] to put a monetary amount on recruitment flyers, because we thought it was a little coercive: "You'll get $20 if you participate." But we've concluded that a gift card for an hour interview is probably not particularly coercive. If you were to say, "We'll pay $600 if we can take blood," that might be a little coercive. So we're trying to decide what the standard is, and how to handle that.

Committees face further challenges deciding how much to pay parents who enroll their children. Committees want to avoid the possibility of parents entering their children into studies for the money, since these youngsters may have little, if any, voice in the matter. As Jaime explained,

> Young minors should definitely not be paid in dollars. So the IRB is working on who should get the money: the parents or the child? The parent is taking the time off as the escort. There should be something for the parents as well. But you have to worry about undue inducement. Sometimes the researcher wants to pay hundreds of dollars to the parents. We'll limit the dollar amount, and talk about what the children should get. It's age-driven: we don't like to put a lot of money into young adolescents' hands. But it's on a case-by-case basis, depending on the nature of the study...the age of the children, and what's involved.... We polled other IRBs if they had a policy. Nobody did.

Given the lack of established policies, IRBs can vary.

These issues can become even murkier when research is conducted in the developing world. Amounts of compensation can range markedly based on established regional practices. Some projects may cover only transportation expenses—either as cash or vouchers—but this practice poses larger questions of whether it is unfair to pay in certain countries and not others. Tensions also arise between exploitation due to overly low amounts, and undue influence due to overly high rewards. Laura said, "I asked one researcher, 'Aren't you exploiting subjects?' He answered, 'It could cut both ways. If you're offering money, it might be coercive because they are so poor.'"

Questions arise, too, when professors require students to participate in research as part of a class: these subjects receive not money or services but academic course credit. They may be given a choice as to which study to enter, yet IRBs may debate whether such participation primarily benefits the students' education or their teachers' careers. As Louis, an IRB chair, said,

> Students can earn that same amount of credit if they complete an extra paper. That doesn't feel like extra credit, [but] coercion. Is it part of their practicum, or are they doing this to satisfy something for a professor?

Participation in a study may take much less time than writing a paper, which takes hours and days instead of minutes.

Conclusions

Committees struggle with defining and applying concepts of risks, benefits, undue inducement, and coercion. IRBs and researchers aim to follow principles, but are often unsure how and to what extent to do so. Compensation poses questions of whether the ideals of scientists should be extended to subjects as well. Scientists dedicate themselves to certain goals—to seeking the truth, by questioning claims about truth—disinterested in money per se, and being universal, communal and ethically neutral.[57,58] But IRBs often appear to feel that these principles should pertain not only to researchers, but to *participants* as well. In general, social groups seek to maintain "purity."[59] Therefore, IRBs may try to keep research as "pure" and unaffected by the taint of money as possible.

But adequate compensation to participants need not sully the purity of research. The larger issue of commercialization of science raises concerns, and should be confronted head on, but not prevent subjects from receiving appropriate payment. IRBs may worry excessively about compensation, misapplying the notion that scientists themselves be "pure." Academic medical centers, built on science, may hold IRBs to this standard—of being objective and unsullied. Yet while many people see science as objective, subjective elements may linger—personal beliefs and financial conflicts of interest may affect researchers' conduct, choices of studies, and interpretation of data.

Desires for objectivity may foster IRB zeal in avoiding coercion. Yet many IRBs appear to use the terms *coercion* and *undue influence* interchangeably. Though Wertheimer and Miller[51] have distinguished between these concepts—arguing that coercion involves an external threat and can often be observed by others, while undue influence is usually inherently subjective (e.g., involving the point at which someone's judgment is no longer entirely rational in following their interests)—critical questions remain.[60] In research, assessing someone else's internal state is inherently elusive. Hence, application of the term *undue* remains subjective and normative, involving questions that external observers may interpret differently—excessive according to whom, how an outsider observer is to know, who should make that determination, and on what external objective evidence? A study subject person may feel $75 is appropriate payment for filling out 1–2 hours of surveys, while an external observer may feel that that amount is excessive. Moreover, participants in a study vary in education, income, job, and personality, and consequently in how much they may be influenced—especially across diverse countries. An individual may feel that he or she is being rational, while an external observer may disagree. Hence, IRBs will no doubt continue to encounter ambiguities and variations in applying these terms.

into their health system, and the subject selection is just. Ultimately, it will benefit the subject population. But sometimes we struggle: *is this really research?*

Uncertainties can remain about whether the results apply to more than one clinic, and the researchers are thus somehow seeking "general knowledge." Laura's IRB wrestled, for example, with whether a study of the effectiveness of an HIV treatment program in the developing world constituted research. Such research, designed to understand how to improve care in a local treatment program—examining, for instance, whether clinics in rural areas perform as well as those in urban areas, or whether female patients are more likely to return for follow-up appointments after they have seen a male *vs.* a female provider—could, however, aid programs in other institutions as well. "We first treated it as research, and then said it wasn't," Laura explained. "But studies use the data or specimens generated." The knowledge garnered could potentially help clinics elsewhere, even if the study is not specifically designed to be generalizable. In practice, generalizability is hard to define since some, though not necessarily all, parts of a study may be helpful to others.

Presumably, investigators will identify an operational research study as such, and ask for it to be exempt from IRB review. A committee, however, may opt to review the study anyway, rather than automatically exempt it, if it involves vulnerable populations or raises other ethical concerns. As Laura added,

> We have sometimes struggled; and to be on the *safe side*, taken operational research involving drugs, a stigmatized condition, and a vulnerable population to full committee—even though it involves only data collection through surveys or medical records.

Treatments and devices that may also be used for humanitarian reasons pose ambiguities for boards, too. In 1990, the Safe Medical Devices Act created the Humanitarian Use Device (HUD) program, allowing device manufacturers to develop apparatuses to benefit patients with so-called orphan diseases—conditions that affect less than 4,000 patients per year in the US. These devices can then bypass the FDA's usual standards of rigor and evidence of safety and efficacy. The FDA requires that IRBs approve the use of these devices, but this use does not constitute research per se.[5,6] "Fast-tracking" thus generates controversy, as manufacturers have charged patients more for expensive new products that are later found to offer no benefit over cheaper existing treatments. This procedure also confuses IRBs. Kurt, the chair, said:

> We've had a few conflicts with humanitarian use devices, which are not well understood by the doctors using them; but are *not* research. They

got assigned to IRBs because the Feds thought that was a good place. But these are *not* experimental.

Federal regulations also exempt from IRB review studies of *educational tests* as long as the data are not linked to identifying information. A researcher may only want to study, for instance, whether male and female students perform equally well in math or chemistry tests in school. IRBs don't need to review such research.

Nonetheless, despite regulations exempting educational studies, some institutions may require committee review because human subjects are involved, even if anonymously. Yet investigators may balk, seeing this requirement as an unnecessary burden. Judy, the physician and chair, reported that some boards "follow the same guidance as for biomedical research—even if the investigators are merely introducing a new nursing or medical school course"—that is, if the faculty are simply developing a new series of lectures, and students complete an evaluation form about it afterwards in order to improve it for the following years' students.

Research conducted by students to fulfill academic requirements for a class or for a master's thesis is rarely published and would thus not constitute research, even if the results were generalizable. Occasionally, however, a student may recognize, only after completing a project, that a journal might be interested in the findings. Many IRBs want to be informed about student research, and end up exempting much of it. For their projects, medical students may also draw blood or perform medical tests on patients, requiring IRB review. Some institutions have established separate mechanisms to handle the large number of student projects they review.

Assessing student research poses challenges, however, since much of it is not scientifically well designed. It may be minimal risk, but weak science. As Judy added, more generally:

> We struggle a lot with how much to intervene in minimal risk research where the research design seems crummy, but there's really no risk. It may not be well supervised, or hasn't been presented very well.

Though the regulations exempt certain categories of research because they are not generalizable, arguably all academic work is designed to contribute in some way to "general knowledge." Many IRBs have adopted the *de facto* operational definition of whether the data are going to be published. But the "publishability" of a study is not always predictable. The importance of the results affects whether a journal will publish a paper. Scientists cannot predict what they will find, and thus whether they will want or be able to publish it. Jeremy, a co-chair, said, "an article got published this past year," based on a prior study, the results of which the researchers had not initially thought would sufficiently justify scientific journal publication, "making this issue blow up at our institution. Someone reported the researchers. It became an institutional mess."

Large numbers of social scientists argue that their research is minimal risk and that IRBs should therefore not have to review it. But as we saw with the Milgram and Stanford prison studies, social science research can pose psychological harms. In recent years, scholars in these disciplines have lambasted OHRP's extensions of regulations from biomedical to social science as "mission creep."[7] These critics argue that the regulations were designed for biomedical, not social science, research and that—unlike invasive medical trials—social science studies do not cause serious bodily harm.[8] Critics assert that federal regulations were stretched to include social science without sufficient consideration of either their inapplicability or the challenges involved with compliance.[9]

Many psychosocial researchers contend, too, that IRB reviews can impede and/or harm their research. In exploratory social science research of complex social phenomena, as in anthropology, the specifics of the design may not be fully knowable at the outset. As Louis said,

> A researcher submitted a protocol on domestic abuse. The entire proposal was about developing partnerships with a local board, a sheriff, and a lawyer. The first year was to develop local competence. The researcher wanted the group to create an instrument together, which would take three years. The IRB sent it back as not developed.

Many qualitative social scientists face difficulties because IRBs may not allow sufficient flexibility in descriptions of certain details of the study. Jeff said of one investigator,

> Just describing in advance all the settings in which he might interview people...if he then had to adhere to that, and never go beyond that—it would restrict what he does. Yet if he were to describe it all in advance, I'm not sure an IRB would find it as acceptable.

Committees are also not always familiar with social science, and this lack of experience can cut either way for the investigator. For instance, a biomedical institution may be more flexible than other institutions, since it is used to doing more invasive studies and considers social science research less potentially problematic. Judy explained:

> We do many risky biomedical studies, so...Our social scientists don't have as hard a time as they do at a university with no biomedical research, where they get highly scrutinized.

An IRB at another biomedical institution, however, might be unrealistically restrictive, using a "one size fits all" approach to all the research they review.

Federal regulations exempt *oral history* as supposedly not generalizable, but at times that exemption becomes a loophole. Oral historians collect narratives of individuals to store as part of the historical record, but may at times write about this information in a way that points toward some larger truth. Anecdotally, it appears that some social scientists now advise each other, "Just say that your research is oral history, and it doesn't need IRB review," even though the research may involve data analysis that scholars then publish, and that claims to be of some wider interest and value. In such cases, definitions of "oral history" can become muddled.

IRBs often have trouble determining whether particular studies are generalizable or not, and if so, when, and why. "Many researchers doing oral histories are going to want to generalize some things, so the research really *is* systematic," Dana, a social scientist and chair, said. "How does that *not* require an IRB application?"

Dana conceded that studies can involve systematic data collection but still be exempt. IRB members, however, often feel that they—not the researcher—should be the ones to make that assessment. "The PI should not determine that," Dana added.

Although she is a social scientist, Dana has adopted a pro-IRB perspective, and thinks the IRB should review all social science research:

> Everybody ought to be talking to the IRB. I say to social scientists: "Actually, I can *make* you. I don't want to. But in the end, wouldn't it be better just to get things checked out, and let the IRB make that decision?" Then you get a formal letter saying, "Don't worry about it."

In studies of groups that engage in illegal and/or violent activities, protection of confidentiality can also prove imperative. Anthony described research on gangs and white supremacist organizations: "If their mates in these organizations found out that they're talking to somebody, they are in a very difficult spot."

Interviewees described some social scientists as in fact *wanting* IRB approval, in part because journals require it. "They're concerned," Robin, an IRB chair, explained, "that they won't be able to get it published otherwise."

Committees differ in how much they fear that psychosocial studies could raise emotional issues and pose more than minimal risks. Jeff, the social scientist and chair, remarked, "[A relative] was interviewed as a Nazi refugee for an oral history. I don't know if she experienced great emotional stress, but others could." He felt that some IRBs treat all social science experiments as minimally risky and therefore expedite their reviews, and that that can be a mistake. He brought up a psychological study about 9/11 to illustrate his point:

Another medical center, whose IRB chair I know well, expedited the same study that our IRB reviewed very closely! They are a hospital, and did not have any psychological studies. So, to them it was expeditable.

Jeff thinks his IRB was right; though arguably, more uniform standards are needed.

Is the Science Good Enough?

The categories above concern the *parameters* of the research that falls under IRB review. But IRBs also face dilemmas of judging the science itself—if they should do so, how, and to what degree.

In recent years, the role of IRBs in evaluating research has become increasingly controversial, though not well understood. Of genetics researchers, for instance, 15.8 percent reported that an IRB had required "substantial changes" to a study design,[10] yet how, when, and why IRBs make these decisions is unclear. Researchers frequently complain that IRBs unnecessarily alter study designs without possessing the expertise necessary to do so, but rarely is the rationale for these decisions explored.

In 2002, the US Department of Health and Human Services (HHS) funded Kathleen Dziak and her colleagues to interview by phone 3,000 patients at 15 different primary care institutions. The survey asked about demographics, health status, satisfaction, and receiving preventive service, and recorded no identifiable patient information. They submitted the study to the 15 IRBs with a letter asking for expedited review and a waiver of written informed consent. But the 15 IRBs varied widely in the length of time for approval (5–172 days), and in how they changed the study. Of the 15 sites, nine permitted an expedited review, but six required a full review by the whole committee. Three sites required that patients be allowed to opt out. Two IRBs gave patients opt-out by phone, and at these institutions, 1 percent and 5 percent of patients, respectively, did so. One committee let patients call or return a card to opt out, and 11 percent did. Another board required that patients opt in by completing and mailing an opt-in card. Of these patients, 37 percent did not do so. Hence, the rates of refusal at these insitutions ranged from 0 to 37 percent, impeding the researchers' ability to compare the data from the different sites. Alterations in approaches to subjects about participating in a study can thus change the scientific design and results.

Yet researchers get annoyed partly because they feel that IRBs should be ethical rather than scientific bodies—that by interfering with the science, committees are straying from their mandate. Upon closer examination, however, it becomes clear that IRBs' determinations involve efforts to ensure that the potential scientific benefits outweigh the potential risks to subjects. Balancing subjects' rights against the potential benefits of the study is hard.

The scientific quality of protocols is tough to gauge. No specific instrument or "gold standard" exists.[11] Several scales have been used to assess the quality of clinical trials, but these measures vary widely. Furthermore, most of them have not been adequately developed or tested for validity and reliability,[12] causing problems. Since scientists regularly try to pool together data from different studies, to conduct meta-analyses, making these comparisons is important.[13] After an article has been published, the number of times it has been cited, and the rating and reputation of the journal publishing it are frequently used as proxy measures of quality.[14] As investigators conduct research, they can also seek on their own to verify their methods, but that does not involve comparing the quality of different researchers' experiments.[15] The number of articles a researcher publishes about a study has been assessed as well.[16] Yet these indices are all post hoc, and do not guarantee validity and quality of the scientific design (as opposed to, say, the importance of the results or the researcher's ease or frequency of writing articles). Certainly, studies should be "well-formulated," "well-designed and executed," and "independent, and balanced,"[17] but applying and measuring these broad, vague standards can be difficult. Better benchmarks to assess the quality of science are needed for funding decisions,[18] too, but no clear consensus or measure exists.

WHAT SHOULD BE THE IRB'S ROLE IN THE SCIENCE?

IRBs wrestle with whether their role is to alter the quality of the science, and if so, when, and how much. As Elaine said:

> If it's poorly designed, does that increase the risk for subjects, and should the study not occur? The other argument is: our job is just making sure they're applying the regulations and treating subjects ethically. Who are we to criticize someone's design? Should it matter if it's . . . more or less invasive?

IRBs thus confront several questions: whether their job is to ensure that the quality is adequate, or to alter or stop inadequate studies; and whether these roles should increase for studies that pose a greater risk to their subjects.

Some committees recognize that their widening scope makes many researchers wary. Maggie, the community member, observed:

> Researchers feel that the IRB often oversteps its bounds . . . going beyond just looking at risks and benefits, and actually dipping in—trying to dictate researchers' protocols. *It's a fine line.*

Separate Scientific Review?

To resolve these tensions, some institutions have established separate scientific reviews, but these vary widely in quality and scope. They may improve the science but take extra time, and IRBs may still raise additional scientific questions if they feel that the science is not worth the risk. As Jack explained,

> I get asked all the time if the IRB's job is to get involved in the science. Investigators first get questions from the Scientific Review Committee, and then proceed to the IRB. It takes a long time—a couple of months. PIs complain, "I had to answer all those questions for the Scientific Review Committee, and now the IRB is also asking me scientific questions. What's the deal?"..."You can't do research for...no meaningful scientific outcome." Our IRB is a backstop. Ultimately: the buck has to stop at the IRB.

Institutions vary in who conducts academic "pre-reviews" prior to IRB submission, and the quality of these assessments ranges from substantive to a mere formality. Departmental reviews are often perfunctory, vouching for a study's logistical support (space and time), but not its scientific merit. Christopher said,

> Department chairs are supposed to review protocols scientifically, but most have never even *looked* at it. They say, "Oh it's fine." We end up spending a lot of time *fighting*...is the study design adequate, is the sample size going to be meaningful? But those should not be IRB issues! It should be vetted already. The IRB issue should be: given that this is scientifically valid, does the consent form explain it?

Scott also observed that department chairs may simply approve protocols *pro forma* without fully reading them:

> Every department chair must sign off on an application. But that's a formality...Most of these sign-offs really exist to acknowledge that the PI will be spending certain time and effort on non-clinical responsibilities, and use X-amount of space. Certain departments have scientific review committees that evaluate the research before we get it. A few chairs actually do look at it. I commend them. I don't know when they come up with the time.

Departmental chairs may be clinicians, not researchers themselves, and thus not have the appropriate training to be evaluating the scientific design. IRBs therefore do not always know whether the fact that a department chair has approved a protocol guarantees that the science is sufficient.

Generally, IRBs feel justified in suggesting or requiring alteration in a study's design if they feel it may harm subjects or not justify the risks. But sometimes those I interviewed also felt that they had a role in increasing the "rigor" of studies and stewarding scientific resources and opportunity costs within a field. As Frank said,

> We're just trying to prevent investigators from slipping through the easiest, least sought out ideas, and wasting a tremendous amount of effort on something that people think is just really not even the direction we should be going.

Yet the specific criteria for assessing such rigor are unclear.

What If Studies Have Been Approved Elsewhere?

Often, protocols under review have already been approved by federal or other institutions. While many boards readily accept such studies, others don't. "Some IRBs won't believe that a study funded by NIH or NSF is scientifically sound," Louis, a chair, commented. "So they'll take it upon themselves to evaluate the science. We try not to do that."

Some IRBs refrain from asking for changes in NIH-approved or multisite studies because of the logistical burden of such requests, or the belief that such changes might not be feasible. When unsure, boards may consider the importance of the changes they desire. As Judy, the physician and chair, said:

> We won't like parts of an industry-sponsored multi-centered study. But if we want to change the design in any way, we couldn't, because it's already at 50 or 100 centers. Then we have to decide either that our objectives are *so strong* that we're not going to let the investigator be part of it or that we can live with the study the way it is. Most of the time, we can't change an industry-sponsored protocol unless it's just at a few centers. A big multi-centered trial isn't going to change the protocol a few times a year for each committee.

Nonetheless, a few IRBs felt justified in requesting changes in studies that had been approved elsewhere (e.g., by the NIH), and appeared to take pride in having detected an important ethical problem that had been previously overlooked. One committee, for instance, was the only one to complain about a multisite study requiring patients to agree to enroll in a registry before entering a study. As Cynthia said,

We were the only IRB that found issue with that—which amazes me. They thought it was not an IRB issue because it was a registry—not a research study. But isn't this an invasion of a parent's right to choice and confidentiality? The researchers then rescinded it. A lot of institutions would have OK'd it.

Some IRB members viewed their review as an integral part of the science. "Many researchers believe that IRB review is just an endless chore," Henry said, "as opposed to an actual *part* of the research." Yet researchers may feel very differently.

HOW GOOD IS "GOOD ENOUGH"?

IRBs confront dilemmas of what standard to use in deciding whether the science in a protocol is "good enough" to approve. Definitions and perceptions of "good enough" science themselves can vary widely. In general, in evaluating protocols, IRBs face tensions of whether simply to follow the federal regulations as narrowly defined (i.e., minimizing risks and ensuring that they are commensurate with benefits), or to go *beyond* the regulations and seek to *maximize* the benefits by increasing the quality of the science. Some IRB members feel that studies should be as sound as possible, or not approved by an IRB. Jack, the rural physician and chair, said,

> A couple of members come down quite hard on clinical research and shut down studies if issues don't look really fixed: "If we can't guarantee that studies are *absolutely perfect*, we should stop them." But studies are never going to be absolutely perfect. There's no such thing as an error-free human system.

Certain committees see themselves as "pro-research" and may therefore be a bit more lenient and forgiving. "It doesn't always have to be great science," Jack said. "In general, we don't give investigators that much of a hard time." This stance can reflect the views of the chair, vocal members, and/or the mission and ethos of the institution. Some universities may be more invested in research, and heavily dependent on research grants. Jack added,

> A study would have to have something really substandard or really bad for *us* not to approve it.... Sometimes, studying a little spin on conventional therapy is fine. We think, "This is not a great comparison," so it's not great science; but it's what the investigator wants to do—as long as it's not *egregious* or really increasing the risk, or giving other potential subjects inferior care.

Yet other interviewees sought a higher standard. Even when committees have deemed a study low-risk, they may think the quality of the science is inferior because it explores "uninteresting" questions, or seems superficial. An IRB may deem a proposed study a "fishing expedition" unworthy of approval. Some boards felt that aspects of certain studies would not harm subjects but were nevertheless unessential, and thus should be altered or not approved in the current form. As Charlotte said,

> We were able to convince an investigator to drop observations of stu-
> dents in a school, because they were completely unnecessary—these
> weren't going to generate the type of information he wanted, and was
> just poorly thought out. We were able to convince him, because the
> two scientists on our board were in agreement. It wouldn't really have
> harmed subjects. It was just unnecessary.

The presence of particular scientists on an IRB can also therefore legitimate a committee's position, highlighting how researcher responses to IRBs can involve both *what* is said, and by *whom*.

Sometimes a study may be exploring the right questions but have too small a scope. IRBs then must decide whether to approve such protocols, if these may nonetheless lead to later, better-designed studies. As Patrick said,

> There's a dilemma: if you're going to need 1,000 patients for this study
> to be effective; and have fewer, but the risk is negligible, should it be
> approved? I want to encourage research, but know [the researcher]
> is just going to get indeterminate results. I wrestle with that a lot, and
> decide case-by-case. I'd like to say, "Don't bother, because it's not
> going to be level one data." But then I think: success builds success.
> If you let someone do a study, maybe they'll do the definitive study
> next. So, if the risk is negligible, I usually lean to saying, "Just do
> it." But that's probably my bias, being a clinician. Others say, "Why
> bother because it's going to be an indeterminate study," or, "It's not
> perfect science." So, studies get squashed. But sometimes the perfect
> study isn't going to get done. It's too laborious or not feasible. Each
> study can't be perfect. Theoretically, there's some happy medium.

Given these conflicts, some committees periodically remind themselves that the design only needs to be "good enough." (As one member put it, "Once in a while, someone says, 'Wait a minute—we're not here to review the science!'") According to this argument, the primary focus of the IRBs' mandate should be the ethical issues involved, but the need for this reminder reflects the complexities involved—that ethics can necessitate review of the science to a certain extent, but that an implicit boundary exists.

Problems can also emerge from a study's presentation. Researchers at times submit sloppy protocols that then frustrate committees. In the end, the IRB may not approve the study because it is poorly described, rather than because it has ethical problems *per se*. As Charlotte explained,

> One protocol was so poorly written, you wondered how this guy got a degree. The science was not harmful, but we had to flesh out aspects of it. When I first read it, I had two pages of questions. "What do you mean by *this*? What's *that*? How many students? Where? How are they doing it? When? This is inconsistent. It doesn't flow logically." Pieces were missing. The PI made some of those changes, but ignored most of them. At the meeting, everybody was confused....The reviewer felt weird going to a respected colleague and saying, "This is a piece of shit. We can't understand it." We approved it, but doing so took a really long time....It was like pulling teeth.

Tensions with Researchers about the Science

An IRB's right to alter a PI's research design may constitute the most controversial issue between researchers and reviewers. As Charlotte said,

> We're not supposed to muck around in the scientific design, except when it begins to affect the subjects' safety. But scientists get pretty antsy when non-scientists start telling them that their science is designed poorly. They just think we don't know anything.

Non-scientists on the IRB may have valid critiques, but their lack of training—and hence their recommendations—may be questioned by researchers.

Committees may try to anticipate and address these conflicts in several ways—though not always successfully. For instance, IRBs may try to have reviewers talk with the researchers beforehand. Yet committee members may not always want to critique faculty directly about a poor design, since doing so may impinge on professional taboos against criticizing colleagues. Hierarchical differences—for example, between senior PIs and junior IRB members—and the institutional atmosphere can hinder such diligence as well. Charlotte said,

> We have sort of an odd culture here. We don't really confront people. At our institute, we're great at giving people lots of strokes, and not really saying, "That is a ridiculous idea."

Such cultural aspects of institutions can thus shape IRBs, hampering the fullest possible ethical review.

To avoid awkward clashes with colleagues, IRBs may simply approve low-risk studies despite their reservations about the science. As Vicki said,

> We used to review proposals for a local college that didn't have their own IRB. Many of their studies were inane. Their methodology was fine, but the studies were just silly. Most of it had to do with early childhood education: they would study kids rolling on balls to improve their balance. We would roll our eyes, but approve it, because it was to get a Master's.

In this instance, the fact that the review was from another institution and for graduate students further softened these critiques.

Student research in particular may be of lower quality, and some IRB members feel that approving such research damages the institution as a whole. As Anthony explained,

> We have had some intense screaming matches with certain departments. I am heartsick that somebody is earning a Ph.D. for a particular study because the science is atrocious. These departments dig in their heels, and say that is not our purview. It's not my charge as chair, but when I see substandard quality of rigor and depth, and somebody's going to earn a Ph.D. from it, I have enormous problems. I have rattled cages—all the way up to the university president—with little avail, because there's pressure to have high enrollment. But then, the quality suffers as an inevitable consequence. One colleague was simultaneously mentoring 22 Ph.D. students!

Consequently, committees must weigh tensions between perceived broader, professional responsibilities to the quality of science and the university's economic needs.

Certain aspects of study design have proved particularly tricky in recent years, such as the use of placebos and the introduction of new technologies and areas of study. Drug companies often want to show that a new therapy is at least better than nothing. An existing effective therapy may, however, be far better than the new product. Some proponents argue that placebos may be used, even if a proven treatment exists, if the reasons are compelling and the use of placebos won't harm the subject.[19,20] A few commentators have argued, for instance, that certain antidepressants are ineffective, and that placebos can therefore be used in studying new possible treatments for depression.[21] An existing treatment may have severe side effects, or a lot of patients with the condition may respond to a placebo. At present, the FDA permits companies to submit placebo studies as evidence, but OHRP and the Helsinki Declaration oppose such use.[22,23,24] Battles erupt.

IRBs thus face periodic debates about whether, for patients who have failed to respond to any treatment, researchers should compare a new experimental therapy against a placebo or "no treatment." As Martin, a researcher and chair, said,

> Most university IRBs would require clinical trials on psychiatric patients to have a very good reason to include a "no treatment" arm. Sometimes companies send clinical trials to private IRBs, which seem to accept those designs.

But Martin felt that *his* board would be less swayed than an independent private one by certain arguments in favor of placebos—such as that "adding risk to [subjects'] lives is minor, because they have such terrible lives to begin with." IRBs at nonprofit institutions tend to see for-profit IRBs as far more ethically lenient. He added,

> The arguments in favor of using a placebo: these illnesses are chronic. This patient has had several relapses. The placebo arm would delay treatment by a few weeks, but not affect the illness long-term. But that argument would not get very far at *our* institution.

Committees may disagree, too, over whether the placebo effect could or should be listed as a benefit. Liza said about one study:

> You can't say to subjects that, as a benefit, there's a 50 percent chance you could be randomized to the active drug. Other institutions said the placebo effect is a benefit—which makes sense in certain psychiatric studies, but not *this* study.

IRBs also face challenges when a study employs a new technology, and no consensus about its use yet exists. Generally, with new types of methods, IRBs are uncomfortable at first. "We spend an inordinate amount of our time trying to fit a certain study into the regulations," Joe, the chair, said. Only gradually will a board tend to feel more at ease with these novel approaches.

For instance, studies increasingly make use of the Internet, electronic medical records, and telemedicine. Questions surface of how to obtain informed consent from subjects, if not face to face. "What would the parents say," Charlotte asked, "if they found out their 11-year-old has gone on our site and answered questions about their illegal drug use? *That* makes us uncomfortable."

Studies involving "big data" also pose quandaries. Despite the Health Insurance Portability and Accountability Act (HIPAA), IRBs are unsure exactly how much to protect privacy. Some studies now collect and examine personal data on thousands of subjects. As Martin, a researcher and chair, said,

> Major healthcare systems are constructing enormous new databases...Most of the faculty IRB members are reasonably comfortable with these databases; but some of the lay, community members are not. They just don't trust large, complicated studies: a commercial entity or group of researchers getting their hands on 10,000 medical records is scary! News stories about somebody's computer at the VA getting stolen with the records of 20,000 veterans don't help. There's...a lack of comfort.

These reservations may reflect wider national worries, as manifested in broader debates about Internet privacy. How long should electronic records be kept? "Some people say data can be stored without a time limit," Elaine said. "Others say no. You have so many ways now, with the Internet, of carrying data with you. Who owns it?"

Long-term storage of biospecimens is also increasing. Kevin, a health care provider and IRB chair, highlighted its complexities:

> Tissue banking is in rapid flux and escalation. The US Department of Health & Human Services and The National Bioethics Advisory Commission agree in most areas, but differ with OHRP. There is little guidance on whether IRBs should be looking solely at protocols that involve tissue banking, or stick their noses into other areas, and review other tissue banks created at the institution. Clinicians may have blood left at the end of the study, and stash it away in the freezer for posterity. Along comes a new super duper test they can use. Should that be allowed? How should the IRB respond?

Innovative research advances science, but also poses threats. Given the rapid growth of science, consensus at any one point may be absent—for instance, regarding the appropriate length and type of follow-up for particular diagnoses. Sufficient expertise is theoretically required on IRBs, but can range across a vast spectrum. A reviewer may be in the same specialty as the PI whose protocol he is reviewing (e.g., oncology), but not subspecialty (e.g., lung *vs.* bone cancer). As Judy, the physician and chair, said,

> One committee might think: shouldn't the follow-up be longer? With this drug, you won't see differences in three months, and need to treat for at least six months. Or shouldn't you monitor with eye

exams? The other IRB might not have picked up on those particular issues at all.

New scientific areas of study, such as biorobotics, may be unfamiliar to *all* members of an IRB, which limits the committee's ability to evaluate the research. As Troy, an IRB chair, pointed out, "It will be hard for us to understand robotic microbes in the blood—mini-cellular devices—and designer drugs that target specific receptor sites."

IRBs therefore must not only evaluate the science, but also manage their anxieties about the science. As Judy, the physician and chair put it, "A lot of research seems very risky and innovative, which is always a big problem for us. It's *scary* sometimes."

Conclusions

In assessing the quality of science, IRBs thus encounter ambiguities. The definitions of "research on humans" can prove hazy: are all studies science, and if not, which do not fit this category? Moreover, the quality of science is hard, almost impossible, to measure a priori. While IRBs may feel that they are justified in altering the science and are thus improving the studies, researchers often think otherwise. Such quality can be hard to evaluate, involving inherently ineffable and subjective characteristics, which exacerbates these strains. Moreover, IRBs that attempt to alter the science due to ethical concerns, but lack adequate scientific background, may inadvertently damage the quality of the study under review. As we saw with Kathleen Dziak's study, for instance, an IRB requiring subjects to opt *into*, rather than *out* of, a study decreases response rates.

Science is advancing, shifting, and unpredictable. The results, and hence value, of a scientific experiment—especially one conducted on human beings—can, by definition, never be known in advance. IRBs require ever more expertise and sophistication to evaluate studies adequately. Alas, many committees sometimes lag behind, causing problems. Though regulations stipulate that IRBs must have sufficient scientific expertise, new and evolving biotechnologies and subspecializations make that very difficult. No one faculty member can have adequately sophisticated knowledge of all of the research in a field. The definition of *sufficient* may be critical here, since a committee member may have some partial knowledge of most areas within a larger field (e.g., neurology), but lack detailed enough knowledge about a particular sub-specialty (e.g., experimental therapies for brain cancers, Alzheimer's disease, or stroke). Yet a particular subfield may include very few individuals, who may then have inherent conflicts in reviewing each other's studies. Indeed, when a subject, Ellen

Roche, died in an experiment at Johns Hopkins in 2001, a government probe found that members with needed experience were not always involved in reviewing protocols.[25] Such tensions need to be addressed.

Some IRBs argue that increasing the quality of the science from adequate to superior maximizes the potential social benefit of the research. But the risks may have already been commensurate with the benefits *without* altering the science. IRBs must then decide whether to suggest these changes to PIs, given that animosity may ensue. Committee chairs and members often have dual goals: as researchers (to advance science) *vs.* as IRB personnel (to protect subjects). In either role, IRB members sometimes clash with researchers over whether these committees have the authority and scientific expertise to make certain changes. Moreover, deciding what standard to use in evaluating a protocol's potential future scientific benefits is difficult, and researchers and IRBs often disagree.

OHRP, the IOM, and other organizations should determine and disseminate examples of studies where such scientific design changes are or are not legitimate, clarifying these boundaries for both IRBs and researchers.

At the same time, researchers may fail to grasp the regulations and tensions that committees confront. PIs should avoid submitting, out of frustration, sloppy or incomplete protocols, as these may very well impede interactions with IRBs. Both sides need to appreciate one another's challenges far more than they do today.

Definitions of science and "good science" also remain murky. Future scholarship should probe more fully what constitutes "less interesting" science, and how institutions, researchers and funders might aim higher. Science continues to grow, but faces constraints in government, university, and at times pharmaceutical industry funding. Hence, developing better assessments of scientific quality in some way, if possible, would have many advantages. Here, too, more development and dissemination of guidance and consensus about these varied concepts can help improve the ethically appropriate advance of biomedical and other research.

CHAPTER 5

What to Tell Subjects

BATTLES OVER CONSENT FORMS

In May 2001, Ellen Roche, a healthy, 24-year-old lab technician at Johns Hopkins, volunteered to be in an asthma study as a normal volunteer.[1] She would receive $25 for each of the first-phase visits, and $60 for each of the second-phase visits, for a total of $365.

The researcher, Dr. Alkis Togias, wanted to understand why patients developed asthma. He hypothesized that it resulted when the neurological mechanisms that kept airways open in normal people stopped working. To prove this hypothesis, he proposed having healthy individuals inhale a drug, hexamethonium, to block communication between neurons, thereby replicating this proposed cause of asthma. The IRB approved the project, and Togias entered Ellen as the third patient. Within 24 hours of taking the drug, she was in dangerous respiratory distress; within a month, she was dead.

Investigations by the FDA and the Office of Human Research Protections (OHRP) criticized the investigator, the IRB, and the institution. As it turned out, the first subject to whom Togias had given the drug had developed shortness of breath and a cough, but he did not report these symptoms as "adverse events" to the IRB until after Roche had been hospitalized. His review of the past literature about hexamethonium had also been cursory, and so he had failed to turn up earlier evidence of its potentially lethality. Previously used to treat hypertension, the drug had been removed from the market in 1972 by the FDA for its ineffectiveness.[2]

The informed consent form signed by Roche and approved by the Hopkins IRB, however, said only that the drug was "a medication that has been used during surgery, as part of anesthesia." After Roche's death, the government investigations faulted the form both for being incomplete—Dr. Togias' review of past studies was careless in his own research—and misleading, because it ignored the fact that the drug was not only experimental but had in fact lost its FDA approval.

In the SUPPORT study on oxygen levels, too, central debate has concerned what exactly the consent forms should have said. The form did not mention the possibility of death—presumably because it existed for the infants whether they enrolled in the study or not. But death might be more likely to occur in the study since more infants would receive lower doses of oxygen (85 to 89 percent) than they would otherwise. Death also differs from other adverse events, and is a relevant and important part of the study, since it is one of the two outcomes being assessed. Even if the odds of death are not greater within the study, respect for persons would seem to suggest that parents have the right to be told or reminded, as they considered participation, that their infant could die from the intervention. Moreover, parents were consented before their child was born, and perhaps did not fully realize the possibility of death was relatively high—1 in 5. Potentially, the form could simply have said that a risk for all premature babies is death. Researchers may not have wanted to include this fact since it might have frightened parents and decreased enrollment. But the interests of full disclosure appear to dictate otherwise.

My father, too, started an unproven intervention in part because of the way his doctor optimistically framed the treatment. To respect individuals who participate in an experiment, the researcher *must* provide the necessary information to make a proper decision. Hence, informed consent is vital. The researcher needs to disclose the information that any reasonable person would want concerning what the experiment involves, and the risks, benefits, and alternatives that exist. This principle seems simple enough, but in reality it causes disagreement and confusion. For some studies today, consent forms are now 45 pages, single-spaced, with complex scientific terminology that many subjects cannot understand and thus do not read. The late Yale law professor Jay Katz, himself a Holocaust survivor, concluded that informed consent was an impossible ideal.[3] Yet many patients start unproven interventions in part because of how the researcher frames the treatment. IRBs wrestle with who needs to sign written consent forms and how much information in these documents is enough—how much detail researchers need to provide, and in what way. In our current litigious society, legal as well as ethical responsibilities complicate these choices.

Yet despite the wide attention given to this and other scandals, problems with consent forms have persisted. Often, IRBs are chastised for including too much information on consent forms rather than too little, and these forms have lengthened over time.[4] Committees are also criticized for spending too much time on the details of these documents and demanding too many changes. No checks exist on how much committees are allowed to "wordsmith" or "nitpick" forms, which frustrates researchers. Although all IRBs are mandated to review and approve consent forms,[5] committees nonetheless vary in the types and numbers of consent form alterations they request.[6] These alterations can not only delay studies but as we saw, also increase refusal rates by potential participants.[7]

Most universities state that these forms should not require more than an eighth-grade reading level, but research has found that 92 percent of these institutions fail to meet their own standard[8]. More pages and complexity can decrease comprehension, undermining the principles of informed consent itself.

Despite heightened concern about consent, participants often misunderstand these forms. Efforts to use simplified forms and multimedia formats have had only limited and inconsistent success. The use of trained consent educators familiar with the study may show promise, but can be very expensive.

The Obama Administration's questions and proposed reforms include as suggestions:

> increased use of brief summary sheets and standardized templates. Limiting the acceptable length of various sections of a consent form...prescribing how information should be presented...such as information that should be included at the very beginning of the consent form...reducing institutional "boilerplate" in consent forms (that is, standard language that does little to genuinely inform subjects, and often is intended to primarily protect institutions from lawsuits); and...making available standardized consent form templates, the use of which could satisfy applicable regulatory provisions.[5]

Yet these goals can be tricky—as seen by the fact that, most of us regularly "scroll down and click I accept" on the Internet, without trying to read or understand the text. Moreover, IRBs and researchers face challenges concerning not only how these documents present information, but what they contain.

Strikingly, however, how IRBs themselves view and make decisions about these conflicts regarding consent forms has remained unexamined.

When and for Whom are Consent Forms Needed?

IS WAIVING INDIVIDUAL CONSENT EVER APPROPRIATE?

Questions emerge of whether consent forms are even needed for certain kinds of psychosocial research. IRBs may struggle to find intermediate approaches, or may lack expertise in reviewing such studies; the lines may also be very difficult to draw. In 2010, two professors from Columbia and the University of Pennsylvania received IRB approval from both institutions to e-mail 6,300 professors across the country, pretending to be a graduate student, and asking to schedule a meeting either that day or the following week. The investigators varied the name and gender of the fake graduate student, wanting to see how professors would respond. Many of the e-mailed professors changed their schedules to make time for the supposed student; when they later learned that they had been duped, a number of them became incensed, arguing that they had not consented to be studied, and that the research was hence unethical.[9]

In the so-called hand-washing study (discussed in Chapter 4), the Hopkins IRB also thought the researchers did not need to obtain individual consent from all patients. But OHRP judged otherwise. In Facebook's experiment with manipulating users' moods (see Chapter 1), the researchers and the IRB at Cornell—where two of the three researchers worked—thought that informed consent was not needed.[10] Presumably, they felt that the study was minimal risk. Facebook originally claimed that its user agreement mentioned that the company might conduct research, but it turned out that the company added this possibility to the agreement only after the study had been conducted. Many users and scholars have since argued otherwise—that these subjects had a right to know. Moreover, online manipulation of users, including children and adolescents, is not necessarily risk free. Some messages received on Facebook have psychologically harmed children. Cyberbullying has resulted in suicides. Facebook's manipulation did not constitute cyberbullying. Still, we don't know the extent to which social-media companies conduct experiments (it may be quite often), or the nature of these studies. Experiments on humans need to be carried out as ethically as possible. These cases suggest the dilemmas IRBs confront when deciding when, if ever, investigators can forego informed consent.

Similarly, in studies of public activities, such as behavior on the street, it is not clear how much researchers must notify subjects. In participant-observation research, the investigator may work in community activities and then want to describe the experience in a publication. An IRB's decision may depend on the population, the questions, and the observees' presumed expectations of privacy. Phil explained,

> Periodically, students work in church food programs. Should they wear a sign that says, "I'm a Researcher"? Do they have to get everyone's individual permission? That could be tricky. Sometimes we really struggle. Do you put in a church bulletin that "a researcher will be studying us. He won't be writing down anybody's name. He's interested in this and that?" Or do you ask that everyone be consented? Our struggle relates to: the vulnerability and poverty of the population, what's being studied, whether the behavior is really public, and whether the participants expect privacy in that particular moment. If you want to study on-line

chat rooms, should you just lurk and study, or have to announce that you're a researcher? If it's a sponsored chat room, you might alert the moderator. Other people argue that it's all public, and there should be no expectation of privacy, so it shouldn't matter.

In emergency situations, when subjects cannot consent for themselves, "community consent" can be valuable. For instance, researchers have wanted to study artificial blood products in emergencies. Car crash victims bleeding to death at an intersection may not get to a hospital in time to receive stored donated blood. Yet they may be unable to give informed consent, and the emergency medical services may not be able to reach a relative by phone. The investigator might hold meetings to inform the community as a whole to seek so-called community consent. Yet such a process can be murky since many individuals may remain unaware of the experiment. Dwayne, a chair, said,

> We're the only big trauma center for a big rural area, so sometimes there's a protocol testing, say, fluid volume resuscitation in the field. OHRP has formally described a process of going out into the community and holding forums, as a way to do research in emergency settings without individual informed consent, because otherwise it's not feasible. You can then do delayed [individual] consent. We're trying to make sure it happens safely.

New situations arise that pose further problems in obtaining consent. For example, a study may include home visits to subjects—perhaps to see how patients are coping in their home environments, as opposed to the hospital. But a researcher may then see domestic abuse (which needs to be reported to the state) before the subject has signed the consent. One IRB considered this possibility, and was unsure how to proceed. Finally, one member suggested a creative solution—having PIs mail or discuss the consent form with subjects before going to the house.

In certain developing countries, forms can impede psychosocial research and even be dangerous. Participants may have low literacy, and be wary of written documents requiring signatures—which usually involve the police. Yet IRBs might be inflexible, ignoring or not realizing these phenomena. Jeff said about a study in a developing country: "The villagers thought this document was bizarre. But the researcher had to go through the full translation, and back translation."

IRBs may even require giving consent forms to illiterate groups. Jeff added,

> At another university, an anthropologist had to present a consent form to an illiterate population she was studying. There are procedures to handle that, but her IRB wasn't doing its homework.

This example further highlights tensions in how regulations are interpreted—strictly and to the letter, rather than in the spirit of the broader principles.

WHOSE CONSENT?

In 1999, a Virginia man opened an envelope addressed to his daughter and was shocked to discover a questionnaire asking her whether *he* had a history of depression or abnormal genitalia. *She* had entered a twin study that inquired information about her family medical history.[11] *He* complained to the OPRR—which oversaw IRBs—that such information, ascertained without his knowledge or consent, violated his privacy and rights. He felt that researchers, wanting to obtain sensitive information about him, should have to obtain *his* consent, not only his daughter's. As a result, the federal agency shut down all research at Virginia Commonwealth University,[10] where the researchers worked.

Consent in genetics studies is particularly thorny, as researchers may want to collect a family history, and therefore ask participants to provide data about not only themselves but other relatives who have not agreed to let the researchers have this information. In many such studies, whose consent must be obtained and under what circumstances is unclear. For example, if the identifying characteristics of a family are kept confidential, does a researcher still need everyone in the family to sign a consent form? This would present a terrific burden. But these other, unconsented family members might not like that researchers have sensitive information about them, such as histories of mental illness. Other gray areas emerge, for example, concerning research on adults with dementia. These interviewees felt that more guidance from the OHRP or other organizations would be helpful.

Obtaining consent from children and adolescents can be particularly problematic. With minors, parental consent is necessary but not always feasible, and it can in fact skew results or cause harm. Committees encounter questions of what circumstances might allow researchers to approach children about research before asking parents. Phil admits that the fact that he himself has children influences his view:

> I'm a parent, so always take the position that parents need to know. But sometimes, it makes sense to approach the kid first, because of the setting. You might not interview them, but say, "Would you be interested?"

Studies of high-risk behaviors among children concerning, for example, HIV risk pose particular challenges. Phil added,

> If you're doing HIV-prevention street outreach, it's not feasible to approach the parent first. If you do approach the parent, you may put the

child at risk. In a school, a principal can send a letter home first. But in some settings, there is no mechanism for outreaching to parents.

Certain committee members are uncomfortable asking minors about sex. Charlotte observed, "IRBs can get real rule-bound—'These are kids. We need parental consent. We're exposing them to risky questions about child abuse!'"

Yet in researching such risk activities, requiring parental consent could in fact bias the sample. "The only parents who will give consent," she added, "are those whose kids are probably *not* engaged in risky behaviors."

Getting parental consent for kids living on the street, for example, may be neither feasible nor appropriate. On the other hand, it can take a considerable amount of time for an IRB to understand and consider the full circumstances of participants' lives. Charlotte gave an example:

> A researcher was studying sexually-transmitted diseases and street kids. There was a learning curve for the IRB about these kids' lives. It took a while because it was about sex, kids, prostitution, and drugs. And no parents. After many meetings, flexibility prevailed. A lot of the kids are fleeing abusive households. It's ridiculous to chase down the parents and get consent.

Steep learning curves may be inevitable. But given these tensions, many saw the need for clarifications of guidelines.

Emancipated minors who are less than 18 (usually 16 or 17) but living independently, and who may be mature in some regards though not others, present quandaries, too. Troy, a researcher and chair, said, "If you're an emancipated minor, you could be dumb as a stone, and not understand English, but be consented as an adult. Comprehension varies by child."

Online surveys of minors pose extra dilemmas of whether and when to waive parental consent. As Charlotte said,

> What if you're recruiting 11- to 18-year-olds for a survey, but the research wouldn't ordinarily qualify for a waiver of parental consent? You can't get parental consent—because you're recruiting on the Internet. Kids are not going to stop and call the researchers, and give you an address, so that the investigator can mail a consent form for parents to fill out and mail back. That *does* meet one of the conditions for a waiver: you can't carry out the research otherwise.

IRBs can waive informed consent in research on adults that is no more than minimal risk, and could not be done otherwise, when the participants' rights won't be adversely affected, and the subjects will receive other information afterwards. Committees can waive parental consent with children when it is not reasonable—for example, with neglected or abused children—if researchers use appropriate mechanisms for protecting the participants instead.[12]

Yet other boards may feel that that justification for a waiver needs to be balanced against other considerations, such as potential harm to the subjects. As technology evolves, committees face new and different questions about how to define "everyday risk." With the ever-burgeoning Internet, for example, adolescents may be exposed to far riskier subject matter, without informed consent, than the materials supplied by the researcher. Growing awareness of this fact is changing attitudes and practices. Charlotte recalled,

> One IRB thought recruiting at adult homosexual websites for an HIV prevention study was OK. But, what if a 13-year-old gets there, and is exposed to this? The committee reasoned: a 13-year-old is going to be exposed to a lot more graphic stuff at these adult websites than by going through this extremely long survey.

Research using social networking sites, such as Facebook, pose further challenges—when kids, for instance, post pictures that jeopardize their confidentiality. Charlotte described some researchers who have a website that promotes "pro-social, anti-tobacco" activity among teenagers:

> The IRB is really skittish about allowing kids to post their pictures and profiles. But the kids actually aren't going to come to the website unless it's cool and groovy and they can talk to each other.

Again, IRBs face tensions over how far to protect subjects while allowing research, and their decisions vary widely. More transparency and discussion about these conflicts can help.

The Content of Consent Forms

IRBs face questions concerning the content of these documents—what is included and *how*. The information should be thorough and understandable. For the induced-asthma study at Hopkins, for instance, the consent form was misleading—only partially correct, leaving out key details. Boards commonly feel that they have pivotal roles in reviewing and frequently rewording consent forms, since these documents may be abstruse, and researchers may underemphasize risks and overemphasize potential benefits. Given researchers' potential desires to downplay risks, IRB examination and revision of these documents can be vital. Some IRB members simply "expect a certain amount of bias." As Nathan said,

> The informed consent should say, "This study will be of *no* benefit to you. It is designed to determine the drug's toxicity levels." But our researchers want to say, "This study may or may not benefit you."

Subtle verbal distinctions can become important, as the wording in the Hopkins asthma study demonstrated. Investigators may write that an experimental drug "is not yet approved by the FDA," rather than that it "was never approved"; or that a drug "has already been given to 15 people, and was generally well tolerated," rather than, it "has only been given to 15 people and no one died."

Yet researchers generally want to encourage, not dissuade, potential participants considering a study. Striking the right balance can be tricky. Nathan continued,

> I want the forms to say: "These drugs are new and have never been tried in humans. In animals, they have been shown to have effects on problems similar to yours. There may be some applicability for humans." That's honest, as opposed to saying, "This may benefit you," but it's not dashing their hope.

Jaime, the IRB administrator, said, "Patients don't hear the specifics—the message, 'This is research'—because they want to believe there's hope." In response to potential subject misconceptions, consent forms have become lengthier, and IRBs scrutinize them more carefully. "I try to make sure that the consents are very accurate," Andrea said, "and that the patient can read it and completely understand what's required." Thomas, too, tries to counter subject misconception, but recognizes that this goal may not wholly succeed: "The participant should be given the information correctly, and the chance to make an autonomous decision. That's the best we can do."

These forms may also be more important now than ever before, since investigators increasingly do not know subjects before the study begins. As Christopher explained, "When more studies were investigator-initiated, the subjects were patients of the doctor doing the research." Patients may therefore have felt more comfortable asking questions. Mutual understanding may have been higher.

WHAT AND HOW MUCH TO INCLUDE

In 2011 the ANPRM asked, "What factors contribute to the excessive length and complexity of informed consent forms, and how might they be addressed?"

"Would the contemplated modifications improve the quality of consent forms? If not, what changes would do so?"[13]

I found that IRBs are aware of the increasing length and complexity of forms, and often struggle with exactly how complete and long these forms should be. In fact, many committees encourage extreme thoroughness, seeing it as a virtue. "Researchers may think our IRB is a little more over-the-top than the regulations require," Maggie said. "We require our researchers to be a lot more thorough."

Yet other interviewees recognized that completeness and comprehension can compete. They feared that the length of these forms—frequently over 35 pages—might mean that subjects were less rather than more likely to understand their implications. Between these two goals, Louis saw a "fine line."

Committees must thus trade off, for instance, informing subjects of *all* instead of only *the most important* risks. A few interviewees complained of efforts to inform subjects of as much as possible. As Andrea said,

> Sometimes the list of risks is almost ridiculous—it goes on and on and on. The patient probably just ignores all of it. Would it be possible to talk more about the *likely* risks, rather than a two-page list? Patients just say, "I can't be bothered with that. I'll sign it."

In qualitative social science studies, on the other hand, investigators commonly aim to generate hypotheses, and cannot always fully predict and describe beforehand all the questions and scenarios that may evolve through the project. For a PI to anticipate and include in the consent everything she or he will eventually ask may be hard, if not impossible. Hopefully, the IRB will permit some latitude, but it may require investigators to list all potential areas to be examined, and not allow them to deviate significantly from these.

Committees vary in their degrees of awareness, concern, and perceived ability to alter overly long or incomprehensible forms. Though Ellen Roche was a young, healthy volunteer who expected no personal medical benefit from her participation in the asthma study, many patients who enroll in studies are far more physically and psychologically vulnerable. Some of the IRB members I interviewed were very conscious of the problems long consent forms can pose, particularly for patients under duress from illness. Patients in ERs, or just diagnosed with life-threatening diseases, may simply not be able to summon the concentration necessary to read them thoroughly. As Christopher said, "Someone can read one page, and say yes or no. But they can't do the eight pages, and you don't want them to." Instead, such patients could be given a "one-pager," or be allowed to take the forms home before signing them—although doing so is not always feasible.

In the end, at times, scientists experiment on people who sign forms without understanding them. Subjects rely on trust of the researcher, which is usually justified, but occasionally may be ill founded or broken. Researchers and IRBs try to increase subjects' comprehension of forms, but do not always succeed. Yet IRBs often ignore the full extent of this problem—or certainly do not test to see how frequently it is the case. Indeed, my study of IRBs in the US and Africa[14] showed that the former were, statistically, far more willing to believe that subjects understood consent forms. In part, subjects may simply decide to trust the researcher (and hence sign the form, even if not fully understanding it) or not.

WHEN SHOULD CONSENT FORMS BE TRANSLATED?

Luckily, my father and family all spoke English, but many patients and subjects do not. IRBs then encounter dilemmas of when to require researchers to translate all consents and questionnaires into other languages. Committees range in the thresholds they use in requiring such translations; some may be uncertain, for instance, if they should require translations of documents even for only a small number of subjects. Given the relatively high costs to researchers, an IRB may require such effort for larger but not smaller studies, yielding to pragmatism rather than pure principle. But where do you draw the line? As Charlotte, the administrator, said,

> Some people say that if you have one subject who doesn't speak English, you need to translate. Our IRB argues about this all the time, because our researchers go into communities that are 11 percent Hispanic. If 20 percent are monolingual in Spanish, do we say: "Sorry, you have to translate"? Our scientists are reluctant to start translating everything. But otherwise, you end up excluding people who could benefit from the research. The Feds should come out with a specific formula or cut-off.

Problems emerge, too, because not all questionnaires and surveys have been tested and validated in other languages. Hence, committees may suggest, but not require, translation. Still, not all IRB members may accept this rationale. As Charlotte added,

> We have a really sketchy rule of thumb. We don't take a *heavy* stand. We just *nudge* toward translation. The PIs are real resistant to it. So, we don't require them to translate, but we'll discuss it a lot with them, and let them know we're not happy about it. Translation will be a *concern* and *suggestion*, not *a requirement....* We ask researchers: what will you do if you encounter non-English speaking people? How many do you expect? We don't require pilot and feasibility studies to translate their documents, because the researchers usually have a very small

budget—though that's not a very good reason. A lot of manualized treatments [written manuals that describe procedures for psychosocial interventions and treatments] in English just don't translate well. We also look scientifically: how would this affect the cost/benefit ratio? How much effort would it take, and how meaningful would the data be? A lot of IRBs say: if a person otherwise meets your recruitment criteria, they should be allowed to be in the study.

Given these vagaries, IRB decisions about whether to require translations may vary and not be wholly objective. As Charlotte continued,

My gut feeling is that you cannot exclude any subject on the basis of language. The guidelines say consent forms need to be written in a language that is comprehensible to the person. We haven't been real rigid with that, but demographics are changing. We're collaborating a lot more with other geographic areas. So a lot of PIs translate a lot of their documents, or have translators available. But we don't say you can't exclude anyone because of language.

These decisions may be among the most difficult that IRBs face, and committees may choose to maintain vague, unspecified cutoffs of what percentage of non-English speakers can be in a study before it must be translated. Institutions with few non-English speakers face particular difficulties—pitting abstract notions of justice against practical obstacles. As Maggie, the community member, said,

The hardest issue that we have faced is: when is translation necessary. Our minority population is very, very small. So the researchers say, "Of 250 subjects, we expect to have maybe five non-English speakers. It's too costly." We basically decided not to make it a requirement for small or pilot studies with a small [sample size]. We didn't specify the number. Resistance from researchers made it difficult.

These dilemmas may be arduous because they require balancing justice and participants' rights against pragmatic feasibility for researchers. In fact, the last time Charlotte's IRB was forced to take a vote on a protocol, the point of contention concerned translation:

A scientist studying children in another city didn't want to translate anything into Spanish. We had a feeling that a lot of people there speak Spanish. He just wouldn't do it, and was pretty upset about it. We voted and barely approved the protocol. We said, "OK, this is a Phase I feasibility study. We'll approve it *this* time in English. But don't expect to come back here for Phase II without translating." He was furious. He thought we had a hell of a lot of nerve.

IRBs may make exceptions for a particular study, but not others. Even when they do feel that they have compromised, though, researchers may still not be appeased.

Concerns arise, too, about broader *cultural translations*—making research practices appropriate, and bridging potentially clashing beliefs. "Cultural competence" has recently been emphasized as important for physicians, but here definitional ambiguities confront IRBs as well. Anthony highlighted these wider concerns:

> A six- or seven-page consent translated into Mayan or Nepali is only part of the problem. Is this going to be meaningful or *culturally appropriate*? Otherwise, the translation is a waste of time. We try to be flexible—not overly rigid saying, "Subjects *have* to sign it. I don't care." But we don't all have experience in those settings. There's *trust*. Maybe key contacts in the community can help us understand what would be appropriate.

Broader cultural differences need to be addressed but can be hard to measure. Anthony fears that individuals in another culture will view Western researchers warily and think:

> "Here comes the white man. You haven't taken the time to understand us, our needs." Or, "You've collected health data on us for 25 years, and put out peer-reviewed publications. But none of this has helped us with the disease."

ARE FORMS LEGAL CONTRACTS? QUESTIONS OF INSTITUTIONAL LIABILITY

In the Ellen Roche case, the SUPPORT study of oxygen levels in premature infants, and the Kennedy Krieger lead abatement study, IRBs and researchers were castigated for insufficiently detailed consent forms. After a subject dies unexpectedly, the legal issues inevitably compound ethical ones: is the institution in question now legally vulnerable? Will a poorly phrased consent form prove to be the chink in the institution's armor?

These challenges reflect underlying tensions of whether consent forms are legal contracts or ethical, informational documents—that is, whether they are designed to protect the participants or instead shield the relevant institutions and funders from the participants.

DIVIDED LOYALTIES, UNCLEAR STANDARDS

As shown in Figure 5.1, I found that in deciding how much information is necessary to inform participants sufficiently, these committees are often caught between competing pressures and input—from government, their own institutions, industry, researchers, and the perspectives of their subjects. Any and all of these interest groups can influence committees' decision making.

These tensions frequently frustrate committees. "We tear our hair out," Judy, the physician and chair, said. She told me of one instance when her committee reviewed a 35-page consent form for sight-impaired subjects, who obviously would be unable to read it.

Those I interviewed often blamed the verbosity of consent forms on liability concerns. Christopher observed,

> There are longer consents designed to indemnify the companies or universities—not protect subjects, or help subjects decide the risks or benefits of the study. There's too much preoccupation on the paperwork.

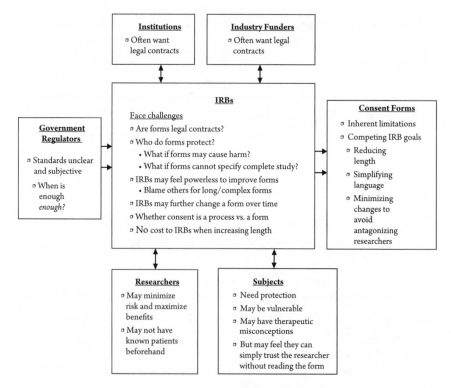

Figure 5.1 Themes Concerning IRB Approaches toward Consent Forms

Other committee members felt there was little alternative. Jeff, the social scientist and chair, said:

> The consent form is a legal document—a contract. There has to be full disclosure of everything that could pose a risk. That makes it very long. Whether people read it thoroughly varies.

IRBs may feel obliged simply to accept the form's status as a legal document—despite realizing that many subjects will not fully comprehend the language.

Many consent forms contain lawyer-supplied templates that do not pertain to the protocol the subject is entering; but removing these sections may be discouraged, or even prohibited. Jeff explained,

> Our university's boilerplate has a lot of wasted language that I'd like to take out, but the attorneys won't let me. The form says, "Before you sign this, you can take it to discuss with whomever you like." But, that doesn't make sense when a patient is about to have an urgent procedure. However, we aren't allowed to take it out! [Researchers] have to delete either the "university, or College of Medicine"—whichever didn't apply. Occasionally they forget, and the IRB would miss it. So, the forms say: "University, or College of Medicine, whichever applies."

IRBs customarily see the protection of subjects as their priority, yet they *can be forced* to take other considerations into account, as well. Jeff continued,

> Protecting the institution definitely conflicts with protecting the subject. [Our committee] had a Compliance Officer and an attorney talk about protecting the university. As chair, at times I would say, "Yes, but that's a different consideration—not ours. That's for *you* to act on." But, at other times, unless certain changes were made, the study wasn't going forward: what would be the point of IRB approval if the Compliance Officer was going to reject it?

Some IRBs may attempt to avoid yielding to the broader legal contexts in which they and their institutions operate—not to succumb too much to input that institutional lawyers might provide—but this goal can be hard. As Nancy said,

> We try really hard not to cave in to our legal or contracts department. They try to get us to standardize consent protocols. It may take us longer

to review studies because we don't give researchers a cookie-cutter form. Our approach is not necessarily efficient.

Trade-offs may thus arise here between rigid boilerplates *vs.* customized forms that are more relevant to the subject, but can also lengthen the review processes.

Committees vary in how comfortable they feel opposing their institutions' legal counsel. Nancy explained,

> We have an outside lawyer on our IRB who's really good. I would put him up against any in-house lawyer. If the institution's lawyer said, "You have to use exactly this language," our whole IRB would resign.

Yet other boards with a different composition may feel less able to resist such pressure.

Some committees struggle to fight legalese, but may not always succeed. Still, some negotiation is at times possible. As Nancy continued,

> We don't like consent forms with a lot of potentially exculpatory language, where it looks like the researchers are trying to protect the institution, and confuse participants. We'd rather err in the direction of protecting the participants, and maybe risking some institutional exposure. Clauses may make perfectly good sense in a clinical intervention, but are confusing in health services research with no intervention—about withdrawing from treatment, and not being compensated if you get injured. Usually these concerns come up when we're cooperating with another IRB. First, we object. Then they say, "I'm sorry, our lawyers will not let us change this." So we say, "OK, you can have it in there if you also agree to include an insert—a Q&A sheet in layperson's terms.

Yet in multisite studies, these forms may then diverge between institutions, and different numbers and types of subjects may agree to participate, skewing the sample, and potentially making the resulting data more difficult to combine, impinging on the science.

Industry Pressures

Industry funders also tend to see consent forms as legal contracts that offer indemnification. Troy, a researcher and chair in an urban institution, said,

> The IRB says, "This is ridiculous: a 22-page consent form." Subjects' eyes glaze over because they're not feeling well. But the company requires it. So, we try to compromise.

Hence, corporations may design these forms to protect themselves as third parties, not subjects or institutions. "Some are a little better than others," Troy added. "Some have their absolutely rigid bottom line: 'This is what you're going to do.'"

Corporations may not be willing to alter forms unless several IRBs complain, and/or do so strongly. Troy continued,

> In a couple of instances, we said, "We can't do this. It's just not right!" Generally, at that point, companies have been responsive if they want the study done. Usually, they get similar complaints from other institutions.

With corporations, as with institutions, these negotiations may be easiest when they occur between two lawyers, further underscoring the underlying legal aspects of these documents. "Our contracts office knows how to work with the company lawyers," Troy explained. "Lawyer-to-lawyer: a lot more gets accomplished."

UNCLEAR STANDARDS: WHEN IS ENOUGH ENOUGH?

The anecdotal perception of IRBs, as out of touch with researchers' concerns, thus contrasts markedly with the reality of being squeezed between many competing pressures. At the same time, committees often struggle with when to stop making small changes in consent forms—when "enough is enough"—and they fiddle with forms in ways that appear excessive. IRBs differ widely in what *standards* to adopt. Some boards try to develop and follow implicit or explicit criteria, such as whether they could stand by the consent form if they are audited by the OHRP. Yet such criteria pose questions whether protocols should simply be "good enough," and if so, what that means.

Several interviewees conceded that IRBs sometimes become too nitpicky. These individuals tended to defend the status quo overall, but thought that obsessiveness about consent forms should be reduced. "The system is good," Liza said. "Unfortunately, we need to change the bureaucracy, and the pendulum-swinging of dotting i's and crossing t's."

Other interviewees felt that over time, their standards for consent forms have in fact risen. As Jeff, the social scientist and chair, said, "I have become increasingly less inclined to feel, 'this looks like a good consent.' I feel more: 'I don't like what it says in this or that phrase.'" As a researcher, he is acutely aware of the trade-offs involved, but believes that changes in forms can help subjects. Still, he struggles to balance these competing goals, and thus aims at least to make all of the changes simultaneously, rather than through repeated iterations.

> One doesn't want to say [to researchers], "OK, you've made these changes. Now, here are six to eight more." Occasionally, "I'm sorry we

missed it, but can you please change this phrase" is fine. But in big complicated studies, it could go back and forth several times.

At the same time, Jeff acknowledged that his committee tolerated imperfections. He continued:

> Yes, the description of the study's purpose makes the main or most relevant points, even if it's not a good objective account of the study. [We] might let a little confusion sit, rather than insist that the researcher makes that completely clear.

These determinations are nonetheless highly subjective—whether the standard should be "perfect" or "good enough," how to decide, and whether a particular form has met the standard, whatever that might be. Jeff's lenient stance is far from universal. IRB chairs and administrators often say "the perfect can be the enemy of the good," but may then make edits that are not essential.

Inconsistencies can ensue both within and between committees. At times, an IRB may even change a consent form it has previously approved. "Faculty say, 'This has been approved for seven years,'" Louis reported. "But the consent is very, very technical. *I* can barely understand it." Changes in the committee composition, a scandal at another institution, or simply a change of heart among the same members can alter their attitudes. Not surprisingly, however, such unexpected obstacles catch researchers off guard and anger them.

THE COSTS OF INTERFERENCE

Only a few interviewees acknowledged the disadvantages of demanding too many changes—the danger that researchers may dislike IRBs more, and therefore respect and respond to IRBs' concerns less. Kurt, for example, tries to avoid "nitpicking consent forms to death"—to curb how much IRBs concentrate on relatively insignificant matters. As a researcher and chair, he said,

> I try to focus on protecting human subjects—not on the more trivial stuff. I won't let us get out of compliance. But the consent document is a relatively small piece of the process. If you had a perfect document, but whip through it at the speed of light and hand it to the subject to sign, it wouldn't do any good. If you take enough time with the subjects, it doesn't matter that much what the consent form says. So, I tend not to pick these forms to death. If they attest to the elements in the regs, are not written only for college graduates, and the major elements...are detailed enough, I let it go.

This attitude results in part from the fact that Kurt himself also conducts studies.

> I myself have submitted research to the IRB, and gotten consents back where every few sentences, the IRB made some stylistic change that's not as good, or they didn't like something. IRBs don't get the investigator on their side that way. Researchers then spend more time on making a nice consent form, and perhaps less time on something more important, like actually consenting the subject.

In Kurt's account, the IRB's interference was not only unnecessary but deleterious to the protocol. He also underscores the notion that time discussing the research with the subject—again, "the process"—is just as significant, if not more so, than the forms involved.

WHEN TO REQUIRE RE-CONSENT?

Researchers often alter a study once it has started, seeing needs to improve it—perhaps adding further tests or questionnaires. Other times, new findings from another study are relevant—discoveries of additional side effects or benefits of a drug. Boards then debate whether researchers need to *re*-consent subjects, and if so, when—how much alteration of a protocol necessitates re-consent, given the logistical difficulties involved. Re-consent takes time and effort, and certain changes such as adding a few more questions to a survey, may be exceedingly minor. Gwen said,

> Even for something as insignificant as a couple of extra blood draws, some members say, "You've already consented them for blood draws. It's no big deal," while other members say, "No, these patients want to know every teaspoon of blood that you're taking. If you're adding three tablespoons, *they want to know.*" It boils down to keeping the patient informed, but weighing that against not wanting to hold up the study too much. That's been *a big back-and-forth.*

FOCUS ON FORMS *VS.* THE PROCESS

Louis and others assert that consent is "not just a form, but a whole process," yet committees generally focus only on the form. As Christopher explained,

> Consenting is not a one-time form, and you're in the study forever. It's: this is what we're doing. How are you feeling? Do you want to stay

in it, or not? Doctors think, "Oh, they signed the form; that means they're in."

At present, committees generally lack resources to ensure that consent *is* more of a process; they have no way to monitor directly the interactions between research-ers and subjects. A more conscientious researcher than Togias at Hopkins, for example, might have taken the adverse reaction of his first subject more seriously, reported it to his IRB, and reviewed more prior literature about hexamethonium before continuing. Unfortunately, the IRB was reliant on him to give the "process" its due.

IRBs may realize these limitations, but see few, if any, options. "The consent form is important. But the process is much more important," Liza conceded. "What can we do about that? You lose the forest for the trees. Better education is needed."

Yet much of the debate in the Havasupai, SUPPORT and hexamethonium asthma studies focus on a handful of specific words in their consent form. Many subjects agree to participate in research without reading most of the consent form. IRBs say that consent is a process, but they then nevertheless treat the informed consent as a legal document, often arguing intensely over the presence or absence of specific words. The researcher would presumably discuss key points verbally with subjects. But in the scandals that occur, the specific wording of the forms becomes key, and closely scrutinized.

Improved researcher training about the importance of engaging subjects in dia-logue could help, and cost less than monitoring consent; but many investigators feel they already have too many competing demands on their time and resources. A recent study I conducted with colleagues found that researchers thought that they would not want to spend more than half an hour with a subject when return-ing his or her whole genome, whereas this task could in fact take hours.[15]

Some may feel that lengthy forms impede comprehension, but the assump-tion that consent *is* a process may help to legitimize overly long and complicated forms. This line of thinking would argue that, since the form is only part of educat-ing the potential subject, a detailed discussion with the research staff will presum-ably follow. In that scenario, the fact that the form is imperfect is less problematic because it doesn't stand alone. But researchers' discussions with subjects may be brief and cursory, not detailed. Full understanding by subjects of relevant details should remain the goal.

POSSIBLE SOLUTIONS

Having Non-MDs Review Forms

Some IRBs discuss and attempt various strategies to ameliorate these problems. To enhance understandability, IRBs frequently have non-physicians—staff, "community" members, or others—edit these documents. Christopher reported that one surgeon has his teenage daughter review consents:

> Our IRB has a surgeon with a 16-year-old daughter. He uses her as a sounding board: "Does this make sense?"...He says that if she can't figure it out, no one's going to be able to. That's a nice metric.

The surgeon's daughter asks questions the committee didn't anticipate—for example, why anyone would want to enter a study: '"What are the real risks and purposes. What am I being asked to do? How long is it going to take? Why would anyone do this?' A lot of PIs don't have answers," adds Christopher. These efforts can help with comprehension, but do not necessarily decrease the length of these forms, and might even increase it. In this particular case, it is also unclear why the IRB does not have a staff or community member, rather than a member's daughter, performing this function.

Shorter or More Standardized Forms

Several interviewees mentioned the possibility of shorter consent forms—such as one-page "summaries," with an added, longer form available. Yet none had yet tried such an approach.

Several critics have also called for more standardized IRB reviews and consent forms,[10] but potential problems surface, including needs for flexibility and adaptation of templates, and questions of what and how much to standardize. Templates can result from institutions' and funders' legal concerns about length.

Yet, in developing such boilerplates, boards confront ambiguities of what particular elements to include or exclude. Certain risks may be possible, but rare. Phil, a social scientist and chair, said,

> Our IRB very often has included in consents information about harm to self and others, and a referral for help if you feel stress as a result of being in the research. But students have wanted to interview professors about these professors' careers. Does it really make sense to talk to them about suicidality?

Still, IRBs may insist on keeping such statements in every form—even if these have little, if any, applicability—due not only to liability concerns, but to anxieties and inertia, feeling that such information might help some participants. IRBs may imagine scenarios in which such precautions may be warranted, even if exceedingly rare. Phil continued,

> It seems absurd for anyone to worry about a clinician, being interviewed about conducting family therapy, suddenly talking about self-hurt or abuse.

> Yet I studied employees at an agency, and one disclosed that they had been abused at the agency and was very distressed. We didn't expect that.

This example highlights, however, tensions concerning real, imagined, and feared possible future scenarios of very low probability. Similarly, for the interview study on which this book is based, my IRB insisted I include a statement that "the alternative to participating is not to participate," which a few of these interviewees felt was obvious and unnecessary. The costs to IRBs of including such additional phrases are low, but consequently, forms grow and may appear to participants to be legalistic and not wholly relevant—often designed to protect the institution more than inform subjects.

To treat every study the same is simpler than having to decide when exactly regulations do or don't apply. But flexibility can be critical. Phil said,

> It's much easier to operate from a universalistic principle: we're going to do this in all these consents, with everyone. Otherwise, everything is a little bit of a judgment call, which makes everyone a bit nervous.

Requiring Tests of Comprehension

To enhance understanding, IRBs occasionally require that researchers test participants' comprehension. No guidance exists on this topic, and a single IRB may change its desires for such exams over time, frustrating researchers. Jeremy, the physician and chair, described his criteria: "We require a test of formal comprehension if we feel there's a higher risk level, a vulnerable population, concern about capacity, or high risk with no benefit." Yet such standards can be hard to assess, leading IRBs to vary in necessitating such exams. Researchers can also "teach for the test" focusing on instilling the answers to specific questions, though subjects may end up not comprehending better the study overall. Jeremy continued,

> PIs send back nasty e-mails: "I had a very similar protocol at the other IRB two years ago, and *they* didn't ask for a test of comprehension. Why are you asking for it? Is there any proof that it makes a difference?"

Conclusions

IRBs face challenges concerning informed consent that can impede simplification, shortening, and subjects' comprehension of these forms. Heightened research complexity, lack of prior relationships between many researchers and subjects, and funders' and institutions' liability concerns lengthen and complicate these documents, and lead committees to differ. IRBs often try to counter these pressures, but vary in success.

Boards seek to enhance these documents and fight researcher biases, but face ambiguities concerning what and how much to include, with what level of complexity, and how "perfect" these forms should be. Dilemmas underlie these questions: whether these documents are legal contracts, and if so, to what degree; whom these statements ultimately protect; and how to improve them. IRBs may seek to "perfect" these forms without fully taking into account the costs to researchers, who alone may bear these burdens. No mechanisms exist to check committees that want to elongate and elaborate these documents.

Frequently, researchers merely hand subjects a 30- or 40-page form to sign, summarizing it verbally in two or three sentences. Subjects decide whether to participate based on these oral comments. Committees may implicitly recognize this discrepancy between obtaining fully informed consent, and the "realities" in the field, and consequently may emphasize that consent should be an ongoing process. Yet committees do not usually promote or monitor "the process," and in fact may undermine it by overemphasizing the form itself, "nitpicking" it, and hence increasing focus on it, rather than on the quality of the interpersonal communication and relationships between the researcher and subject.

The inherently subjective nature of these quandaries leads to variations and frustrations among researchers, and often IRBs themselves. Committees may be aware of, and wrestle with, these tensions, but still be unsure how to resolve these conflicts, and need further guidance.

In response to the questions raised by the Obama Administration and others about why consent forms are long, these interviewees suggest several factors. These documents constitute one of the few aspects of researcher interactions with subjects—a very downstream process—that committees feel they can control. Many committees thus feel obligated to exert as much control as possible over these forms and the written protocols that PIs submit, though these efforts can clearly become counterproductive, adding pages and hence decreasing comprehensibility. Many interviewees also felt that researchers, institutions, and funders, and not boards themselves, are often responsible for excessive length. Yet anecdotally, many researchers appear to think that it is the IRBs who want lengthy and detailed forms. Each side may blame the other. Questions emerge about the legal status of these documents among not only IRBs, but institutional officials, too, who frequently also want these forms to be as thorough as possible. Clarification of these contrasting views can help.

Though the Obama Administration and others have proposed "prescribing appropriate content" for these forms, questions about *how* information should be presented involve both form and content. The ANPRM seeks templates, but avoidance of "boilerplates"; in practice, however, the distinction between these two can blur.[5] Templates may reduce variations between IRBs, but be applied too fully and rigidly by certain committees. Boards may require inclusion of parts that do not apply in particular studies.

One-page summary forms are also possible and can help, but ambiguities need to be addressed concerning what exactly these abstracts should include. While the proposals also suggest presenting information at the very beginning of the consent document, questions remain, too, about the *content* of the language to be used there—the complexity and amount of detail—that also need to be addressed. Lawyers representing industry funders and institutions may not feel comfortable with or permit such abbreviation; thus, subjects will still have to read and understand the longer forms, too. Shorter, one-page summaries can potentially aid subjects in grasping the longer documents. Concerns arise that in practice, researchers and subjects may view such shorter summaries as replacing, rather than merely aiding comprehension of, the longer documents. These recommendations for change are valuable, but heightened recognition of the complexities that emerge here must be tackled.

The degree to which consent forms are legal contracts also needs to be determined. Until then, attempts to shorten these forms may have limited effectiveness. In certain ways, these forms appear to be *both* legal and informational documents. But the boundaries and balance between these two models and respective expectations then need to be addressed. Institutions, courts, and others may see these forms as potentially legal; and to ignore that view is unrealistic. That viewpoint and tension needs to be acknowledged and addressed rather than denied in order to bridge these potentially conflicting perspectives.

The OHRP and others should also develop and promulgate standards of when exactly "enough is enough." IRBs should acknowledge far more fully the costs of nitpicking too much. Checks and balances should be established. Such feedback loops are critical. Presently, IRBs have little incentive to shorten and simplify forms. The ANPRM suggests that IRBs report to the OHRP how often they go beyond certain other proposed changes. Requiring such reporting for instances in which committees exceed length recommendations can help motivate IRBs to follow these limits more fully.[5] OHRP could also require that these forms be publically available and posted online (e.g., at the US government website, www.clinicaltrials.gov,[16] which lists all drug and device studies), with redactions if needed, to increase transparency and feedback.

These data also highlight several subjective aspects of consent forms that will, no doubt, continue even with recommended changes—the exact extents to which subjects should be informed, and what and how much information to include. In deciding when a form is "good enough," IRBs also confront underlying tensions between giving subjects all information *vs.* having them understand the relevant issues—how much subjects should be informed *vs.* comprehend. Subjects may receive large numbers of details (presumably fulfilling researchers' objections to disclose information) but not understand these.

Even if more tests of comprehension are used, questions persist of what they should include—how much detail subjects need to grasp in order to pass—and whether such tests should just be given once, immediately on entering a study, or repeated over time. If the latter, it is unclear what should happen if subjects forget key parts or comprehend less over time, as may well be the case.

Questions about whom these forms in fact protect reflect larger quandaries of whom IRBs' primary clients are—participants, institutions, funders, PIs, or the IRB itself—and how committees should determine and balance their responsibilities and roles.

Though the Obama Administration and others have also suggested excusing certain studies from IRB assessment, these committees can in fact potentially be important in tempering potential biases in consent documents.

IRBs' input to researchers also emerges here as varying across a spectrum from heavy to light—from requiring changes to expressing "concerns," suggestions, and "unhappiness" about aspects of a study. These differing types of communication suggest varying levels of expectations and negotiations. Researchers may not all understand these differences, and may instead feel that all committee "suggestions" are mandatory.

The OHRP and others could nonetheless develop standard consent documents, addressing not only the *form* but the *content* of these documents, and IRBs can be trained to use these, to gain a sense of acceptable and appropriate boundaries and lengths. Yet recognition of the limitations of such forms, and the ongoing needs for flexibility and subject comprehension of other details would remain critical. With use of shorter summaries, future questions will persist of how much comprehension of a study suffices. IRBs have also developed "rules of thumb," or best practices that may be effective, and can potentially be shared to help reduce these tensions. Enhanced patient education about science and research—from randomization to placebos—is also crucial. In an ever more globalized world, determining how best to explain complex scientific concepts and terms will be ever more vital.

CHAPTER 6

From "Nitpicky" to "User-Friendly"

INTER-IRB VARIATIONS AND THEIR CAUSES

■

As we saw in Chapter 4, Kathleen Dziak and her colleagues wanted to survey patients at 15 institutions about basic demographics, health, treatment satisfaction, and preventive services received, without recording any identifiable information. The 15 IRBs involved not only varied from 5 days to about half a year to approve the study. But while nine committees allowed an expedited, administrative review, six required a full review by the entire committee, three mandated that patients opt out, and one required that patients specifically opt-in, by filling out a card (which over one third of the the patients didn't do). These differences altered the researchers' ability to combine the results from these various sites, hampering the science. Certain groups may be particularly wary of research, and thus refuse more commonly, impairing the generalizability of the data.

This example is important, since multisite studies are becoming ever more common,[1] and response rates to surveys have been declining in general.[2,3] Moreover, the study does not seem on the face of it to be ethically troubling or complicated.

Seemingly small IRB decisions can thus significantly impact scientific research, yet IRBs tend to defend, ignore, or downplay not only these variations but also their costs to science. Overwhelmingly, these boards claim that they come to different decisions because of differences in their local community values, justifying the discrepancies and the power that each individual committee possesses. As one IRB member, Sharon Kaur, argued in an essay, "How IRBs Make Decisions: Should We Worry If They Disagree?" in the *Journal of Medical Ethics*:

> The fact that IRBs proffer different opinions . . . should not on its own be viewed negatively. IRB membership should reflect as much as possible the diversity of the communities in which the research is carried out,

and this will inevitably result in members coming to the review process with different ideas about coercion and undue influence. What is significant is whether decisions taken by IRBs are consistent and coherent given the similarities and differences of the communities in which the research is being carried out.[4]

Yet no data have ever been published supporting this assertion that these discrepancies are due to differences in local community norms. In addition, studies documenting variation[5,6] have not examined *why* exactly IRBs differ in their decisions.[7] Rather, I found that IRBs even within the same community and institution often differ widely.

Many protocols are straightforward, but others prompt discussion and at times debate. Dwayne, a rural researcher and chair, explained,

> 30 percent [of studies], basically sail through—"Everyone who is for it say 'Aye.'" For the other 70 percent, there's something to discuss. And out of those, about half have something serious to discuss before voting. With 10 percent, there's a problem. Rarely do we actually reject a protocol outright. But we have recently done that more. An industry-sponsored study in children looked at a very benign condition, and the drug had a lot of side effects.

Estimating the proportions of studies in each of these three categories of IRB responses is not easy, and may differ between IRBs.

Interviewees discussed disagreements within their board, but often minimized the importance or implications of these. Jack, a rural physician and chair, said,

> A third of the time, there's some substantive disagreement. In general, we come to agreement pretty easily. But *everyone has their own little biases*. A couple of people are *much tighter* about procedural issues. Some focus on *language*. But it's rare that we have really opposing views on the ethical issues. People generally come to consensus pretty quickly.

Yet differing views of language often reflect varying views, interpretations, and evaluations of ethical concepts. Moreover, although members on any one IRB eventually achieve consensus, different IRBs can reach very different conclusions. Several boards may agree on broad ethical principles but interpret these differently, defining key terms in various ways, potentially impeding research. Although each of these committees may see their process as routine, these inter-IRB variations can feel obstructionist to researchers.

Interviewees may acknowledge "minor" variations among IRBs in "fine-tuning and nuance," but in fact the contrasts can be far greater.

Where Variations can Occur

DISAGREEMENTS BETWEEN INSTITUTIONS

As we have seen, IRBs commonly disagree on a variety of topics—from what is research and when a study is scientifically "good enough" to whether the risks are acceptable and what exactly the informed consent forms should say. But how do IRBs themselves look at, and understand these variations? Do these committees see these discrepancies as problems and why or why not?

DISAGREEMENTS WITHIN ONE INSTITUTION

IRBs often say that differences result because of variations in their local community values, but in fact discrepancies occur even within a single institution in a single community! Many institutions have more than one IRB, and these committees can disagree. In one academic medical center, multiple scientists may be participating in the same study, yet each may submit it to different IRBs within the same institution, which then evaluate it differently. As Judy explained,

> Protocols may not all go to the same committee, and we're really not consistent. The investigators get very upset: "How come you let so-and-so do it here, and they didn't have to change the consent or do this?"

The committees in one medical center in a single community can range considerably in several personal and social ways. As Christopher described it,

> Different IRBs at our institution feel totally different. One chair is very obsessive and particular. His IRB can spend an hour going over a consent form. In the IRB I run, everyone participates, and says what they want....We very much use our lay people, and empower them a lot more than some of the other IRBs do. It's whether you're going to be a committee that *really* discusses things, or a *Robert's Rules of Order* kind of committee. We have both, and sometimes when we don't have a quorum, people move around, and are on other IRBs, and are astounded that that we're at the same institution!

He distinguishes between the letter *vs.* the spirit of the regulations (i.e., *Robert's Rules of Order vs.* "really" discussing issues). He sees his own approach as justified, and as implicitly better than that of other committees (e.g., "we" can "empower" unaffiliated members, while another chair is "obsessive").

Occasionally, chairs within the same institution will come together to try to reduce these variations, but such efforts do not always fully succeed. Christopher added, "A steering committee of the IRB chairs meets monthly, so there is some oversight and attempt to get some consistency, but not much." One chair may remain adamant about particular risks, and have significant sway. As Olivia said,

> When the chairs get together, there are definitely differences. The primary chair of my committee is very concerned about pain and suffering—*very* concerned—and really takes it to heart when there's the slightest indication that subjects may experience what he determines is suffering. It's caused a lot of problems.

INCONSISTENCY WITHIN A SINGLE IRB

Even single IRBs can vary over time. Anthony said,

> Investigators feel we are flip-flopping: "You never made me do this in the past!" Or, "I used to do this all the time, and you never had any problems with it." Sometimes, we've had changes in impressions from OHRP or elsewhere, and we have no choice. But in other cases, they're right! We go back and look through, and really can't justify why. It appears willy-nilly.

In part, these changes may be due to the fact that members of an IRB rotate periodically, which in turn alters the committee's dynamics and decisions. As Elaine, an administrator and member, explained,

> The membership can change. PIs say, "You approved this consent form a year ago. Why, now, are you saying it doesn't make any sense?" I don't know a solution. Because if you had the same people on forever, there'd be burnout.

A committee may also review the same protocol differently when a recently appointed chair or member raises new issues about a study that the board had previously approved. The IRB may suddenly challenge and not reapprove the protocol. As Dwayne described,

> Along comes a new [chair] like me. I'll question something, and the PI sends me back a nasty e-mail: "Why is this not being approved

now? It was always approved in the past!" I think that's good. Because you always want fresh ideas. For example, a hematologist has recently joined our committee. None of us had thought of bleeding with a specific drug, because none of us knew enough about thrombosis. We didn't really think about it. She did. So, if this protocol had come through before, it might have gone through as smooth as silk. But now, with this person on the committee, it was a stumbling block. That's OK.

In this instance, the change results from additional scientific expertise on an IRB—which presumably should have been sufficiently present beforehand. IRBs may thus see such differences as beneficial. Yet these changes can antagonize researchers. Consequently, committees may need better to explain these alterations to angry investigators. Dwayne added,

> I do see PIs' frustration on "the other side." We just need to communicate as best and honestly as we can about the issues. I would just explain: we overlooked the issue last time.

Some IRBs also try to reduce these mid-course changes to only significant ones, but such restraint is hardly universal.

INCONSISTENCY IN AN INDIVIDUAL MEMBER

Even a single IRB member may shift his or her stance about an issue over time. A person may judge each protocol on its own, but then express seemingly conflicting concerns about different studies. Jeremy reported,

> One member is one of the fiercest critics of IRBs running amok and constantly beating down investigators and coming up with new things. He says we focus on trivial minutiae, and are blocking progress. But frequently he will also call for a test of comprehension, or doing extra things...He comes to a conclusion based on the case at hand....Even within this one guy, there is a pretty wide range!

Elaine admitted that she herself has also changed her mind about certain points while serving on her IRB. "The committee is made up of people," she explained. "*People change*. I can look at something one day, and then the next day: what the heck was I thinking?"

Types of Variation

Rarely do IRBs fully approve studies with no changes at all,[8] but committees differ in the stringency of their standards. Christopher said,

> The issues tend to be how picky one IRB is going to be *vs.* the other. Some will table a protocol for a typo. Others will give specific minor revisions. It's rare that a protocol gets tabled by one IRB and fully approved by another, but it is interesting when issues keep coming up at one IRB, but not another.

Christopher's latter observation suggests that the discrepancies may reflect features of the IRB rather than the protocols *per se*.

Some committees see themselves as being relatively more "conservative"—meaning, specifically, cautious—than others, which can delay approval. As Joe said, "Our IRB has tended to take a more conservative approach. So it takes longer for investigators to get those types of protocols reviewed and approved by the IRB."

In contrast, several committees pride themselves for being more "research friendly," user friendly, and "congenial." Committees can differ, for instance, in how much they imagine possible problems that may arise in conducting a study in the field. IRBs may fear unrealistic "worst case" scenarios and vary significantly in accepting or challenging such statistically unlikely outcomes. To conceive of future potential risks involves imagining fears of the unknown that may not be wholly empirically based. Yet no built-in checks or brakes on such anxieties exist—no tests of how *reasonable* or unrealistic such speculative harms may be. A few IRB personnel may attempt to remain "reasonable" when considering such risks. "When we get into fear-mongering, and talking about worst-case scenarios," Charlotte said, "we do a pretty good job of coming back from the edge." But this sort of "reality checking," can itself be difficult, and may not occur.

The Causes of Variations Between IRBs

CLAIMS THAT DIFFERENCES IN "COMMUNITY VALUES" ARE THE CAUSE OF IRB DISCREPANCIES

The original justification for local, as opposed to centralized, IRBs was the assumption that the ethical values of subjects in protocols would vary widely between communities, and that committee members should consequently come from the same locales as the subjects. A national IRB could not reflect these local differences. As Greg, the social scientist and chair, said,

> IRBs can use their local flavor, *their local community view* of things, and it's reflected on how the protocols are reviewed. It's good: *you've got the moral standards of a community,* reflective of the populations you're going to be sampling.

But do IRBs in fact disagree because of local community values? Or for other reasons? In the 40 years since these regulations were developed, many aspects of research have changed, and much has been learned. In the United States today, though, many hospital and university staffs consist of professionals from all over the country, if not the globe, and—as discussed earlier—even an IRB community member may not accurately represent the subjects in a particular protocol. Yet, IRBs continue to justify variations between them as due to cultural and racial sensitivities.

Recently, for example, in response to a paper I published, drawing on these interviews and illustrating how differences in local community values do not account for differences in committee decisions, Douglas Diekema, an IRB chair at Seattle Children's Hospital, defended deviations between committees. He pointed out that the Native American communities may differ from others in important ways, citing in particular the research scandal involving the Havasupai Indians to make his point.[9] But this scandal was not a situation in which IRBs differed due to variations in local community values. In fact, the researchers knew that the tribe would not like studies on rates of mental illness within their community. But these investigators nonetheless chose to deceive the tribe; and the IRB knew the investigators' plan to study schizophrenia and approved the consent form that did not mention any psychiatric diagnoses. The researcher recognized all too well how the tribe would view these studies. Hence, this case does *not* serve to illustrate the need for local IRB reviews.

Certainly, some groups within a community may look at issues differently. But no examples have ever been provided of how this reason is the cause of IRB inconsistencies. Rather, researchers working closely with these groups generally appear to recognize how different groups may perceive relevant issues, and these investigators tend to work hard to address these concerns.

A rare few interviewees thought that this commonly stated explanation for discrepancies was only *part* of the reason. Phil, a social scientist and chair, said,

> The *stock answer* is to say that the IRB is supposed to consider community conditions, and that it's possible that what we do here and what you

do there would be different—because of the population, because of who we are as researchers, the community setting, etc. That's why we have community members. To some extent that's a *piece* of it.

But, as we will see, other factors—including different "comfort levels" and toleration of uncertainty and anxiety among certain IRB personnel, rather than local community variation—in fact fuel these discrepancies.

COMPARING ONE'S OWN COMMITTEE TO OTHERS

Strikingly, IRBs turn out generally to have little sense overall of how exactly they differ in their decisions from other boards. Many committees operate in relative isolation. Occasionally, chairs become aware of discrepancies through multisite studies and investigators who switch institutions, but such grounds for comparison are rare. Greg, the social scientist, said,

> Researchers come from other states, and say that *that* IRB would've easily approved this or expedited it, or, "You guys are way easier than University such and such." But you don't get too many of those.

In fact, IRBs appear to vary for several reasons.

PRIOR RESEARCH REVIEWED BY THE COMMITTEE

It turns out that several other factors, such as a committee's own past expertise and experiences, fuel variations between these committees far more than do differences in local community values. For instance, an IRB's views of and comfort with risk often depend on the types of risk that it has permitted in prior studies. Implicitly, committees may hence weigh the potential dangers of a particular study in relation to other research they have approved. In part, comfort is shaped by the highest level of risk the IRB previously vouchsafed.

Familiarity with a type of study can get established over time, and an IRB's amount of experience can either facilitate or impede an assessment. For example, a particular type of cancer research may have been previously reviewed by some IRBs, but be new to other committees. Or certain IRBs or members may be more comfortable with social science research because they have reviewed many social science protocols in the past. IRBs less familiar with a particular type of investigation may be more cautious. As Charlotte said,

> I've seen hospital IRBs overreact and get incredibly conservative and careful when reviewing a behavioral study because they just don't really

know how to treat it. It's new and different. They know they've got to do something, and are a little worried, so they get incredibly rigid and rule-bound. We might expedite a survey of kids that asks about physical activity habits. Whereas a hospital IRB that never sees a behavioral survey like that might feel the need to have all their experts sit down together and review it. Conversely, we would probably do the same thing if *we* got a clinical drug trial. We'd freak out, and not know what to do.

An IRB may have its own norms and accepted practices—particular ways it has come to interpret, see, and exercise its role. An IRB's past decisions and practices thus tend to shape its future views and choices. Elaine said,

Urban myths are out there—things that the committee has interpreted in the past that are not regulations but are just comfort levels. Our IRB says, "You should say 'fill out,' not 'complete,' a survey. 'Complete' is coercive." But that's not in the regulations. Our IRB also likes consent forms to be on institutional letterhead.

Elaine's phrase "urban myth" suggests how power can irrationally accrue over time around such habitual responses.

IRBs vary, too, in whether they think they should "go beyond" the regulations, and if so, how, and to what degree. "Federal guidelines lay out a foundation," Louis said. "Institutions should have the right to go above and beyond." He elaborated:

Our standards are probably a little bit more stringent than another institution in protecting the right of the individual person—changing wording to make it clearer to the subject exactly what they're going to be asked to do.

Yet such changes may impede a multisite study, since one committee's stringency (*vs.* leniency) is another's obsessiveness (*vs.* user-friendliness).

"Good Catches": The Effects of "Many Eyes" Reading a Protocol

Discrepancies arise, too, because studies entail complicated logistics and implications that may not be obvious during an initial reading. IRBs can thus vary in the degrees to which committee members have fully anticipated all on-the-ground possible scenarios and details.

One IRB or member may be the only one to "pick up on" a particular problem. In detecting potential defects that others have overlooked in reading a protocol, IRB members cited "good catches"—a term used by physicians. Researchers themselves may have overlooked these details. Cynthia gave an example:

An investigator was surveying homeless individuals, and was going to mail postcards. We pointed out that these subjects are *homeless*! We all laughed. But if you just use a template, it's a normal standardized method: "We will send everybody a postcard, reminding them of their next visit." The researcher had to think of another method—giving subjects little items to keep in their pocket.

Such details are often missed, highlighting the all-too-human aspects of the review process. As Liza added,

> A protocol randomized subjects and then gave them the informed consent for the arm they were randomized to. It went right through the IRB. But I said, "You're randomizing people before their informed consent!" "Oh, are they doing that?" Sometimes the principles just get lost.

When "many different eyes" view a protocol, one reader may spot a problem that others have missed. This process may be inevitable, but not systematic. At a meeting, only one person—such as a specialist in a particular field—may perceive certain problems. Therefore, his or her absence or presence at a meeting, easily reversed by happenstance, can alter the committee's decision, fostering discrepancies. Dwayne, the rural researcher and chair, said,

> A protocol had a drug that can cause bleeding. [The] hematologist on the IRB brought up a very important issue that none of us had foreseen: how to monitor for bleeding in an emergency. If a subject has trauma, how are you going to *reverse this drug*? We tabled the protocol to have this hematologist discuss the problem with the PI. They came up with a monitoring plan.

Variations between IRBs may thus reflect the availability of particular experts.

Cynthia's IRB was the only one to complain about a multisite study requiring patients to agree to be enrolled in a registry before they could be in a study. She elaborated,

> The researcher wanted to have a national database where any parent would have to have their child's name entered before they would be eligible to go into a clinical trial. If you disagreed with putting your child's name into this national database, you were not allowed to enroll in any trials. I said, "You cannot take away people's right to enroll in a research study if they say, 'I don't want to place my child's name in a national registry.' You've suddenly made registration an eligibility requirement." We

were the only IRB that found issue with that—which amazes me. They thought it was not an IRB issue, because it was a registry—not a research study. But isn't this an invasion of a parent's right to choice and confidentiality? They then rescinded it. A lot of institutions would have OK'd it.

Again, unique discovery of these points reflects the value of having multiple people viewing the protocol.

Boards were generally proud of "catching" points that other committees had not. In part, doing so seemed to justify boards' independent existence. Yet while chairs have contended that an advantage of local IRB review is that they alone have caught a particular problem, questions then arise of whether this advantage is worth the redundancy of effort and expense, and how much the current system significantly reduces harms to subjects: would a more efficient system necessarily be less safe? How many reviewers are necessary to discover points not found by other reviewers is not clear. In a multisite study, far fewer reviewers may be needed than are now engaged in IRB reviews at every institution.

"Sniff Tests": Individual Attitudes and Beliefs

Members' own personal views, beliefs, values, comfort, and anxiety can also affect their decisions. They confront quandaries not only as members of particular socioeconomic or professional groups (i.e. related to gender, social class, race, or being an MD or PhD, or a community vs. regular member), but as individuals beyond these labels alone. In confronting difficult decisions, many interviewees drew on their "gut feelings" and "intuition" about a proposed study, at times using "the sniff test," and their personal knowledge and impression of the investigator rather than careful "ethical analysis," per se.

Moral judgments can be hard to describe. Indeed, recent research on the roles of emotional processes in moral decision making suggests that our brains process moral decisions far differently than we think we do.[10,11] We develop quick feelings about moral issues that we then try to put into words. Psychologist Jonathan Haidt asked study subjects what they thought of a brother and sister having sex once while using a condom, with her using birth control. Subjects universally felt disgusted, but then had trouble explaining exactly why.[12]

To grapple with and try to convey their moral standards and judgments, interviewees used a range of metaphors. For example, Cynthia, the administrator, described how IRBs "frowned" upon bad protocols, and discussed whether researchers had "any black marks against them," evoking the specter of a strict and disapproving headmaster. In this instance, the interviewee's language suggests a possible moral issue with the researcher as well as the experiment itself. These metaphors can reinforce the stereotype that many researchers have of IRBs as harsh, disapproving authorities that must be appeased.

At other times, committees felt anxious about being too lax. These individuals described being "worried" about aspects of protocols, and sought *"peace of mind,"* at times deciding between competing ethical options based on their visceral sense of comfort or discomfort. Frequently in the end, IRBs' "peace of mind" becomes a de facto standard. But what exactly that phrase means and when it is achieved is not always clear. Committees vary in how and to what degree they weigh their anxieties. "Occasionally, we approve a protocol that makes us a little uncomfortable," Judy, the chair, said. "Probably not more than five times a year."

Due to the importance of focusing on precise details of protocols, IRBs may attract personnel with certain personality traits. Some individuals may be very cautious a priori, which can be important. "Some members would take these things apart with a fine-toothed comb," Gwen, an IRB member, said. "On page five, you said two micrograms, but on page 25, it says two milligrams. Which is it?" Personal psychological issues and traits mix with background and training, each affecting, or contributing to, the other. As Joe observed,

> Individuals who are a little more cautious, or come from a more compliance background, are more likely to be conservative than individuals who are investigators. A whole host of *temperamental* issues play a role as well.

INDIVIDUAL MEMBER CONCERNS AND PET PEEVES

The fact that a diverse group of individuals compose each committee also molds decisions. These personnel may have concerns or biases regarding particular areas of research or investigators that can affect the board's discussions and decisions. Some of these individual perspectives are legitimate and important—providing necessary scientific expertise. For instance, Jack, the rural physician and chair, said that a member who is "the only oncologist"

> may be the only person who has little nagging irritations about the subtleties of what constitutes a weak comparator of a chemotherapy regimen. Many other nagging irritations come up from other people's perspectives. The community members will often come up with something that the medical people just don't think of.

But individual members vary in how thoroughly they ferret out potential problems, fueling variations between committees. "Certain committee members are better at this than the rest of us," Dwayne said. "One member will call the phone numbers on the consent forms to make sure they work. Sometimes they don't!" Hence, having many eyes examining a protocol can provide benefits, but may not be systematic. Moreover, legitimate points (such as checking phone numbers) can, arguably, also be included in a checklist that IRBs could share.

A vocal member with strong views can potentially influence an IRB, furthering inter-IRB variations. Members' senior faculty positions can help legitimize their arguments, even when they don't have expertise in the specific area of a protocol. Elaine said,

> One member with really strong views against the study can sometimes sway the committee—one power-tripping jerk, wanting to tear everything apart. Our old IRB chair just let such people go on—"They're tenured faculty."

In such cases, advocates for a study might push back, although with varying success. Olivia, a health care provider and chair, said,

> [A vice] chair has gotten a lot of members biased about sleep studies—where subjects are kept awake for 60 hours at a time, hooked up to EMGs, EEGs, EKGs, and rectal thermometers. The remuneration is abnormally high: $6,000–$10,000. The committee had a lot of misunderstanding about who was going to participate—worried that it would only be really poor people with no other way of getting money. But most participants had alternative lifestyles—ski bums or artists who do these types of studies for a couple of weeks, and then go off and ski in Utah. The desperately poor were ruled out immediately because they would usually not be able to comply with the study anyway. That information persuaded some members. Not everyone.

The fact that reviewers' perceptions of a study's risks may be based solely on written descriptions, without knowledge or experience, can also foster unrealistic conceptions of potential harms, overly increasing or decreasing concerns. Olivia added,

> The IRB thinks it must be terrible to stay up for 60 hours. The rectal thermometer probe is everybody's greatest concern, but participants say it's the thing they get used to most quickly. Our community member was beside herself because of the description of the actograph. It looks like a wristwatch, and measures movement. But the protocol made it sound like it was a significant risk.

When IRB members fear possible bad events that are not realistic or *reality-based*, additional information, and even at times visits to the research site, can potentially help. After this anxiety took hold within her committee, Olivia tried to educate the members:

> We went to the site to actually *see* the physical surroundings, and what people go through. It's great—not nearly as horrible as it sounds... One member got an actograph. Some still weren't convinced. The *bias* is so strongly imbedded now; it's going to be very hard to get rid of.

Still, even as a chair, Olivia was not entirely successful in countering her committee's bias. An open-minded leader can attempt to mitigate such obstacles, but other chairs may not even make the effort.

Questions arise here, too, of why written descriptions alone don't convey certain information—in this case how little discomfort a rectal thermometer actually causes. This particular example involves a socially awkward topic (rectal sensation). Clearly, reliance of paper forms has limitations—highlighting an illusion that these documents can convey "the reality" of studies. The fact that one community member saw one of the devices but remained biased against the study poses other challenges. Again, however, the resistance here involves an individual's fears, not unique community values, per se.

For personal reasons, chairs and members may also be predisposed against a particular researcher. Occasionally, in such instances, a chair or administrator can arrange for another IRB to review the investigator's studies. Olivia added,

> A vice chair and a PI did not get along. If it's just getting personal, *that* cannot affect the way a study is reviewed. Finally, we decided at an administrative level that those studies could *no longer come to our committee*. We did that very quietly. The vice chair is a wonderful physician, very well known in his field, but could not get over this fight.

A chair or member may possess many virtues, but wrestle with issues—consciously or unconsciously—that can affect IRB reviews. Olivia ran interference.

> Everyone has biases, but *some are more easily overcome than others*. This personal bias is a combination of having to work regularly with this other physician, and not liking the kind of research he's doing.

Researchers' personalities can cause and exacerbate problems. The investigator in question is from another, non-Western culture in which he isn't used to being challenged. Olivia explained,

His whole cultural attitude is: "I, as a physician, should not be questioned."
He doing is important research. But everything he submits is very sloppy.
It's very irritating, and takes a lot of time to fix—usually, two or three times.

Several problems can thus exacerbate one another. The option of having a different committee review an investigator's protocols is not always available, depending on whether a university has more than one IRB[13] and whether an enlightened
chair or administrator recognizes the benefits of a switch. Smaller institutions
may lack such an alternative.

PRUDISHNESS

Studies involving sex or sexuality, in particular, can also make IRB personnel
uncomfortable, affecting responses to protocols. Elaine described a "conservative" chair who got "weird" about studies involving these topics: "He would just
see a title about LGBT, and say, 'That has to go to the full board.' No, it doesn't!"

Studies examining sexual behavior—for example, concerning HIV risk among
adolescents—can become particularly fraught. As Eric said,

> For some studies, it's almost like the Supreme Court: you pick one side
> of an argument, and the other side of the room picks the other side. It's
> very hard to get the two sides together. Members put their views of the
> world into it. It gets harder when it's around teenage girls, because the
> school board becomes involved. Parents give consent, but a small group
> on the IRB always hesitates.

Such topics invoke deeply felt beliefs and fears. Greg felt his IRB "was a little
bit Puritan," and "didn't like asking juicy, sexual questions."

Yet an individual IRB member may be "prudish" based not on the community's consensus as a whole, but on his or her own *personal* discomfort. Such
attitudes no doubt exist among many individuals but do not necessarily represent the entire community. One doctor I interviewed, who was an IRB member in the developing world, said that he thought his teenage daughter would
be uncomfortable with questions about sex in an HIV prevention study. Other
committee members thought that his view reflected his own discomfort more
than that of members of the community. He was insistent, and the committee eventually yielded to him—because he was a senior male physician—and
asked the researcher to remove the questions. Indeed, no mechanism exists
for systematically ascertaining and incorporating views of the majority of the
community.

Uneasiness about sexuality may manifest itself implicit and indirect rather than
explicit and direct ways. For instance, at an institution in a relatively conservative

area, some IRB members resisted protocols that asked students about their attitudes concerning homosexuality without fully informing these subjects in advance that this topic would be explored. Louis said,

> A professor wanted to study students' perceptions of homosexuality. That, in itself, was not an issue. But the informed consent said the study was about their beliefs related to "culture and their attitudes," and never specifically said what the survey was really about. It went from expedited to a full-board review. The reviewers were not comfortable making that decision alone. The researchers had to change it.

Louis claimed that the problem here related to deception, not homosexuality. "It had nothing to do with 'the topic.'" But in this conservative region, the IRBs' uneasiness may have partly reflected its fear that students would feel awkward responding to questions about homosexuality, which may or may not be correct. IRBs' perception of local cultural values may thus stymie research, and not be wholly accurate. An IRB's views of differences in community values may not necessarily be correct, or supported by evidence, as opposed to reflecting the fears or concerns of one or a few members, rather than represent the views of most of the community.

The few examples provided by interviewees of purported differences in local community values between IRBs concerned sex—and appeared to reflect the personal prudishness of a few members, rather than different views or approaches toward research ethics per se, and in no instance necessarily represented the community as a whole.

The committee members generally discussed perceived variations as if these were based on population mores, even when their own testimony contradicted this assertion. Olivia, for example, explained variations as follows:

> Here in a big city, we are much more comfortable than in more conservative regions with certain issues that aren't a big deal for us to talk about, but I'm *sure* would raise eyebrows in other places, and be more difficult. So it's to be expected, and not a bad thing to have some variation based on community standards.

However, she then segues into explaining divergent opinions within her own IRB:

> But even our own committee isn't consistent all the time, *depending on who is and isn't there that day,* and how discussions go. Sometimes, somebody will get hung up on a small thing, and it will be blown out of proportion. Get enough people going on it, and it will become more of an issue than it should. [Emphasis added]

In a few instances, certain differences may indeed exist among communities. Yet Olivia provided only one example of such topics—studies of "gay, lesbian and transgender...sexuality and HIV." She suggests that large cities may differ from isolated rural regions in attitudes toward HIV studies among gay men. But among these large cities, community attitudes may not differ significantly. Moreover, all IRBs that review research in these areas are required to have relevant expertise. Additionally, in most research, even such variation—for example, concerning attitudes related to HIV research among gay men—does not seem to occur.

Strikingly, her justification (being in "a big city") does not fit the case she describes of differences *within the same* community. Specifically, all of the IRBs at her institution are located in the same big city, yet at times disagree in substantial ways. Hence, the interinstitutional differences she describes appear to be related *not* to the local community (being in an urban *vs.* other area), but to the personalities and preferences of individual members. Still, in the end, she accepts, and does not seem very bothered by these differences.

MYTHS ABOUT COMMUNITY DIFFERENCES REDUX

Despite the reasons for variations between IRBs explored above, members tended to justify the existence of local rather than central boards, and variations in decisions between boards, by maintaining that differences existed in the values of the local communities in which these IRBs resided. At times, these justifications got blurry. Jack, the rural physician and chair, said:

> The concept of local IRBs was to get local cultural input into the review
> of studies in a particular community. I suspect that that's less of an issue
> in very white and affluent areas like ours. It might be a very big issue in
> Alabama. I think Tuskegee could have been very different. So, the basic
> philosophical premise of local IRBs is very good.

Yet today the Tuskegee study is recognized as egregious universally, not just by the local community in Alabama. US government researchers conducted the Tuskegee study before IRBs existed, and the local community did not know the relevant details.

While the Obama Administration and others have proposed more centralized IRBs, many interviewees disagreed, citing, as justification for local review, their belief that IRBs reflect local community values. Charlotte, an administrator, said,

> A centralized IRB system for multi-site studies *sounds* like a good idea,
> but the local research context and the *community attitudes* towards

research still need to be checked. I'm *torn* about that, because there's tension. It would be good and efficient to have one body with all the information, providing oversight and monitoring. But somebody out there in Timbuktu could screw up, or do something inappropriate to that culture, and nobody would know. You wouldn't have a local community member saying: "This will never fly in my community." So, a centralized mechanism doesn't get you away from the problem of having to go through multiple hoops.

Charlotte cites the importance of contrasting community attitudes but invokes the notion of "Timbuktu," an exotic foreign locale, to suggest that domestic differences also exist, and therefore justify local IRB review in the United States. *But clear differences in local community values or local laws do not appear to account for inter-IRB variations.*

In fact, it was striking that *interviewees here suggested possible discomfort about sex, but none provided clear evidence of even this factor causing discrepancies in decisions between IRBs; or clear instances of differences in local community values or laws per se as doing so.* Occasionally, interviewees offered examples of what they felt were community differences. Dwayne, for instance, a chair in a rural area, believed that people in rural and urban areas had varying perceptions of research. Patients in his community were more likely to decline study participation:

> It is very difficult to recruit people for anything invasive. In the city where I trained, we did the same level of invasive studies, but people just kind of understood this research: I'm volunteering. *Here*, you have to explain yourself more: this is what research means, this is the importance of doing it…it just takes a little more effort to give them the confidence that it's OK. A lot of it has to do with it being a rural community—less of a big city. Here, everybody knows each other. But research just isn't understood as in a big urban center, due to exposure in everyday life. Here, the newspaper has articles about farming and, on a far distant page, about science.

Yet, the differences Dwayne is suggesting here appear to result from contrasts in awareness and education rather than in underlying community *values*. Rural and urban regions may also range in logistics. He continued,

> There's sort of an identity here of rugged *individualism*, but I *don't* think that's what gets in the way. It's just lack of awareness, exposure, and understanding of the importance of research.

Perceived variations may also arise from geographic factors. Dwayne added, "Part of it, though, is that some people would have to drive three hours to get here, and that's just not feasible." It is also possible that the same proportion of the population may be interested in research in both locales but rural areas simply have fewer patients overall; hence, more populous regions have higher absolute numbers of interested participants.

How Much Inconsistency Is Ok?

INCONSISTENCY IS GOOD

Not only do committees generally feel untroubled by the apparent relativistic aspects of these phenomena, but indeed as we saw, IRB personnel, authors such as Susan Kaur see these discrepancies as "good."[4] "Each of our IRBs has its own feel or flavor," Christopher, a chair, said. "That's good." Jeremy concurred:

> These differences are healthy. The analogy is somewhat the political process: you have a continuum, and generally the solution in the middle may be the best; or best balances out everyone's needs.

Yet, especially given more multisite studies, consistency is needed between IRBs, and committees should seek such harmonization as much as possible.

Moreover, as we saw, IRBs may develop their own "urban myths" and norms, including interpretations of regulations with which they may then compel all protocols to comply.

However, many committees are also wary of attempts to reduce interinstitutional variation, seeing these efforts as in fact potentially harmful. Anthony, a researcher and chair, explained:

> I am interested in consistency much more within an institution than between them. In some cases, *local cultural differences* might influence how committees make decisions. If we constrain committees too much to make them clones—it could do more harm than good.

He also recognizes that at times, his IRB will simply decide to change its mind. Yet he and many others do not mention the *costs* of such inconsistency.

Moreover, when they do notice intercommittee differences, IRB members generally feel that their decision is the better one—whether it is more rigorous or more user-friendly. Such interviewees may even disparage other IRBs, and take pride in either having "higher standards" or being more flexible. An IRB may recognize that it is "hard-assed," but see this machismo as a virtue. Andrea said, "It's our responsibility to protect the patients here. Just because something is OK *elsewhere*, doesn't mean it's OK here!" Conversely, Charlotte criticized *other* IRBs as too rigid:

One group of PIs had 13 IRBs, and spent most of their time just trying to get through all the IRBs. The PIs pointed out that the research was really minimal risk, and could be expedited. But the IRBs said, "I don't care. This is the way we do it. We don't expedite things like this. That is our procedure—that everything like that goes to the full board."

Other interviewees applauded the way the regulations allowed for different interpretations over time. "I'm amazed at how flexible the regulations are," Liza said. "25 years later I can pull out the regulations and read the words *differently*, and see things that we didn't realize." She does not mention the potential disadvantages of such subjectivity. A tension may thus be inevitable. Case-by-case evaluations are thus needed; but, so, too, are rigorous efforts to be as consistent as possible, and avoid idiosyncrasies. *Courtroom judges may interpret laws differently over time, too, but publish, reference, and build on prior judicial decisions.* That is not the case with IRBs.

Interviewees may recognize that these discrepancies suggest subjectivity in the review process, but these individuals usually legitimize these differences. They argue that protocols have to be reviewed individually on a case-by-case basis, which is correct, but does not by itself justify the lack of attempts to harmonize or standardize decisions, and reduce idiosyncrasies. IRBs also tend to see their decisions, once made, as definitive, a belief reinforced by the fact that no external-appeals process exists. This absence of such a mechanism fuels divergence and a lack of attempts at concordance.

THERE SHOULD BE MORE CONSISTENCY

In their views of the acceptability of these variations, interviewees differed. A rare handful of interviewees felt that more congruency was important. "I worry most about making sure we are *fair*," Olivia said, "doing everything consistently—not picking out one particular thing with one PI, and letting the same thing fly with someone else." Yet she was almost unique in her concern.

Some felt that consistency should be the goal but would ultimately be limited. A few interviewees acknowledged that IRBs inherently involve gray areas, and that more consistency should exist; but they questioned how much, and how to attain it. As Jaime said,

> There should be *some* kind of consistency. But circumstances can be viewed differently by different people sitting around the table at that time. There should be some kind of decision tree.

Dana, in fact thought that research integrity *necessitated* attempts at consistency, "to make sure we have standard ways of looking at studies—that we're not saying 'OK' for one study, and 'not OK' for another." Her social science training contributed to her attention to, and questioning of, the process.

Others felt that IRBs should actively seek more consistency, but that this goal would probably in the end prove elusive. Robin, a lawyer and IRB chair, said,

> One IRB says a study has to go to full board because participants have a mental illness, and another IRB says it's an anonymous survey, so is exempt. We should be able to do a better job than that, and get in the ballpark. There might be slight variations of interpretation, but we ought to try to get it as consistent as we can. If everybody applied regulations in exactly the same way, we wouldn't need IRBs. We're never going to have a computer program that would spit it out, but at least we can have *some* more consistency. Part of that's training.

She accepts that variations are inevitable; but as a lawyer, thinks that committees should nevertheless seek a standard of "reasonableness." She accepted that IRBs are not "literal" interpreters of law, but she felt that as a standard, they should at least be able to defend their position.

> As long as I feel that I can *justify* what we're doing, my judgment is *reasonable....* If it doesn't fit the rules exactly, then as long as we can justify it, I'm willing to sit down with a federal auditor and say, "You may disagree, but this is reasonable."

A handful of interviewees described themselves as "IRB critics," citing flaws in the *status quo*; but in the end, even these relative skeptics tended to defend the current system. As Kevin, a chair, said,

> The whole IRB system is a mess. There are now over 5,000 IRBs in this country, and if you are a company trying to place your protocol in individual institutions, that can drive you nuts. It's terrible.

Ultimately, however, he supported a local rather than centralized or regional system, to maximize the *quality* of reviewing and protection: "The closer you get to the actual subjects, the better review you get, and the better you can protect the rights and safety of the subjects."

Even a few of those who value consistency feel it can somehow go too far. Judy, for example, after saying that her committee had "decided to at least *try* to be consistent," immediately added, "But we don't want them to be *totally* consistent." In this case, consistency seems to be equated not with rational decision making, but unthinking uniformity.

Dwayne expressed a similar sentiment:

> It sounds arbitrary, but has to be taken case-by-case...Practicing medicine is the same thing. We try to be consistent, and have therefore developed lots of guidelines, but every protocol is so different, that flexibility is built in.

However, inconsistencies arise regarding not only different protocols, but the *same* protocol, suggesting that the cause of variations is not always the nature of the "case" or protocol—but rather the particular individual reviewers. IRBs tend to see their decisions, once made, as definitive, feeling that these deliberations reflect local population mores and are thus essentially incontestable.

INCONSISTENCY AS MINIMAL

A few interviewees felt that IRBs are gradually becoming more consistent, though studies have not supported this notion.[14] In part, IRBs may differ in how they define "consistency," exacerbating problems. "We don't disapprove studies that often," Jeremy said. "That is an example of *consistency*." Yet his definition of consistency—"not disapproving" studies—represents a relatively low standard, and ignores many crucial types of variations that concern not simply *whether or not* a protocol is approved, but *what specific changes* are requested.

IRBs may also misunderstand the scope and types of inconsistencies that exist. "We all have to follow the same policies and procedures and guidance documents," Olivia said, "so *at least we are making decisions in the same way*" (emphasis added). Yet given the wide *variations that exist in interpretations and applications* of these principles, this view seems somewhat philosophically naïve .

Most IRBs minimize discrepancies and the problems that might result. IRBs may acknowledge that institutions vary, but only slightly. Dwayne said,

> The *phrasing* of the consent form might be formatted a little differently, but the main elements are the same. Locale shapes it somewhat, but in the fine-tuning, not the major components.

But in fact the differences are frequently far more significant.

DISCREPANCY AS INEVITABLE

Many interviewees felt variations were simply unavoidable. Jeremy said,

> Somebody is going to take the conversation in direction A, rather than direction B, emphasizing certain points, and you are going to come to

a different conclusion. I think PIs understand that you can't eliminate that. It is just the way a peer review is going to happen. For journal articles, one reviewer loves your piece, another thinks it's crap—from *the same journal at the same time!*

Yet peer-review of journal articles and NIH grants focus on science—not ethics—which presumably has more objective standards, for instance including enough participants so that findings are not, statistically, due to chance alone.

Ethical decision making involves interpretations of attitudes and values, and certain variations are thus unavoidable. Nathan said,

> Anything that deals with ethics is an endless discussion, without concrete things like an integer—one or two. All these things are works in progress. Leaders can be flawed. Perfection is elusive.

A few interviewees recognized not only that ethics is a contextualized, subtle, and unpredictable human activity, but also that perceptions of "ethical appropriateness" can be historically contingent, and develop over the years. Martin, the researcher and chair, said,

> Ethics are a moving target. What we considered ethical ten years ago, we don't necessarily today. Ten years from now, we will decide that things that we do today shouldn't be done. It isn't static. *It's a human activity, involving human judgment.* I am always amazed when there's *any* agreement.

In these decisions, discernment and intuition play vital roles, but are inherently subjective. As Laura, the lawyer, said,

> IRB work is complex, requires a lot of judgment, and is hard to teach—there are rules, but also *judgment*, because we are always balancing, and dealing with exceptions.

But the importance of such judgment and balance is rarely mentioned or taught—ignored rather than explored. In fact, many of these interviewees did not express much awareness of how much they are interpreting and applying terms in ways with which others might disagree. Similarly, although physicians in clinical medicine know factually that many treatments once commonly practiced—like leeching, say—were subsequently rejected, they often fail to see that this evolution suggests that our contemporary practices may also be flawed or in flux. IRBs know that ethical problems were, in retrospect, handled poorly in the past; but they demonstrate little awareness of how much their own processes and practices are part of a historical continuum.

Some thought that "reasonableness" rather than consistency was in fact sufficient, and should be the standard. "You try to select the right group of people," Nancy said. "They are all governed by the same regulations. I don't know if consistency is in the picture."

Increasing Consistency and Knowledge of other IRBs' Decicions

Just as more contact among IRBs at the same institution can be very beneficial, so, too, can wider contacts between IRBs from different institutions and parts of the country. As Charlotte said,

> I often come back from a conference with *validation* about the way we're doing something. Because we all work in isolation. You compare notes and realize: we're on the right track. Everybody's struggling with this issue. We're proceeding appropriately.

On the other hand, input from conferences can be very unsystematic, depending on how the meetings are organized, for what specific purpose, and who attends. National meetings can powerfully affirm the difficulties of confronting gray areas, but anxieties and uncertainties can persist.

Increased documentation of areas of agreement between boards and of precedents can also be beneficial. "Maybe case studies or protocol summaries, and breaking those down to fit into a flow chart, would be useful," Greg, the social scientist and chair, said. Yet some IRBs worry that inter-IRB communication would breach confidentiality. Examples with details redacted can overcome this objection, but some IRBs may still resist—arguing that intellectual property may be threatened, or that overly redacted examples lose important nuance. Phil said,

> It is very difficult to post on the Internet: "Here are the ways we've struggled with this, and what we came up with." Once you abstract things too much, reasonable struggles start to seem absurd. It gets very difficult to put in enough detail to make the struggles vivid and understandable.

Arguably though, a middle position exists that would allow presentation of underlying issues while preserving confidentiality.

Conclusions

"We just look to check off the box," an NIH program officer once told me, "to indicate that, 'yes, the researcher has IRB approval.'" It is a formality. What matters is that it is done—not how it done—not the details involved.

But this attitude ignores the complications that are often involved. I discovered in my interviews that IRBs range widely not only in how they interpret, apply, and balance key principles and terms (concerning risks and benefits, undue inducement, research, scientific benefit, and informed consent), but also in how they perceive these differences among themselves. These committees vary in "flavors" and "colors" from flexible to rigid, and pro- to anti-researcher. Discrepancies between them result from the ways each IRB struggles to define, interpret, and gauge abstract terms, and how it imagines and fears uncertain future possible risks and unpredictable scientific results.

Unfortunately, most IRBs are not sufficiently sensitive to the existence, causes, and costs of these discrepancies to researchers, and have no incentive to act more uniformly. A few IRB members feel that they "try their best," given limited resources, and that that alone is sufficient—suggesting that they sense they do not always fully succeed. They work hard and with commitment, but questions linger, due to the inherent subjectivity of some of these reviews, and of what constitutes an ethically "good enough" review.

Though IRBs' dedication is impressive, in the complex human endeavor of interpreting abstract principles, institutional cultures and personal idiosyncrasies almost inevitably influence decisions. IRB members may not only be "self-taught" in ethics,[15] but use "gut feelings" and the "sniff test," not careful "ethical analysis." Hence, even within one institution in a single community, IRBs differ due to personality and other factors. Members also range in their abilities to imagine possible future logistical problems in conducting a study. Yet remarkably, these interviewees do not seem surprised or disturbed overall by these differences, and instead tend to see these variations as inevitable and even desirable. Rarely did any mention the high costs to researchers. Furthermore, the lack of transparency and an appeals process often make the group feel uncontestable. "Right" becomes synonymous with "what those of us in this room right now all feel is right." Some IRBs argue that these individual peccadilloes, views, and predilections (e.g., being "obsessive" or have "pet peeves") reflect those of a larger community, but that does not generally appear to be the case here.

Interviewees frequently ascribed these variations to differences in "community values or predilections," but the evidence did not support such assumptions. Instead, it seems that this phrase is a crude and inaccurate stand-in for differences in *committee* values—that is, each IRB is, in essence, its own mini-society, with its own idiosyncratic characteristics on any given day.

Few interviewees here admitted that their decisions were in any way open to different interpretations by others. They tend to see their job as applying the regulations correctly, and appear to feel that ultimately there is one absolute "right way" for their board to do so. Though ethical debate, consensus, and standards continue to evolve, committees tend to think that at any one point their decisions are right and justified.

These data raise questions of whether and to what degrees such variations can be diminished, or are inevitable—how much consistency can or should be expected, how to obtain it, and what to do if it is lacking. When policymakers set up the current system of local IRBs in the 1970s, multisite studies were very rare, whereas today cross-institutional protocols are widespread: the SUPPORT Study, for instance, included 63 separate institutions.[16] The regulations' authors do not seem to have seriously considered an alternative to making these committees local. Policy makers assumed that relevant differences in community values existed, yet no data supported this supposition, and none exist today. Certain laws may vary between states, but these do not appear to be the cause of differences that arose here between IRBs (e.g., in interpretations of "good enough" science and consent forms).

The fact that many of these interviewees displayed little concern for these inconsistencies, or awareness of the consequent costs to researchers, is striking. Few interviewees here admitted that their decisions were in any way open to different interpretations by others. They tend to see their job as applying the regulations correctly, and appear to feel that ultimately there is one absolute "right way" for their board to do so. Inconsistencies cannot be wholly eliminated, but they emerge here as wide and of many types, and can and should be reduced; and far more efforts are needed to do so. At several institutions with more than one IRB, the chairs meet periodically to try to harmonize the decisions of the committees in their institution. But even here they often don't succeed—though all located in the same community. A few chairs may seek uniformity in response to a particular protocol that more than one board within their institution happens to review; but such efforts are needed on a much more systematic, ongoing basis for all studies where individual, idiosyncratic committee attitudes may prevail. Such consensus, meetings, and conferences could be established at national levels. This indifference fuels critics' desires for more centralized IRBs. Yet almost all of the interviewees here opposed such centralization.

While IRBs do not now bear any of the costs of discrepancies, these boards must somehow be encouraged and even incentivized to reduce these idiosyncratic differences. Though ethical debate, consensus, and standards continue to evolve, boards tend to think that at any one point their decisions are right and justified. Many see themselves as "simply following the regulations," and believe that their decisions are inherently valid, and essentially incontrovertible, because these reflect local community values rather than constituting subjective interpretations.

At the same time, in arguing that high levels of idiosyncratic discrepancies are acceptable, and that local rather than central IRBs are needed, IRB members may be revealing inherent conflicts of interest. Much is at stake—their jobs—but that alone shouldn't prevent efforts to improve the future functioning of the system as whole as we enter the new millennium. The critical questions, in part, are how much variation is acceptable, and why, and how to determine that. Heightened awareness of these variations and their costs, and increased efforts at consistency, are crucial.

IRBs *VS.* INSTITUTIONS

The Contexts of Decisions

CHAPTER 7

Federal Agencies *vs.* Local IRBs

Repeatedly in recent years, the Office for Human Research Protections (OHRP) has blasted IRBs for being too lax—in the hand-washing and SUPPORT oxygen-to-preemies studies, and shutdowns of all research at Duke, Hopkins, Virginia Commonwealth University, and the Los Angeles VA. As IRBs are the group in charge of ethical concerns at local institutions, it is inevitable that, in a sense, "the buck stops" with them. These committees have a federal mandate, and a lot of autonomy. Yet, while conducting these interviews, I soon saw how these committees in fact also reside in dense institutional webs that can in turn powerfully influence their decisions. Hence, if we are to understand them and how they address their work, it is vital to grasp the larger contexts in which IRBs operate.

I found that four sets of relationships can affect these committees: their interactions with federal agencies, industry funders, local academic medical centers, and researchers. This section of the book—the next three chapters—explores the first three of these interactions. The subsequent section will examine committees' links with the investigators themselves.

The federal government brought IRBs into being, and continues to shape them profoundly. At the same time, in this arena—as in many others—political and practical questions arise as to how much and what regulation is desirable and effective.

In recent years, scholars have emphasized the importance of seeing institutions not as static, but instead as engaged in dynamic relationships.[1] Systems theory has explored how complex social systems like health care function and develop feedback mechanisms.[2,3,4] Managers in an academic medical center[5] work in intricate ways to enforce, for instance, environmental safety regulations concerning chemical toxins and radioactive waste. But the fact that IRBs similarly operate in such dynamic contexts, and how and with what implications, has not been systematically examined.

As illustrated in Figure 7.1, I soon observed how multifaceted direct and indirect relationships with federal agencies, particularly OHRP and the FDA, can

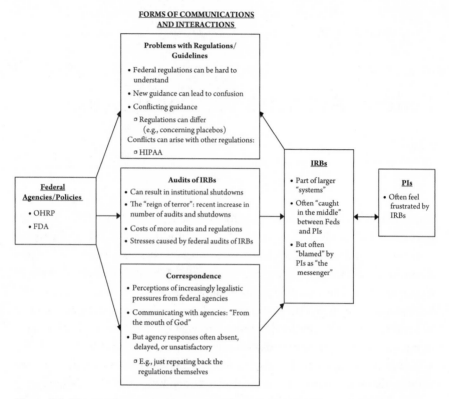

Figure 7.1 Themes Concerning Interactions Between IRBs and Federal Agencies and Regulations

powerfully mold IRBs' views through audits, guidance documents, and other communications. Yet each of these interactions can pose problems for both committees and investigators. Researchers often blame ethics restrictions on IRBs when in many ways IRBs are merely the "messengers."

Federal Regulations can be Hard to Understand

OUTDATED CATEGORIES

As we saw in the hand-washing and the SUPPORT studies, figuring out how to apply the regulations can be hard. A central part of the IRB's job is to interpret, apply, and "translate" the regulations, but many of today's protocols do not readily or easily fit the federal guidelines' pre-established categories, which were written 40 years ago. Unfortunately, federal agencies generally do not provide clarifications as much as committees would like, even when IRBs request it, prompting confusion and discrepancies. Laura said,

For prison research, the IRB has to choose one of four categories that fit the study. But...we always kind of stretch it a little bit to fit the research into one of these categories. We hold our breath and say, "Oh well, it's sort of A or B." Generally, OHRP wouldn't disagree. *It's almost a wink and a nod, because both sides know that this stuff stinks to work with. It just doesn't fit.* [Emphasis added]

NECESSARY VAGUENESS?

Laura's experience suggests that the guidelines are out of date, but also that agencies and committees jointly acknowledge that regulations must be capacious to have any hope of accommodating all research. In other words, the government may recognize the clumsiness and "absurdities" of the regulations, but choose not to supply corrections or clarifications. In fact, many laws and regulations need to be vague to allow for a wide variety of circumstances in which they will invariably be applied,[6] and clarity may therefore remain illusory.[7] Current "minimalistic" regulations may thus always burden the IRB precisely because these cannot explicitly address all the questions that surface.

Nonetheless, in other realms, mechanisms exist for clarifying such ambiguous federal regulations. In the law, for example, judicial decisions are documented and published, establishing legal precedents; and the judiciary system and appellate courts regularly resolve further disagreements. In the end, the Supreme Court can adjudicate disputes. But for IRB regulations, none of these structures exist, leaving committees to struggle with ambiguities, often with little guidance.[8]

For instance, many committees are still unclear as to what research can be either exempt from IRB oversight or expedited by the chair or a de facto administrator, rather than requiring full-board approval. Laura, the administrator, was glad that OHRP had agreed with "a wink and a nod" to her interpretation of the regulations concerning prisoners, but she remained troubled by the fact that these elaborations did not always follow the letter of the regulations themselves. Nancy sought, for example, "some really clearly detailed examples on use of extant data." She also wanted guidance about how to estimate the likelihood or magnitude of risk in social and behavioral research. The risks of these studies are generally less than those of invasive biomedical investigations, but still exist. She desired, specifically:

how to handle that cross-culturally or internationally. What's the standard? OHRP should bite the bullet. It's a really touchy ethical question, but somebody needs to handle it, otherwise everybody's playing a guessing game.

IRBs may thus disagree in their interpretations of the same regulation. For example, the NIH allows survey research to be exempted from review if subjects cannot be identified, or may be identified but would not be at risk if the information were disclosed.[9] Yet, Nancy said, "We have collaborated with institutions that just don't exempt *any* research if it involves interacting with human participants in *any* way." Such IRBs may treat federal regulations and guidance as a "floor," and choose to be even more stringent than required.

Questions emerge concerning not only definitions of major terms such as *risk* and *benefit* but also about other areas that the regulations do not explicitly address. For example, with large multisite studies, other institutions will ship researchers blood samples, which can trigger quandaries. Investigators "involved" in research must obtain IRB approval. Presumably, researchers with significant responsibilities will get approval from their IRBs. But what if a researcher at another institution is only minimally involved? What if a doctor merely sends a tube of blood to a researcher elsewhere? Does that doctor need to obtain IRB approval from his or her IRB? Liza explained,

> Investigators study rare diseases, and want multiple doctors and researchers to send them samples, as a favor. I'm not going to comment if someone sent them a sample, and [that researcher's name] happens to get put on the published paper. But I'm having problems: OHRP considers that "engaged in research" because they're getting recognition. But we can't get IRB approval from that person's institution. Samples come from all over the world. I would find input useful.

Questions about these procedures can consume much of a chairperson's effort and concern. Liza added:

> I spend more time thinking and worrying about specimens, and researchers going into patients' records in ways that are probably not a risk, *vs.* things that I would like to be spending time on.

Many interviewees noted that researchers frequently complain that IRBs focus on small details, but this problem may arise in part because the committees aren't sure which of these details the government expects to focus on; IRBs thought that concrete examples of cases from federal agencies might be especially helpful. One agency released such a document on expedited review, providing specificity that filled cognitive and pedagogical needs. Nancy found it especially useful:

> The regulations are hard. You have to make it more concrete. The National Science and Technology Council—not OHRP—put out a

little pamphlet, a guidance document, about expedited review in social and behavioral research. They gave examples of studies where you might want to consider using this expedited procedure.

IRBs struggle to interpret and apply abstract terms and definitions in specific cases—partly because no published precedents exist as they do in case law.

NEW GUIDANCE CAN ALSO CONFUSE

Periodically, federal agencies do new guidelines, documents, and regulations, but these can also generate additional questions. As Joe said,

> OHRP needs to get together a large number of very helpful guidance documents. They've started to do that, but these vary in their helpfulness. OHRP needs to think about what IRBs do—and what daily problems we face.

Moreover, when OHRP does post new "guidance" (as opposed to official, binding "regulations"), committees can be unsure if it all needs to be followed. As Jeff said,

> OHRP gives out a lot of guidance, and often creates a problem: the regulations say one thing, and the guidance says much more. Are you obligated to live up to the guidance or not? The regulations don't say. But if a problem comes up, you are going to be asked: why didn't you follow *all the guidelines*?

Some IRBs may therefore see guidance as mandatory, whereas OHRP may view it as nonbinding, and merely of potential help. Kevin felt:

> Guidance is really a double-edged sword. If OHRP puts something up on their website as guidance, most IRBs are going to feel they have no choice. The guidance has to be followed. OHRP expects you to do it.

FEDERAL AGENCIES SHOULD ENCOURAGE MORE FEEDBACK

When OHRP does release new statements, IRBs must react without much negotiation or communication, even when the new directives seem perplexing or counterproductive. This exacerbates stress. Christopher, the chair, said,

> OHRP and other agencies put out new guidance, and IRBs are jumping around to modify things to fit. There's not a lot of give and take

in terms of: Is this reasonable, or helping? It's just mandated.... That's not good.

Many interviewees found federal agencies sometimes rigid in this regard—doubtlessly reflecting constraints that these agencies themselves confront. Still, especially given the potential grayness involved in ethical interpretation, more flexibility can be beneficial. Christopher continued,

> New regs are hard because they need to be implemented and operationalized in the real world but are not always clear; and there is little opportunity to discuss or negotiate these problems with OHRP.

In many ways, IRBs are hence caught in the middle, having to translate, implement, monitor, and enforce these federal dictates with specific local investigators. He added,

> A lot of the regs don't make sense for scientists in the trenches. Policies sound nice, and I'd agree with them, but how do you *implement and operationalize* them...how do we get the *spirit* from this cut-and-dried, yes-or-no kind of rule?"

Bilateral more than unilateral communication could help, given these intrinsic complexities.

Mixed Signals from Above

Federal agencies can also disagree with one another, creating tensions— particularly in controversial areas such as whether a study can include pregnant women, and when the use of placebos is acceptable. Christopher described conflicts regarding, for instance,

> whether to exclude women who are of childbearing age and pregnant but seriously ill. NIH keeps saying, "You need to include women, and can't discriminate against them." But FDA is pretty clear: most trials exclude women of childbearing potential, unless they are sterilized and have quadruple birth-control methods—pretty nutty stuff. If women are being excluded, how generalizable is the data? We struggle with that a lot. It would be nice if FDA said that for certain kinds of studies, it's silly to exclude women of childbearing potential. If you get a pregnancy test, does someone need to be on birth control for three months to get

a one-time injection of a study drug? Why? It would be nice to have it clear. When?

These problems become exacerbated, too, because certain restrictions apply in research but not in clinical settings. IRBs may thus see agencies differing on certain issues, in part due to their varying priorities (e.g., gathering health data to aid the population as a whole *vs.* gauging the toxicity and benefits of possible new drugs). Women can make certain decisions for themselves in clinical but not research environments. Hence, some critics feel that to deny women access to a drug because they may get pregnant is unfair. Christopher added,

> If the only way to get a drug is through a trial, are you excluding patients because they happen to be pregnant? In a clinical situation, a patient could say, "Yes, I want to go ahead." Whereas, because it's research, she can't. Patients don't have access to a lot of experimental drugs, unless they are in a trial. It'd be nice to have some clarification....

These conflicts reflect in part larger differences in standards between clinical *vs.* research settings—the fact that patients are now generally more vigilantly protected in research than in clinical care.

DIFFERENT REGULATIONS CONCERNING PLACEBOS

IRBs perceive differing views among agencies about placebos: while drug companies frequently like to use them, and the FDA often indirectly sanctions their use, OHRP does not.[9] Martin, an IRB chair, said,

> One of the better ways to get through the FDA is to have single control data. So, one branch of government sets a bar that requires placebos to get control data. Yet another branch has made it relatively clear that in the US, it's really not ethical to expose people to placebo as a treatment. The solution is to do things elsewhere that wouldn't be considered ethical in this country. The FDA has no problem accepting those data from abroad.

The FDA does not stipulate placebo use per se, but some interviewees felt that the agency implicitly encourages it—permitting placebos when demonstrating a drug's effectiveness might otherwise be difficult.[9]

Nonetheless, agencies experience obstacles trying to reconcile such conflicts. The fact that 17 separate federal agencies endorsed 45 C.F.R. 46, the regulations governing IRBs, creates barriers in changing it. Laura, the lawyer and administrator, said, "Nobody wants to take it on because it's a lot of work to get so many different agencies to agree."

Hence, researchers who want to use a placebo may conduct the study abroad. "The favorite place to do these now is either South America or Eastern Europe," Martin said. Yet using this loophole poses ethical conundra—a double standard—when US researchers are involved.

CONFLICTS INVOLVING OTHER REGULATIONS: HIPAA

IRBs confront difficulties posed by other federal policies as well, particularly the Health Insurance Portability and Accountability Act (HIPAA).[10] Passed in 1996, this law aims to ensure the privacy of certain "protected health information." Originally intended to protect patient privacy in billing and insurance paperwork in clinical settings, HIPAA is now also supposed to pertain when institutions are "involved with research" as well. In this complex ever-evolving world, though, seemingly simple or straightforward determinations of that phrase can become confusing. For instance, does the law cover all research records, and if not, when doesn't it? As Christopher said,

> HIPAA is complicated about what really is personal information. What's in a medical record, or purely for research? If someone comes to a substance abuse program to be in a *study*, they don't really have a *patient* chart. So, if you collect data from research charts, is it "protected health information" or not? I would say no, but it *is* personal information, so it raises issues.

Additional vagaries emerge concerning applications of HIPAA to social science research. Greg, a chair, said,

> HIPAA may be more of a medical billing issue, but when researchers are looking at local schools' student records—health issues associated with their success in public schools—is that covered under HIPAA?

Committees often remain unsure.

The "Reign of Terror": The Consequences of Federal Audits and Shutdowns for IRBs

Federal decisions to shut down all research at several institutions, primarily in 1999–2000, sent shock waves across the country, unsettling universities and their

IRBs—many of which have grappled to restructure and improve. As Stephen, an IRB chair, said,

> Prior to the shutdown, we basically had one committee with 50 members. We didn't pay as much attention to certain things as the regulators wanted us to. Our continuing review process was much less substantive than now. As we've re-engineered ourselves, I've learned a whole lot more about human subject oversight. We really weren't doing it right.

Government investigations can be triggered by complaints by subjects or researchers (including whistleblowers), or even the investigator's own IRB. While some complaints are justified, others prove frivolous. A single grievance can prompt a federal audit that costs millions and finds little, if any, evidence of wrongdoing. "The investigator was cleared of the original charges," Henry said about one such case. "But it was a long, multi-million dollar investigation." The historian Daniel Kevles examined charges against the Nobel laureate David Baltimore and found that federal officials and journalists may eagerly seek evidence of misconduct even when none turns out to exist.[11]

Dissatisfied or mentally ill subjects and faculty members can also prompt audits. Laura, the lawyer and IRB administrator, described one faculty member who sent OHRP a report claiming that an international collaborative study in a foreign country had not obtained informed consent:

> The accusation was made by a disgruntled former faculty member here who, by other folks' accounts, has some mental health issues. He was driven to try to "take down" this PI. He wrote a 25-page complaint, and named 10 to 12 studies, and threw in a couple with an American PI—apparently just to make it look like it wasn't racist. He wrote to the university president: "You should build health care clinics for all the poor people there, and if you want I'll come and run them for you." Then, he applied for the money himself. With that kind of big, 25-page complaint, OHRP thought, "Well, this person has credibility," so they needed to take it seriously. They asked a lot of questions, and with that many studies, the back-and-forth took a lot of time. OHRP perceived this foreign country's government to be coercive and dictatorial. Patients were not being herded into a study, but that's what he accused. OHRP found no evidence that these claims were true, but it took *four years*! We ended up getting out of it with a clean slate—mostly just with small administrative stuff—you didn't include this or that in the consent form. But *there was no finding of any harm to subjects.*

Complaints can thus have little or no justification, but get taken seriously, and create burdens. In this instance, however, Laura's IRB ultimately received more resources from its institution.

THE STRESS OF FEDERAL SCRUTINY

Olivia, a chair and health care provider, said that in one year the FDA audited her institution 14 times—seeming to targeting researchers who received the most industry support.

> The FDA does about a thousand visits per year nationwide. They tend to pick us because we have a huge amount of industry funding. So, the FDA was here 14 times—very often to see the high-end rollers. The FDA says that lots of industry funding isn't a criteria for who gets audited, but we know it often is. Most researchers did fine, but a couple did not, because they didn't have things in the correct order.

This metaphor of "high-end rollers" suggests gamblers, cash, and risk; and with large amounts of money come higher risks of something going wrong. She also distinguishes between the substance *vs.* the form (i.e., "order") of documentation, and suggests that only the latter, not the former, was deficient. The threat of future federal action still looms over her institution. "They've told us they will be back," Olivia said, sighing. It is unclear whether her institution was, in fact, audited this many times—although her impression that it was is nevertheless important—and whether this use of government resources is optimal or ineffective.

Whether, when, and how federal agencies will respond to an audit's findings is also uncertain, creating stress for IRBs. Concerning "one routine audit," Stephen said:

> There were some findings which we responded to. We never even heard back whether those findings were appropriately addressed or not. Then a few months later, we got the letter that basically we were *shut down*! In some ways maybe we were an example, because there were many other IRBs ... going through the same thing at the same time.

Government agencies often evaluate exceedingly small details—just the sort that PIs accuse IRBs themselves of paying too much attention to. As Olivia added about the FDA,

> They give us anywhere from 24 hours to a week's notice, and will look at everything—all the documentation ... that amendments, adverse

events, or violations have been noted. Individual study files: that the EKG is within normal limits, and that there's a copy of that EKG. They will pick up on the slightest thing.

But whether this level of detail helps or hinders overall IRB effectiveness is not obvious. Again, these interviewees' statements may be seen merely as complaints, but reflect these individuals' views and experiences.

In responding to these agencies, both IRBs and researchers can easily get defensive, but committees have to be very cautious not to do so. Olivia explained,

> You have to just listen to what they say. They submit a letter, and you have a right to respond. You have to be careful how your letter is worded. Some FDA inspectors are very easy to work with; others are very strict, following the letter of the law. It can be nerve-wracking. We've had some very difficult experiences over very minor things. Every institution has. If the investigator gets defensive and angry, it can ignite a fuse, and can get out of control.

Differences arise in how much particular agency personnel follow "the letter" versus the spirit of the law. At times, federal audit citations can seem "petty" and "ridiculous." As Greg said, for example, auditors may note that the number of IRB members voting does not match the number in the room—"because someone went to the bathroom."

Some antagonisms may feel personal, but these problems occur within a larger context of cumbersome federal or state bureaucracies, further confounding matters. Troy, a researcher and chair, admitted,

> The system is hard to work with…Not just with the OHRPs perceived vindictiveness to nail people…It's trying to work a system that's difficult and complicated.

VALUABLE LESSONS

Nonetheless, audits may ultimately yield beneficial outcomes. Even Stephen, whose IRB was shut down, credited the investigation with sparking necessary reorganization and change. Beforehand, his institution "basically had only one committee":

> The quality of our minutes and how we documented our votes was very poor. For greater-than-minimal risk studies, we were doing our continuing reviews inappropriately—not doing them at the full board level. We

completely reengineered our whole review process. We now have four panels, and a full-time member who just does exempt and expedited reviews.

Stephen feels that the federal investigation was painful, but ultimately effective:

It took the two-by-four hit between the eyes for the institution to realize they needed to commit the resources, the expertise, and the energy for doing this right. It probably took the shutdown to get everything in place.

PRESSURES TO BECOME MORE LEGALISTIC

Some interviewees felt that, increasingly, government agencies have been shifting their focus on to assessing forms more than protecting subjects. In the past decade, many IRBs have become accredited through the Association for the Accreditation of Human Research Protection Programs (AAHRPP), and other committees debate whether to undergo the process. Yet some saw such accreditation as further emphasizing paperwork without necessarily protecting subjects more. Christopher added,

New regulations may also not really help the patient. With OHRP, and accreditation bodies like AAHRPP, the focus is much more on: Do you have the right forms and policies? Not: Are patients really better off now than 10 years ago? My sense is no.

Critics have argued that the heightened focus on paperwork since federal shutdowns of institutions in 2000 might not protect subjects better.[12] In the end, such regulations and guidance could potentially even impede patient protection. More regulations can also increase IRB expenses in ways that agencies may not recognize, diverting resources away from aiding patients' health. "It's always costing more and more money to run the IRB," Christopher added, "because there are more and more levels of regulation."

Over time, due in part to legal pressure from these government bureaucracies, IRBs have become more formal, as well. Jeff, a chair, said,

The process is now very different than what was originally intended, because of pressure coming down from OHRP—which, at this point, lawyers heavily staff. Historically, IRBs were to be a committee of colleagues with community and non-scientist members, to make sure this research was on the up and up, and not simply [researchers] scratching each other's back. The reviews were very collegial....Now, the scrutiny is very different. I'm not sure if it is fruitful. We get letters back from a lawyer going through consent forms line by line, complaining about some specific phrasings. IRBs are getting drawn into [the] legal process.

Hence, efforts to reduce the lapses of a few researchers create more of a burden for all investigators and IRBs. Unfortunately, the few wrongdoers cannot be accurately and readily differentiated from the majority of researchers who follow ethical guidelines.

Concurrently, of course, many segments of society have become more legalistic and litigious. As Jeff observed, "This is part of a larger regulatory drift in America." Not only federal agencies but trends within the broader legal system can affect IRBs. And even a frivolous lawsuit can involve IRBs and their members and cause stress. On a few occasions, IRBs have been named in lawsuits.[13,14,15] Jeff continued,

> A patient was consented on the gurney, outside the operating room, and subsequently had a stroke, and sued. His attorney interviewed a former IRB member who was the primary reviewer. They questioned the detailed wording in the consent form—why the approved wording differed from the model in the university guidelines.

Such perceived legal liability can heighten committee anxieties.

FEDERAL MISSION CREEP IN SOCIAL SCIENCE RESEARCH

Many social scientists castigate OHRP for increasing oversight of their research. As Jeff argued, these rules are "intrusive and inappropriate." Compared to biomedical studies, social and behavioral research tends to involve fewer invasive interventions, less money, no deaths, and fewer multisite projects. Critics thus assert that IRBs should not push these regulations into these academic disciplines, or should do so in much attenuated ways—that the regulations have been expanded too aggressively and too far. Such research may be minimal risk, and thus warrant expedited review, yet IRBs may vary in these decisions because they fear being reprimanded by OHRP, frustrating many social scientists. In July 2011, the Obama Administration suggested excusing all research that investigators feel is minimal risk from IRB overview; but whether this proposal will be implemented and if so, how, and when, where these boundaries will be drawn, and what unintended consequences might ensue, remain highly uncertain.

Several interviewees thought that the current regulations have evolved beyond their initial intent. Phil, the social scientist and chair, said,

> Federal folks who developed the regulations seemed shocked at how far these have been extended. They didn't anticipate these

consequences—where institutions, to protect themselves, err on the side of being more inclusive. One of the authors of the regs said, "We never expected people to make this cover *everything*. It says it only has to cover federally-funded research." But a lot of institutions look at *all* research. *The regs have a life of their own!*

This increasing encroachment has incensed many social scientists.[16] The agency has said that IRBs generally review social and behavioral science quickly, using only one person, not the whole board. But Jeff, a social scientist, felt that boards frequently did not follow these limits.

I've found OHRP communications to social scientists to be dishonest. A couple of times, the previous head of the OHRP spoke at social science meetings and said, "You're all complaining, but almost all your studies are easily expedited. It's just a few pages of paper work. Why get excited about it?" If you pointed out to him that many social scientists do research on prisoners, juvenile delinquents on probation, or mental patients, and would require attention since those are vulnerable populations, he'd say, "Oh, that's true," without real discussion of the implications. OHRP does not have a rich understanding of how ethnographic research would be done. The regulations don't match up very well with how social scientists actually work.

Communication between Agencies and IRBs

UNSATISFACTORY RESPONSES

The fact that federal agencies at times communicated in limited, incomplete, or frustrating ways appeared to compound these problems. Committees may request clarifications from OHRP and the FDA, but find the answers "unhelpful." Interviewees said that sometimes the agencies simply didn't respond; and at other times, did so unsatisfactorily, merely reiterating the regulations without offering clarification. "If they don't want to say much," Liza said, "they'll just repeat the regulations in five different ways."

In not issuing definitive official opinions, federal agencies leave committees to wrestle alone with these vagaries. Working in this interpretive vacuum without guidance can generate stress and discrepancies. "The Feds often seem to back away from taking a stand," Troy, the chair, reported. "They'll turn it back to us, and say, 'It's up to the IRB.' They'll come in and criticize us *later*." Stephen concurred:

Many times when you call for advice, they essentially just read back the regulations. You basically have to make your own decision, which is great, until you have an audit, and then you're told you didn't make the right decision.

Chairs frequently thus feel frustrated and disappointed with federal responses that refer IRBs back to the language of the regulations rather than clarifying or elaborating guidelines. Joe, a chair, explained,

We want to hear it from *the mouth of God,* and don't get that. We get vague generalities. That's not what IRBs need—because all of us have a certain way of doing things. We may think that we handle things optimally, but may be inconsistent with what OHRP wants us to do.

Moreover, when these agencies do respond, they often refrain from doing so in *writing,* or say that the clarification does not apply more generally. Joe added about OHRP:

They have not been forthcoming. In fact, it has been very difficult to get any kind of opinion from them, which is very disturbing. If we write to them for an opinion for a very specific situation, they make it very clear that their opinion is relevant to this very specific question, at this specific time, for this particular institution, for this particular subject—they are not providing any general rules or guidance or algorithms. And they rarely will put anything in writing.

These interviewees raise questions that further research needs to investigate further of how prevalently these agencies in fact communicate only verbally, rather than in writing; how agencies make these communication decisions; and whether the content of these two different types of communications differ, and if so, how, and why. Through the form of their communications, agencies may hence foster variations between IRBs, though not generally seen as doing so. In the end, this reticence can thus impede optimal IRB functioning.

DELAYED RESPONSES

Agency feedback can also be extremely long in coming. Pam, an administrator, said,

Of all the letters we sent, I just got a report back last week saying they have accepted our changes from *two years ago!* I have not gotten anything back from more recent reports. We've *never* gotten anything back from the FDA. We have very tight time limits for reporting, and 10 working days to make a decision. When it takes them two years to get back to us, it is annoying. Not everything gets back in two years. We have not gotten back things from *three* years ago! Maybe they were fine with those things, and didn't feel they needed to correspond back. If we got something back, it would give us validation that we did it right. Somebody said once that if there really were problems, you would hear from them. But how do we know?

In the interim, IRBs presumably allow these studies to continue, but OHRP may or may not later criticize the committee for its decisions. Interviewees felt that OHRP, in responding to IRBs, may not even acknowledge these perceived difficulties. As Liza said, "The response I get is: it's in the queue."

Agency Constraints

But without additional or timelier federal guidance, IRBs are often afraid and may be hesitant to alter their approaches or stances toward researchers. Liza continued, "Until something happens at that level, IRBs are going to be scared and *very resistant to change*."

Lack of consistent agency guidelines can exacerbate discrepancies between committees. "They don't want to make mistakes, or appear like they are being overly prescriptive," Pam, the administrator, said of these agencies. "But IRBs all need to be doing the same thing."

Agency staff members may wish to assist IRBs more, but not do so—either because they perceive limitations in their mandates or because they feel overwhelmed by their current responsibilities. "It's a stalemate down there," Liza added. "They genuinely want to help. But there's so much to do that they do nothing."

Some interviewees sympathize with problems OHRP itself faces because of low staff. Though regulations are "clunky," agency employees may be limited in their ability to interpret or clarify these formal policies. As Laura said,

I was really struck by how incredibly careful they are in the compliance oversight division not to overstep their authority. They really *sweat* the determination letters—whether they are going to give feedback on certain issues.

With sensitive decisions involving potential harms to subjects, agency personnel may themselves thus need to feel "comfortable," highlighting the roles of subjectivity and emotion in these decisions—even at the federal level. Liza "made sure that OHRP was feeling comfortable with anything we recommended." Hence, federal officials themselves face tensions, the amelioration of which may require shifts and improvements in not only formal policy, but appreciation of these obstacles. As we will see, some IRBs maintain an "open door" policy, encompassing face-to-face and phones communications and interactions with researchers. So, too, a policy of personal interactions, sensitive to affect, not only logical formal written arguments, might abet relationships with OHRP staff. Yet agency staff may themselves be caught between desires to help IRBs interpret the regulations, and the limited unalterable language of the regulations. The assumption seems to be that the regulations are straightforward, but as we have seen, that is often not the case. As Laura added, "They stick very closely to their regulatory authority."

These bureaucracies' responses (or lack thereof) can instill apprehension among IRBs. Yet, due to fear, committees may be reluctant to be more flexible. "IRBs are scared," Liza added, "and until OHRP says it's OK, no one is going to change." In addressing these issues, OHRP may need to take clearer, more direct and assertive stances.

FEAR OF SEEKING AGENCY CLARIFICATION

Sometimes, IRBs may avoid approaching these agencies because the guidance subsequently given can be binding, not elective. Receiving feedback from agencies can be a double-edged sword. "Once you go to them," Liza said, "you've got to be prepared for their response. You may not like what they say. So, don't go to them unless you're prepared."

Some ethicists and IRB chairs have wanted federal reforms. In 2001, the Secretary's Advisory Committee on Human Research Protections (SACHRP) was created to recommend improvements in the regulations. OHRP may read and reflect some of this input, but still hasn't formally made major changes as a result. Liza said, "OHRP hasn't issued the guidance yet. It's been three or four years!"

Interviewees felt that agencies could be more open to such recommendations. Liza continued,

> If they would just show some effort to say, "We are listening. Advisory committees are important to us...We're doing this, or changing that as a result," it would make IRBs feel easier.

In fact, a few interviewees thought that recently, in responding to IRBs' questions, OHRP has begun to improve slightly, suggesting awareness of these tensions. Committees sometimes received helpful answers. For instance, Liza needed clarity about whether or not IRB review was needed if a patient wanted blood drawn at one institution to be sent elsewhere:

> Our IRB had a whole hubbub: do we need to review that? There's conflicting information and guidance. I said to OHRP: "This is ridiculous." They came back and said: "You don't have to review it."

Several interviewees also felt that agencies had started responding more promptly. Liza said:

> In the last five to ten years, they are much more approachable. Recently, I emailed them a couple of questions. It took them a month and a half to get back to me. But years ago, I wouldn't get *any* answer or *anything* in writing, or they would talk to me on the phone, but put nothing in writing.

Improving the quantity and quality of communication in other ways could be beneficial as well. Louis, a chair and social scientist, suggested, for instance, an "OHRP hotline" to help IRBs. "A place where I can call would definitely be helpful—a hotline, not just FAQs…just to call and say, "Hey, does this qualify for an IRB review?"

The IRB industry

As IRBs have struggled to respond to federal regulations and agencies, they have also interacted and networked with each other to form their own industry, with their own journals, national meetings, and commercial vendors. IRBs have grown, as Phil suggested, to have their own culture. He described his entrance into "the IRB world":

> IRBs are now an industry, building itself. It was quite an eye-opener. People are making businesses as IRB consultants and members for pay. You create constituencies for regulation. That starts out of good intention. But then, like any other industry, it's going to work to keep itself alive. It's less about human subjects than about the industry. I respect many of the professionals in it. But once you have an industry, it starts to feed itself in unpredictable ways.

As a social scientist, he felt somewhat removed from biomedicine and was therefore more wary of IRBs' widening purview. Other chairs, who were biomedical researchers themselves, tended to be less critical.

Conclusions

IRBs operate within larger, complex governmental contexts, generating challenges. Committees interact with federal agencies through audits, guidance documents, and other communications. These bonds can shape IRBs' reviews of protocols; but how exactly boards operate as part of interactive systems in relation to federal agencies and regulations has received scant attention.

The legitimacy and constitutionality of IRB regulations have been criticized as law,[17,18] and these men and women illuminate how IRBs struggle to work effectively within this environment, highlighting problems in both the nature and implementation of these regulations. Variations in local institutional implementation of *other* types of government statutes have been explored.[8] IRBs are each very cautious, but nonetheless vary widely in their decisions, in ways that have been shown to impede science.

Researchers often blame frustrations that they feel on IRBs.[19] Yet these boards essentially serve as the "local face" of federal agencies and regulations. IRBs are therefore commonly "stuck in the middle" between regulators and researchers, implementing and monitoring regulations they did not devise. While investigators may see IRBs as possessing considerable power, these committees generally see themselves otherwise—as stressed and constrained. Criticisms of IRBs thus need to be seen in these larger contexts. Variations exist in how much committees seek, receive, welcome, avoid, and/or fear federal input, and also how frequently and in what ways these agencies interact with these boards.

Researchers may in fact "blame the messenger," rather than "the message," but that does not excuse IRBs if they apply regulations in unjustified ways. Appreciation of the actual contexts in which IRBs operate and the pressures they face can, however, help to facilitate agencies, IRBs, and researchers working together and addressing the tensions that arise. This "systems perspective" can potentially help in understanding and addressing limitations and misunderstandings IRBs confront, and in improving the *status quo*. While many systems have effective feedback loops, the forms of feedback here are often inadequate and/or inefficient. Scientists gripe about IRBs to policymakers and others, potentially shaping federal regulations, as seen in the recent ANPRM, which grows out of PIs' complaints.[20] Yet federal agencies do not always reply as fully or timely as IRBs would like, exacerbating frustrations.

These data highlight the importance of not only clarifying what the regulations consist of but also how exactly they are carried out at micro-institutional and person-to-person levels—how individual IRB personnel feel about and approach agency staff. Both structural and attitudinal interventions could be developed to improve these interactions. For instance, agencies could be required to respond to IRB communications, and to do so within a set period of time (e.g., three months), rather than allowing two to three years to pass without answering, if ever. Federal agencies may at times now be starting to answer IRBs more quickly; but how long they take to respond, what they communicate, what challenges persist, and why, needs to be more fully examined. Other mechanisms for communication (e.g., perhaps more rapid, online forums between IRBs and federal agencies) can be beneficial, too. Increased awareness of these problems and frictions among agency staff and leaders, IRBs, institutional officers, and PIs can also help. More frequent and specific communication from OHRP and the FDA can improve IRBs' relationships with agencies, and hence enhance committees' interactions with researchers to optimally benefit science and society, and protect subjects.

Researchers complain about the stress, and focus on paperwork involved in audits by IRBs, yet these committees experience similar frustrations and stress in being audited themselves. These two sets of audits may be related—harshly rigid focus on documentation by agencies may fuel similar concerns by IRBs. Both types of audits could potentially be conducted less stressfully.

These men and women also pose critical questions concerning when and how frequently agency audits do and should occur. Agency resources may be too limited to interact with IRBs optimally, but agency support should then be increased. Studies should examine how agency staff see their roles, what tensions they face, and how they make decisions, and seek to resolve conflicts. These agencies could potentially serve as *de facto* appellate courts—negotiating disputes between IRBs and PIs—but do not now appear to see themselves as fitting this role.[9] These interviews highlight the importance of seeing IRBs in as full a context as possible—that is, as embedded in complex social dynamics with federal regulations that can shape committee functioning, decisions, capabilities, and comfort. IRBs are not static, but shift in response to various external factors.

Future studies can explore more thoroughly how IRBs operate in these complex and dynamic milieus—how committees vary in their perceptions of these agencies and of their own roles as local representatives of these external authorities. Future research can probe these *ecologies of ethical decision making* further—how committees differ in reacting to these pressures, what factors are involved, and how boards may approach researchers differently as a result. Subsequent research can examine more fully, too, how IRBs may react to these agencies differently due in part to past experiences and psychological traits of chairs and/or vocal members.

IRB chairs, members and staff, researchers, policymakers and others should see these committees far more as working in these complex interrelated systems, and realize that these close interactions can affect the quality, effectiveness, and efficiency of human subject protections. Committees should recognize that dissatisfied investigators may complain to federal officials. Researchers would benefit from understanding more the complexities of these systems, and neither blame the IRB alone for the regulations, nor seek to avoid these regulations because of frustration with, and perceived unfairness of, an individual committee. Perhaps most importantly, federal officials and policymakers should become more aware of how they themselves affect IRBs, and how added guidance and clarification can reduce ongoing problems.

CHAPTER 8

The Roles of Industry

In 1999, Jesse Gelsinger, a healthy 18-year-old volunteer, died in an IRB-approved University of Pennsylvania study designed to see if a new gene therapy, contained in a virus, was safe. The researcher, a leading figure in the new, much-hyped field of gene therapy, had suspected problems with the laboratory-altered virus, but continued to inject it into subjects anyway, including Jesse. The researcher turned out to own part of the company making the therapy, and stood to gain millions if it worked.[1]

Yet industry plays an ever-increasing role in research. In 2007, the pharmaceutical and biotechnology industries spent $58.6 billion on biomedical research.[2] In comparison, the NIH budget that year was $29 billion. Moreover, when controlled for inflation, the NIH budget has in fact been decreasing—22% from 2003 to 2014[3]. During this period,funding from industry, though decreasing for a few years due to the 2008 recession, has nonetheless increased more than did that from government.[4] The growing number and proportion of industry-sponsored studies is shifting the relationship between scientific knowledge and financial gain, and straining the guidelines established to keep research ethical. The Bayh-Dole Act of 1980[5] allowed universities to reap profits from discoveries made using government funds. Since then, medical centers have encouraged researchers to seek patents—often in conjunction with corporations—and to obtain industry funding. As a result, not only government and local institutions but also pharmaceutical and biotech companies shape the challenges and decisions that IRBs and researchers confront.

Industry has funded much good research, but recent scandals involving studies funded by large pharmaceutical companies raise many questions, including what the role of IRBs is and should be in such instances. IRBs may confront not only the conflicts of interest (COIs) among researchers and institutions but also their own conflicted motives.

Corporate financing and ethics can clash in several ways—especially regarding corporate practices and COIs. Industry money can affect researcher's choices of topics to study, and restrict their discussions of results with colleagues.[6,7] In randomized clinical trials, for example, it has been found that industry sponsorship is associated with "pro-industry" conclusions. Drugs have been found to work better in studies sponsored by the drug company than in studies funded by others (e.g., the government, foundations, universities, medical centers).[8] Study results that indicate that a new drug is better than its competition can raise profits. The opposite results hurt profits. These divided loyalties can potentially distort the analysis and publication of studies, severely harming scientific integrity. And yet public trust in science is crucial both to continued governmental and public support of research, and to the adoption of medical discoveries.[9]

Since Jesse Gelsinger's unfortunate death, such conflicts of interest have increasingly been decried among researchers as well as IRB members. COIs are defined as "conditions in which professional judgment concerning a primary interest (such as a patient's welfare or the validity of research) tends to be unduly influenced by a secondary interest (such as financial gain)."[10] Large companies, for example, may compensate researchers who are also IRB members and chairs. Federal regulations prohibit IRB members with such conflicts from participating in reviews, except "to provide requested information,"[11] but only a handful of studies have examined how IRBs actually handle these issues. Hence, many questions persist about the nature, extent, and management of these strains. Most major academic medical centers have COI policies,[12] but many nonacademic community hospitals have less rigorous policies and now conduct research as well, raising additional concerns.[13]

Unfortunately, most publications about these strains have been theoretical (generally commentaries), with relatively little data about these phenomena. But the few existing prior studies in this area, which have tended to be quantitative, have highlighted several concerns. For instance, despite the potential threats to integrity, 36 percent of IRB members have financial relationships with industry; 23 percent of those with a COI had never disclosed it to an IRB official; and 19.4 percent always nonetheless voted on the protocol.[14] IRB members with COIs are not addressed in the federal regulations but should presumably recuse themselves. One-third of academic medical center IRBs do not, however, require that members disclose financial COI, and one-third of IRB chairs do not always arrange for members with COI to leave the room when the protocol is discussed.[12] In fact, some have argued that IRB members should disclose COIs, but still participate in IRB deliberations, as they may have relevant expertise.[15] How IRB chairs in fact navigate these tensions is unknown.

Several particular industry practices also cause problems for IRBs. Once the FDA approves a drug, and more patients take it, awareness of side effects may increase. The IOM has emphasized the need for postmarketing (so-called Phase IV) studies to heighten understandings of side effects over time.[16] Yet some companies now design "seeding trials," paying physicians to switch patients to expensive new drugs rather than less costly alternatives, ostensibly with the goal of collecting long-term, follow-up data but with the actual purpose of encouraging doctors to begin to order these more expensive new treatments.[17,18] The scope, definitions, and acceptability of such postmarketing studies pose quandaries for IRBs.[19] Some critics argue that IRBs and researchers should "just say no" to these seeding trials, which not only squander valuable resources of money and research subjects, but also challenge ethical standards.[20,21] Despite these concerns, such studies continue.

Pharmaceutical companies also fund "me-too" drug studies, in which companies "tweak" drugs to create new ones in order to patent and market these new medications—often when the patent on the existing drug is expiring—hoping that these more recent variations may prove to be slightly better. Yet in me-too drug trials, the social benefits are usually *low*, which poses ethical dilemmas. For instance, in a study of such an experimental variant treatment *vs.* a less expensive generic drug, the risks and benefits may appear reasonable and balanced and be presented clearly to the patient, but the company stands to benefit far more than either science or society because an equally effective treatment is already available for less money. Federal regulations dictate that IRBs should ensure that "risks to subjects are reasonable in relation to anticipated benefits, if any, to subjects, and the importance of the knowledge that may reasonably be expected to result," and that subject selection is equitable.[9] It is generally understood that social benefits should not outweigh risks to the individual—we don't want, knowingly, to force subjects to suffer for the greater good—but whether these social benefits should receive *any* weight, and if so, how much, presents quandaries.

Critics have called for better regulation of industry-sponsored studies in general.[22] But the FDA has been underfunded and accused of being too closely tied to industry.[23,24] Several warning signs—such as a study's lack of a control group—can help IRBs identify problematic industry studies. Nevertheless, we know little about whether IRBs even look for this evidence, what challenges they face in doing so, and how they view and weigh these issues if they discover them.[8]

Interviewees spoke openly about their struggle with the "gray areas" when vetting these industry-funded studies, reviewing protocols that "strain integrity"— me-too drug and postmarketing studies, questionable research practices (such as the awarding of "incentive fees" to physicians to push their patients into studies), and the use of contract research organizations (CROs), which are freestanding, for-profit research companies, usually unaffiliated with universities.

The IOM[25] recommends including certain basic information about COIs in consent forms: "that more information about the conflict and its management is available on request." But ambiguities arise as to who would supply this added information (e.g., the researchers, the COI office, or the IRB), what exactly would be provided (e.g., how much detail), how often subjects do or would in fact request it, how they would understand it, and whether such an approach would be sufficient.

Many unexamined questions thus remain concerning whether IRBs have a role here; if so, what; and how these committees view and respond to not only researchers' COIs but also their own. I focus on IRB relationships with industry in this chapter, and committees' interactions with academic institutions and colleagues in the next chapter. Industry funding can profoundly shape both sets of relationships.

Increased Industry Funding and Conflicts of Interest

FILLING THE FINANCIAL VOID

"Researchers are desperately looking for money," Christopher said, "since the university has cut their salary." Especially with the decreased NIH budget over the past few years, more researchers work on industry-sponsored studies that have low scientific or social value. Many universities are also encouraging their faculty to become more entrepreneurial with industry, complicating the roles of IRBs.

Committees themselves have varied and complex relationships with industry. Boards generally support colleagues in seeking and obtaining industry funding. Unless a researcher has financial investments beyond a predefined objective limit, or acts egregiously, many committees try to tolerate a degree of strain, negotiating rather than seeking to eliminate COIs.

Drug companies may give institutions and researchers more business if the IRB quickly and readily approves protocols. While some interviewees are leery, others feel these practices do not necessarily reduce the quality of the reviews. Scott, the director at an institution that has been involved with a CRO, said,

> Pharmaceutical companies will throw more research at you if you have a proven track record. So, from a business perspective, faster turn-around pays off....As long as you don't sacrifice the quality of review, but turn studies around relatively quickly, everyone benefits—clients, human subjects...and the pharmaceutical companies. They get their approvals quickly, and we get to enroll as many subjects as they need.

As Scott's language here suggests, some IRBs may indeed see themselves as an integral part of a profit-making enterprise. "Most PIs have good business experience working with us," he added, "and are satisfied with the 30- to 40-day turn around."

Institutions may set up their own private, for-profit clinical CROs that run trials for drug companies or essentially become CROs, with separate IRBs to attract profits. Researchers at a medical center may thus have a choice of where to submit and conduct research—either within their department at the institution or within its CRO. Several institutions may together establish a research organization that becomes a de facto CRO. As Scott described such an entity, it was originally designed to bring clinical trials to its host institutions and had its own IRB:

> Since then, it evolved. It is similar to a CRO, but now generally reviews clinical trials for all investigators. They are large now, handling, managing and reviewing clinical trials all from industry. Its focus is *industry*.

He feels that the IRB within his institution's CRO has advantages: "They're quicker...we're not as equipped. They have more resources: 40–50 percent of the school's clinical trials go there...it's a one-stop shop."

Given contemporary economic constraints, smaller institutions may face added challenges, exacerbating these problems. "There's a push," Elaine said, "for institutions to become more research-intensive: Places that haven't been as research-y in the past are trying to get that way."

Recent government cutbacks may heighten institutional pressures to obtain outside funding. Industry may try to take advantage of this situation, pursuing smaller institutions with less-experienced, less savvy IRBs. As Andrew, an IRB chair, said,

> Some commercial sponsors go directly to these small places. Pharmaceutical companies...see these smaller places as wonderful if it's for a common disease—diabetes or hypertension. They can get a lot of subjects in a short period of time. And no one is going object very much to what they propose....A lot of these community hospitals are out there. They do research, usually under some sponsor, clearly for the money.

In part, smaller institution's IRBs may be less well staffed or vigilant. Andrew continued,

> I don't think the IRBs there work very well. They usually have an IRB staff of one...I'm worried about how great the compliance is. They are certainly poor at keeping records. The IRBs tend to be rubber stamps. Bad things can happen.

HANDLING RESEARCHERS' COIS

IRBs are often unsure how to respond to the COIs of researchers conducting indus-try-funded studies. Committees realize that many PIs and institutions require indus-try funding; they are also concerned about COIs. In reviewing protocols, however, board members are often uncertain how to define "COI." For researchers it funds, the NIH set a cutoff of $5,000 as the amount they can receive annually from indus-try.[26] Yet this commonly employed measurement may not be ideal, since that amount might be much more valuable to a junior than a senior researcher. As a result, IRBs may be uncertain about what threshold and standard to use. In the field of corporate compliance with government regulations even the "appearance of impropriety…can undermine confidence."[27] I was once part of a grant application to NIH, to which the reviewers felt that there should "not even be the shadow of an appearance" of a conflict. Yet interviewees tended not to invoke this higher threshold.

COIs can also be indirect and ambiguous, relying not on immediate or short-term financial compensation but only on the potential for future gains that are not readily detectable. For example, university researchers may conduct a particular study in the present to increase prospects of ongoing work with the same company in the future. Committees may *sense* such indirect financial COIs, but not be completely sure whether these are present—and if they are, how to proceed. Boards then grapple with how to define, detect, and view such indirect COIs, and how high their institution's ethical standards should be. Jack said,

> Studies that are not great science *strain integrity*. Our researchers think: "We can make good relationships with this drug company that has a good pipeline. The company might be able to help us out with interest-ing drugs five years from now; but we first have to make a name with them. So we will take on these ho-hum scientific studies now." It's more "political posturing" kinds of research for the occasional researcher for whom research is a way of spinning wheels rather than advancing sci-ence—another slight variation on a combination of ho-hum drugs.

Because such potential *future* conflicts may be implicit and indirect, many researchers may not even mention them on the COI reporting forms they submit. In such a situation, many IRBs are uncertain what role—if any—they should play.

IRBS' ROLES CONCERNING RESEARCHERS' NONFINANCIAL COI

Presumably, Dr. Togias at Hopkins enrolled Ellen Roche into the induced-asthma study not for direct financial profit, but to advance his study and hence his career.

While researchers' financial conflicts are generally assessed through forms with established financial limits (e.g., owning not more than $5,000 in a company), researchers' *nonfinancial* COIs are more elusive and harder to gauge. IRBs usually acknowledged that PIs have to accrue some gain for their careers (e.g., publications, promotions, grants, and awards). Consequently, the academic culture of "publish or perish" inherently produces conflicts, yet assessing these tensions is hard.

Researchers can face tensions, for instance, between benefitting themselves *vs.* their subjects. "Are we conducting research for the sake of *our own vitas*," Louis asked, "or for the whole community?"

Nonfinancial COIs can also manifest themselves in researchers' excessive aggressiveness in enrolling subjects. Such COIs may be widespread, since ambition drives many scientists. Nathan pointed out that large numbers of clinical trials are conducted to enhance the investigator's "academic standing and prestige in the nation and around the world." He continued:

> They're thinking about the next presentation in Brussels. Even when their financial statements are completely disclosed, they have no conflict of interest, and the informed consent is completely transparent, we know how much money they're paying participants, and what they're saying to the participants, *it still is a conflict of interest because the PI wants to enroll a patient.* He actually doesn't have this ultimately neutral, mythological person out there describing the study to a patient and not caring whether the patient enrolls. Even if everything else is OK, the PI has a vested interest in the study, so is not completely conflict-of-interest-free, because he's trying to sell the study to a patient.

These so-called nonfinancial conflicts can in fact represent indirect financial COIs. As Troy said, "Researchers have their own egos and money involved."

HOW INVOLVED SHOULD IRBS BE?

Committees face questions of exactly *how much* to monitor and respond to investigators' COIs. Researchers generally disclose their financial conflicts to a COI office or committee in the institution, but IRBs often do not see this information or the institution's responses to it. In 2005, HHS urged institutions to use "audits or other techniques to monitor compliance," and to set up a "hotline" for anonymous complaints. Since then, many institutions have been developing research compliance programs that monitor misconduct, but what these offices do and how they relate to IRBs varies widely.[28] Many chairs I spoke with had little awareness of, or interaction with, COI committees, or knowledge of these committees' decisions, and thus felt that these offices communicated inadequately. IRBs do not always even know about possible researcher COIs. One board only knew of a major PI conflict because it shared an office with the grants department. As Judy, the physician and chair, said,

> If PIs declare they have a conflict, it goes to the COI committee to manage or eliminate. But the committee usually doesn't send us back a report. They…send a letter saying, "Yes, we are taking care of it." But we may not know the details of how or what's happening.

When a separate COI committee exists, the IRB may know that a plan has been put into place without being given the details. "We just get told there's a conflict, and now a plan," Christopher said. "It's clear when there's a change of PI. We figure that's how they're resolving the issue." Yet many times, IRBs have no idea how the conflicts are being handled.

With relatively low-risk studies, too, IRBs struggle with whether and how to manage conflicts. One investigator, for instance, studied a low-risk nutritional product that posed COI questions. Dwayne, the rural researcher and chair, said,

> He held interest in a company promoting a nutritional product he was studying. It was very low risk, so would probably have had no consequences, but *didn't seem ethically right*. So we proposed that the data be collected and analyzed anonymously.

At smaller institutions with fewer faculty, collecting researchers' personal financial information can cause additional difficulties for IRBs and other officers. There, individuals who review these sensitive data may know these faculty members fairly well, threatening or violating confidentiality. "Some things are *too personal*," Cynthia, the administrator, said. "I wouldn't want to be responsible for keeping that confidential." Organizational structures may also be less formalized or elaborated, reducing potential oversight. At larger institutions, many IRBs don't receive PIs' personal financial information because it is felt to be too sensitive.

Resolutions of COIs, however, are often not always straightforward. Simple structural approaches (e.g., making a PI a mere co-investigator) may not wholly eliminate the underlying conflict or its potential effects. IRBs may also need to know how a COI has been handled in order to include information about it on the consent form.

Nonetheless, most interviewees felt that their IRBs were already too burdened to be more responsible for COIs. As Judy said, "We are already in charge of so much."

COI forms

Some IRBs, feeling that existing institutional COI forms were inadequate, developed their own, separate COI form. Laura, the lawyer, said,

> The university's system for annual COI disclosure is only on-line, and not very good. So, the IRB looks on its own at protocols to see if there's any conflict. Every now and then, there is.

Hence, IRBs may require that researchers fill out a long, extra COI form—in addition to university reporting. But these, too, rely on PI self-disclosures, which may not always be accurate. "We count on the researchers telling us," Judy said. "It's fairly reliable, but not perfect. They might not perceive a conflict that we do." Significantly, individuals may not think of themselves as having COIs when they in fact do. These conflicts may in part be unconscious, or not seen as problems. "A lot of times, if you ask, 'Do you have conflicts of interest?' people will say no," Elaine said. "Everyone *else* thinks they do, but they say they don't." Indeed, research has shown that many doctors deny COIs that exist. For instance, physicians carrying pens from a drug company in their pocket does in fact affect their prescribing patterns.[29] Researchers (as well as IRB members and chairs) may similarly underappreciate how these conflicts affect them, feeling immune from, and hence minimizing, these conflicts.

Investigators may also actively resist or refuse disclosing financial information to an IRB, which they see as "wanting to know everything." Indeed, IRBs sometimes learn of a researcher's COI not from the PI but from other, external sources (e.g., the NIH). "One PI doesn't always disclose that he's funded by private companies that make the devices he works on," Katherine, the administrator, said. "Usually, we find out from another source." Even in a case such as this one, however, for reasons of confidentiality, such financial information could potentially not go to the whole IRB committee.

COI forms may also fail to capture "real" COIs. Any bureaucratic cutoffs (e.g., $5,000) are ultimately somewhat arbitrary. Jack, the rural physician and chair, chastised these guidelines as gauging relatively unimportant potential conflicts of interest—of emphasizing the letter rather than the spirit of the law:

> We see fairly trivial conflicts of interest. A PI gave a lecture for a pharmaceutical company, and the IRB has to worry about a potential COI. That is vastly different from the investigator holding the patent for the research. We know our researchers well enough to know that they don't have any real substantive malfeasances in their work.

Jack's last assumption, however—that his IRB has sufficient in-depth knowledge of its researchers—may not necessarily always be correct.

IRBs may also be more conservative than the institutions' COI committees, having a "zero tolerance" policy concerning financial conflicts and a greater power to restrict PIs. "We're more stringent than the med school," Liza said. "We can do whatever we think needs to be done."

At one institution, PIs submit *both* institutional and IRB forms, yet the information provided in each document turns out to differ in about one-sixth of cases. Generally, the discrepancy does not result from dissembling; rather, the researcher has usually already addressed and managed the conflict, and then forgotten to revise one of the forms. "Investigators mark the forms incorrectly 15 percent of the time," Pam, the administrator, said. "It could be oversight. Or, the PI had managed and gotten rid of the conflict and just not updated the database." This essentially duplicative reporting can also create more additional paperwork for researchers and more confusion for various offices.

Some IRB members sensed that their institution as a whole could monitor potential conflicts better, even in minimal-risk research. "COI are in all types of research," Cynthia, the administrator, said. "*We shouldn't overlook COI because the study may be minimal risk.* Most mini–mental status scales are copyrighted"— that is, researchers have copyrighted many standardized psychological surveys, and earn royalties for other investigators as a result. Cynthia suggests that these financial arrangements may affect how researchers design studies and choose questionnaires.

Financial conflicts can also be cloudy because the future profitability of an investigational product is unpredictable. For surgeons developing devices, for example, the potential conflicts may still be unclear, and not be perceived or self-reported by PIs. Judy, the physician and chair, said, "Often, surgeons don't realize that developing equipment they might eventually sell, or have some interest in, is a conflict. They are not getting money *currently*."

Additional gray areas arise as some IRBs ponder whether they should look "beyond" the immediate source of money alone to the ultimate funder. Doctors are required to take Continuing Medical Education (CME) courses, and many are held through professional organizations. Yet for many years drug companies sponsored such classes that, not surprisingly, emphasized the benefits of the company's products. Such practices are decreasing due to ethical concerns about COIs but continue to some degree. Still, if a PI is paid through a professional organization's CME course, and hence only secondarily by a sponsoring company, IRBs may be unsure whether to consider the arrangement a COI.

WHEN RESEARCHERS SHOULD DISCLOSE COIS TO THEIR PATIENTS

Institutions and IRBs now often require researchers to disclose COIs to subjects in the consent forms that the latter must sign. A COI committee may mandate some of these disclosures, but IRBs frequently do so as well, and differ in how and what they ask researchers to divulge. IRBs often recognize that including COIs on informed consent forms may decrease enrollment. Hence, they debate how to present this information on these forms, and with how much detail.

Committees wonder, too, whether these disclosures are sufficient; how to know; and how study participants understand these declarations. Mention of funding alone may not adequately convey to study subjects the potential impact of the researcher's COI on the study. Many if not most participants doubtless do not know how to evaluate these disclosures.[30] Indeed, these individuals may be more, not less, trusting of a researcher who receives pharmaceutical company money, thinking that the investigator must therefore be well respected.

Research with Perceived Low Social Benefit

Industry funding can create strains for IRBs not only because of the conflicts of interest that may result, but also because of the particular types of studies and practices involved. In certain industry-sponsored studies, IRBs are often unclear how to weigh the fact that the perceived social benefit is relatively low. The interviewees I spoke with frequently believed that their IRB's purpose was to ensure that the risks and benefits in protocols were reasonable and commensurate. In many industry studies, however, particularly me-too drug and postmarketing research, the science—and, hence, social benefit— is relatively weak, even though the balance of risks and benefits to the individual participant may appear acceptable. Some industry studies may also be inadequately conceived, with suboptimal design, using poor comparisons. Committees then struggle with whether to approve such trials. Christopher said,

> These studies tend to be less interesting scientifically, and the consent forms tend to be much more legalistic, and not very informative or useful. It's not clear why anyone would want to be in the study, comparing the 43rd to the 41st ACE [angiotensin-converting-enzyme] inhibitor. What is the purpose? Why do it? We wrestle with those a lot.

As with the SUPPORT Study, researchers may overemphasize the benefits and underemphasize the risks in order to recruit subjects.

"POSTMARKETING" STUDIES

Postmarketing studies can pose several problems for IRBs. Here, committees may question whether universities should even engage in such studies. As Martin said,

> Questions come up about the motivation of the protocol: is it to add to the body of science, or to *market a product*—for the university to assist a pharmaceutical company in increasing its market share? Is that appropriate for a university? The protocol might jump all the hurdles, but questions still linger. Our IRB says there *has* to be a scientific benefit…But there have been some *gray area studies*. The purpose of the study is to give the drug to clinicians free, so they can enter five or 10 subjects from their practice. Some kind of data is collected—usually very naturalistic data. But the *true purpose* of the study is to *prime the pump*—get the drug into clinical use—*to assist with marketing*. The company doesn't really care about the questions they are asking.

Several other industry-funded research practices pose additional ethical concerns. For instance, industry-sponsored protocols may *alter* diagnostic criteria for disorders, which will assist in boosting company sales but reduce the study's clinical validity and utility. As Christopher explained,

> A company was trying an anti-nausea drug out for social phobia. They changed their inclusion criteria to include people that were nauseous when they were public speaking, which isn't a DSM [*Diagnostic and Statistical Manual of Mental Disorders*] criterion. But how relevant is that going to be, even if it worked—which it didn't? So there are concerns when the researchers are changing their clinical criteria for a sponsor to make the drug look better…and such a participant is probably not the same kind of person that you'd see clinically with this disorder…*The companies are not following disease categories*! You then have the ethical issues about putting people at risk, if it's not going to be useful or generalizable knowledge.

IRBs wonder whether certain industry-funded studies even constitute research, as opposed to clinical care. For instance, certain new devices are developed and may help patients but remain expensive. The company that manufactures the device pays a lot of money to the hospital for each patient on the device. Hence, the hospital gets funds from the company, but patients on the device also need to have insurance help cover the costs. Yet the device remains officially "experimental," and consequently, hospitals only get reimbursed if IRB approval exists. Use of the device, however, may represent clinical care more than scientific research per se that has the primary goal of discovering new knowledge. Christopher continued,

> Hospitals are interested in industry-sponsored device studies of the new stent, pacemaker, or implantable defibrillator, because the hospitals get big bucks for the procedures. But hospitals are not allowed to be reimbursed by Medicare unless it's a study. A lot of these protocols actually aren't really studies, but just demonstration things. So should they even be reviewed by the IRB? Hospitals are told that they need IRB approval or won't get funded, and the hospital puts pressure on the IRB to approve it.

Industry may sponsor trials of new products, and use randomized clinical control studies, which are employed to vigorously compare two approaches, but the companies will compare their new product against an existing treatment that is not the best one currently available, in order to make their new drug look as good as possible. These studies may not constitute "bad science" per se, but be suboptimal. Such research may, as Jack said, compare a new drug to a "standard" regimen:

> But they either design a standard regimen badly, or use a really inferior one, trying to tweak the comparator so it's more likely to be a good outcome. You get a feeling there is a little bit of *underhandedness* here.

Ethical problems may thus be subtle (e.g., "underhandedness"), rather than gross ethical violations.

Other industry practices can present additional strains—for example, giving physicians incentives to enroll their patients into studies. Patients "don't want to be roped into a study because a doctor makes money," Christopher said. "Is this science or money-making research? It gets messy." In their responses to this practice, IRBs vary. As Dwayne, a rural chair, said, "Industry will pay if you reach certain recruitment goals." His IRB decided that this is unethical. "Some PIs resisted," Dwayne added, "but overall, we're sticking by our guns." Still, not all committees may be as cautious.

At institutions with more than one IRB, investigators may also engage in "IRB shopping," submitting protocols at certain times in order to have a study reviewed by certain committees rather than others—based on the researchers' sense that some particular boards will view the project more or less favorably. Companies may also engage in IRB shopping among institutions.

IRBs also face controversies concerning so-called non-inferiority trials, in which a study tries to show that a new therapy is not necessarily *better* than an existing one but is simply *no worse*, and may have fewer or different side effects, or require less frequent doses. For example, perhaps a new product has to be taken only once, rather than three times, a day. Some critics decry such trials as "unethical,"[31] yet companies and others counter that at times these new drugs can prove helpful.[32] Other observers feel that such trials may potentially aid certain patients in small, limited ways, but are often poorly designed.[33,34] Some interviewees are concerned that drug companies may seek to conduct such studies primarily to market a new product—even if it is not better than an existing one.

IRBs may find such trials far more acceptable for adults—who at least can comprehend the inherent limitations—than they do for children. With minors, IRBs may weigh additional factors. Troy, the researcher and chair, said,

> You don't like to see a kid stuck with a needle for no clear reason, especially in non-inferiority studies—where a company wants to show that a new drug is no worse than the existing drug. The company wants to show that their drug is at least as good as a standard-of-care medication. If it has fewer side effects, it's superior. So the researchers are just looking for a similar side-effect profile and equal effectiveness. Those do not go through our IRB very easily, especially with little kids. Researchers have to show some benefit. There's discomfort with torturing kids too much. Our IRB would probably approve that for adults, but not children.

Such a study may be permissible for adults since they would understand. Still, some IRBs struggle over whether to seek a higher standard than mere "non-inferiority."

IRB Responses and decisions concerning Industry

A study's science may appear adequate in several regards, but be "boring" or "not great." Committees then have to decide how to assess and weigh these shortcomings against individual benefit, and whether to disapprove certain studies. Generally, boards will not approve protocols of unclear, equivocal design (e.g., not enough subjects to draw conclusions statistically). But the quality of studies still falls across a wide spectrum.

For these studies, IRBs may vary in how they see their roles, and—depending on the specific protocol—focus largely on the informed consent, ensuring that it fully and accurately presents risks, benefits, and alternatives. For instance, in the case of a study of an expensive new drug, a committee may seek to emphasize to patients that a cheaper, proven generic medication may be just as effective. Olivia felt that:

> It comes down to *making sure the subjects are very well informed* about exactly why the study is being done, and what their alternatives

are—particularly that they can maybe obtain these drugs outside the study. These experimental drugs may be just new variations of a drug that is soon going to be a generic—the company is coming up with a new slightly different formulation of it, so that they can still charge a lot of money. We want to make sure that patients understand that an alternative, FDA-approved drug may help them just as much.

In pursuing these goals, however, members or committees may remain troubled. "Those are upsetting studies, because what can we do?" Olivia continued. "Personally, I wouldn't be the investigator doing that study, but that's the nature of *the game*"—that is, to procure funding that may be essential for one's salary. Academic medical centers generally require that researchers obtain grants, which may thus be seen, in part, as involving a "game," with strategy and rules that must be followed to succeed.

Yet while some IRB members may feel that they should merely ensure that subjects are fully informed about the risks and benefits, others seek a *higher* ethical standard. Several interviewees feel that relying on informed consent alone is simply "passing the buck" to subjects who then have to decide what to do. Instead, such interviewees believe that IRBs have a role—that committees should require that studies not only avoid harming subjects, but also have scientific benefit. Jeremy, the physician and chair, said,

There may not be much scientific good or social benefit to the study when it's just helping the drug company.... There's a role for the IRB—determining whether a study gets put in front of a prospective subject. Informed consent is crucial, but not the *only* consideration. Our protective role is to stop studies that should never be before a subject. Informed consent is a flawed process.... So we have a duty to keep those sorts of studies from even getting to that spot in the first place. *Bad science is bad ethics.* A bad study that's not going to tell you anything—even if it doesn't expose people to risk, but only inconvenience, and takes time, just to facilitate marketing—doesn't make any sense to me.

Still, questions arise of *how much* scientific advancement is necessary and sufficient, who should determine that, and how. Even if a study entails only minor risk, participants may still *expect* benefit because of therapeutic misconception (in which participants believe that they will benefit therapeutically from a study even after they have been carefully told that that is not the case).[35] In such an instance, then, when participants do not necessarily gain, an IRB may decide that *some* social good is therefore necessary. Still, on these issues, IRBs can be very divided. Jeremy continued,

> Committee members who voted to approve this protocol said, "It's not hurting anyone. The subject is being paid, and has the choice.... Who's being harmed?" But some risks were involved, even if minor. It's ethically flawed if you're going to take up people's time and expose them to whatever risk there is, even if only minor. A number of subjects feel that if they're in a study, *they're going to benefit*—they're expecting benefit, which they probably won't get. Or you're never going to be able to tell them, because it's designed so poorly, you're never going to contribute anything useful to the field.

Such studies can also erode public trust in science.

Two notions of IRB roles clash here: reducing risk and informing subjects adequately about these *vs.* ensuring a certain level of social benefit. Ordinarily, IRBs focus on the former. But for certain studies, some interviewees believed that the latter was necessary—even if the regulations do not explicitly discuss it.

Assessing limitations in the scientific benefit of studies and detecting whether the protocol may primarily benefit the funder more than science is not always easy. As Jeremy described,

> The IRB recently had a pharma-sponsored protocol in which we couldn't really see a strong, sensible, meaningful study design. An investigator more experienced than me who had interacted with the PI said it was a *marketing study*—gathering data to promote their marketing. We ended up disapproving the study, because there was some risk to subjects, and we didn't think any meaningful information would come out of it that would advance the field.

All IRB members may not always be able to detect that a protocol is in fact a marketing study; sufficient expertise in the type of study may be necessary. A committee may not, however, always possess such expertise.

Board members can vary considerably in how much they are generally "pro" or "anti" industry. Some members tend to be relatively suspicious of pharmaceutical companies. Yet other IRBs may review nonfunded protocols *more* rather than less carefully than industry and government-funded studies, since outside funders do not assess the former. Scott said,

> Departmental projects, not sponsored by NIH or industry, are generally not of the same quality because the PIs are not applying for money,

which vets them.... So, our members need to take a second look at non-sponsored new studies.

IRB members may hesitate to question a study too much because the industry sponsors might then simply "pull out" and take the funding to another institution, thereby impeding their colleagues' careers. Especially as government financial constraints limit NIH funding, some PIs increasingly need drug company support. Jeremy's IRB, for instance, was divided about a marketing study, and eventually turned it down.

> We had a split vote, disapproving a drug marketing study. The majority of the board felt this should not be approved. But a strong minority felt we weren't being consistent: "We approve studies like this all the time. There's not much risk." Perhaps money coming to the institution was part of the reason. That was never explicitly stated.

The disagreement here may stem in part from the fact that despite apparent lack of benefits to society at large, researchers and the local institution may accrue valuable resources. This conflict pits pursuing ethics against loyally assisting one's institution financially, which IRB members may also value. Perhaps this is why, at many institutions, marketing studies often go forward, despite suboptimal design and lack of committee enthusiasm. As Jeremy added,

> We are approving most of them, even though we are not *enthralled* with the study design. Usually, we conclude that the study design is not *horrible*. It's not optimal, but the risk is low, so we let it go.

In the end, IRBs may accept a range of standards—from "not horrible" and/or "not optimal" to "good."

These interviewees rarely described their IRBs as completely and definitively blocking a protocol; instead, these committees tended to give the PI a chance to change it. "It is really unusual for our IRB to disapprove a study," Gwen reported. "That was the first one in three months. We usually give PIs an opportunity to fix it."

In responding to IRB concerns, corporations also vary. "If we bring these things up," Christopher said, "some companies give us a hard time, some are pretty flexible. There's a wide variety."

IRBs may negotiate with industry concerning not only initial reviews of protocols but ongoing monitoring over time. Several of the chairs told me, however, that their committees tended to rely on industry monitors for compliance and integrity, since these companies were obviously invested in managing their data well and avoiding noncompliance. "For clinical trials with FDA involvement, drug companies' monitors are pretty good," Christopher added, "telling [researchers] what to do." An outside observer, however, might question whether industry-arranged and industry-financed monitoring is necessarily superior to independent university oversight. Pharmaceutical companies also evaluate adverse events, but have inherent COIs in doing so—as this chapter's opening anecdote so chillingly indicated. Hence, some interviewees felt that another system might be better. Jack continued,

> Most sponsors have responsible people looking at these events. But there is a potential conflict in the sponsor: not wanting to disclose everything. [The]...system would be better if it could be more transparent, so we could trust it, and have some non-conflicted oversight.

Industry funding can be more problematic in settings with relatively fewer resources—whether in the US or abroad. Especially in the developing world, wide gaps in health and resources can raise concerns about exploitation and lack of social benefit for the local country itself. In some of this research, drug companies may use a for-profit, independent IRB, which worries some US IRBs. Laura said,

> Pharma can be very destructive—for example, in India or Eastern Europe—if it is not working with an academic institution that has certain investment in high ethical standards. The company is basically going to be hiring a CRO, and *shopping* for the most convenient, cheapest, easiest population in which to do research. It's dangerous because—not to derogate some of the independent IRBs—in some places, the oversight system is weak. There may not even be IRB review, because they can get away with it. Maybe it's not going to be FDA-regulated. Or the study could be from some middle-income country that can manage to market a product without IRB approval. With Pharma, there's always a danger: the profit motives outweighing other concerns.

Conclusions

IRBs maintain varied, complex relationships with industry-funded research, assessing COIs and other corporate practices. Corporate funding is a double-edged sword; it can foster science, but also cause tensions. Industry money can threaten to distort research and its ethical conduct and assessments of its benefits and risks. These tensions are inevitable, and need to be carefully handled. Unfortunately, many IRBs are not well set up to address these pressures optimally. Often, committees support colleagues at their institution who are seeking funding. At other times, these boards are unsure about whether to be warier of industry-funded than of other studies, and if so, how much. Many IRBs will try to tolerate these strains and negotiate conflicts, unless a company's or researcher's behavior appears wholly egregious.

Studies may test me-too drugs, or engage in questionable research practices that undermine the experiment's potential social benefits. Some trials may appear adequate in many regards (e.g., having adequate statistical power), but ask "uninteresting" questions, or use unconventional diagnostic criteria or weak drug comparisons. Such suboptimal design may reflect desires to have these studies promote funders more than social benefits. Yet IRBs may not always identify these problems. In part due to competing interests and financial needs of colleagues and institutions, committees are often in a difficult bind.

Boards differ in how they balance these issues and weigh social *vs.* individual benefits. As we saw earlier, IRBs are expected to distribute the social burdens of research among different population groups to avoid overly burdening any one group. When a study appears to have low social benefit relative to industry gain, however, committees face different questions of justice.

Given the widening health disparities in the US, IRBs often wonder how much to weigh social *vs.* individual benefit, but remain unsure. The degrees to which IRBs should take into account these considerations of low social benefit are unclear. These committees are mandated to ensure that the risks are commensurate with benefits. The Belmont Report includes justice as an ethical principle, but the regulations themselves do not explicitly mention it.[36] In fact, these regulations state that IRBs should *not* include a study's long-term effects in public policy as risks. Clearly, high social benefit should not trump individual risks or low individual benefit, but how and to what degree these committees should consider *low* amounts of social benefit is unknown—whether and how much it should matter if individual risks and benefits appear fairly well balanced.

Ultimately, social benefits can aid individuals, but they are not always predictable. Drug companies may argue that even "me-too" drugs can potentially assist some patients, and thus society, more than currently marketed compounds. Academic medical centers may also benefit from industry-funded research that builds infrastructure. But key questions arise as to how much potential social benefit is realistic and sufficient, and how IRBs should know and assess it.

Chairs, members, and administrators vary from being pro- or anti-industry, reflecting broader political attitudes and institutional priorities, but all of these positions can generate strains—in both the committee and the institution. COIs can be indirect, subtle, and even unconscious. The degree to which these other agendas may influence these boards demands further investigation.

Though IRBs are not optimally set up to address these concerns, other institutions may not be able do so, either. IRBs as a whole need to work and communicate more closely with COI and other institutional offices and researchers themselves. The practice of some COI offices of not telling an IRB how an investigator's conflicts are being managed prevents appropriate inclusion of the information in the informed consent. The process at some institutions of requiring researchers to complete two sets of IRB forms is grossly inefficient and can presumably be streamlined.

How social benefits are and should be measured and weighed also needs further attention. Metrics do not exist for assessing studies' long-term social and other benefits. Some protocols may have little social benefit now but potential long-term rewards. These questions hover, requiring ongoing robust discussion and clarification.

As corporations are gaining more political and economic sway in the US and abroad, these issues are becoming ever more critical. More information through public documentation of how IRBs are confronting these challenges would be enormously useful. Governmental and/or professional groups such as OHRP and IOM should provide more guidance and efforts to reach consensus concerning these issues as well. COIs pose increasing problems that need to be addressed to benefit both science and subjects.

CHAPTER 9

The Local Ecologies of Institutions

In 1989, Nancy Olivieri, a physician at the University of Toronto's Hospital for Sick Children, began to study the use of a drug, deferiprone, to lower iron that accumulated in patients with thalassemia. She thought the drug could help these children, and in 1993, she helped persuade the Medical Research Council and a pharmaceutical company, Apotex, to launch a formal drug trial. Two year later, however, she noticed that in several patients, the treatment was raising, rather than lowering iron. Apotex told her *not* to disclose this risk to patients in the study. Troubled, she then went to the IRB. But the company contacted the IRB, too, shut down the study, and threatened her with legal action if she spoke to the subjects. Olivieri nevertheless told them of her findings. As a result, she was harassed, and fired by the University. It turned out that Apotex had discussed giving the university over $20 million. The university had also lobbied the Canadian prime minister on the company's behalf. Olivieri's supporters received intimidating anonymous letters that turned out to be sent by a scientist who continued to receive funds from the company. Eventually, after several years and wide media attention giving her support, Olivieri was reinstated.[1]

IRBs work within the contexts of not only federal agencies and industry funders but also their own local academic institutions—primarily universities, medical schools, and hospitals—which can have competing agendas. Money can corrupt science—in industry obviously more than universities. But academic medical centers are not always successful in avoiding the effects of industry funding, and institutions and their IRBs may unfortunately be swayed by monetary and other factors. Past research has tended to view these committees as isolated entities, leaving many questions about how IRBs and these larger institutions in fact interrelate. After all, institutions are both varied and often themselves in flux.[2,3]

Financial constraints in health care and the rest of the economy are squeezing many aspects of academic medical centers, including how much money and attention they give to the ethical aspects of research. The amounts of resources IRBs receive from their institutions range widely,[4,5] often based in part on the number of protocols they review a year, but many IRBs have been shown to be underfunded.[6] How exactly these parent institutions influence their IRBs, however, remains unclear. Surprisingly, prior studies of IRBs have not systematically examined whether financial pressures at local institutions affect IRBs, and if so, how and to what degree.

The ways in which IRBs are situated in, and receive resources from, their larger academic institutions can mold and potentially bias these committees. My interviewees described how IRBs confront not only financial COIs but *nonfinancial* ones, too. IRB members themselves frequently "wear many hats," being institutional employees and often researchers as well as committee members; as such, they can encounter COIs due to their relationships with industry as well as their employers and fellow faculty. At times, these members do not want to create problems for their institution by erecting too many obstacles for researchers. Explicitly or implicitly, IRBs may try to assist, and avoid impeding, PIs or the institution itself.

Broad Institutional Characteristics

The culture and size of an institution and the amount of research funding it receives are often interrelated. These general characteristics in turn affect the IRB's work.

SIZE OF INSTITUTION

"Here, everybody knows everybody," Kurt, a chair, said. "That makes it harder for a researcher to be defiant, or a cowboy." Several chairs suggested that committees at smaller institutions may be more likely to know an investigator's work, ethics, and character. As Charlotte explained,

> I see everyone almost every day. I know these people. They are always dropping by my office, and can talk things out before submitting a protocol. So, there's a high level of trust. If we were bigger, we would need to add layers of bureaucracy. The IRB would need more employees, more form-checkers. Unfortunately, in this business, you really shouldn't assume too much. You have to make the investigators write everything down and document it. You can't just *assume* they're doing the right thing. We make scientists write everything down, but I just know they're doing the right thing—because I can see it.

Charlotte feels that the small size of her organization fosters both the letter and the spirit of the regulations. Documentation is important—"You can't just *assume* that they're doing the right thing"—and yet the high level of communication and openness encourages a similarly high level of compliance and cooperation, thus facilitating trust. Whether she is actually privy to all that researchers do is unclear, but her belief that that is the case is of note.

Kurt had a similar impression, but also acknowledged that perhaps he simply couldn't recognize his (relatively small) institution's weaknesses:

> Researchers tend to be honest with us—what their problem is or what they want from us. It's cultural, though. I've worked here so long; maybe I am just blind to our problems. I don't know what other institutions' cultures are like.

At smaller institutions, heightened knowledge, and hence trust, of PIs can also trigger more flexibility. Charlotte said,

> Because we're small, we can be fairly nimble. Our investigators collaborate with large university hospitals whose IRBs are pretty rigid about the format of their consent forms, which are written for very serious drug trials, when we're just doing a survey about smoking.

At such smaller institutions, trust and familiarity may foster welcome informality; a closer community might also produce social pressures to conform more. At the same time, bureaucratization can impede trust, making researchers frustrated and wary. Charlotte added,

> At one hospital, if you change the format—just the way the consent form looks on paper—you have to get it reviewed. Because we're small, I just say, "Just give me a copy for my files." If you change the text, you have to submit a modification. But if you just change the way it looks, that's ridiculous—a waste of everybody's time. People are too cautious because they don't know what to do. They don't know, or are not employing the flexibility that the regulations allow.

This institution's adaptability may also be due to it being primarily nonmedical rather than small *per se.* She added about some larger IRBs,

> They have a 15-page consent form that is just silly in readability. You can tell the lawyers have been all over the form. There's always the boilerplate language about injuries—that the university won't pay—which probably doesn't need to be there for a really minimal-risk study.

If some interviewees felt that their counterparts at larger institutions were too alienated from PIs and bogged down in IRB bureaucracy, others thought that the committees at smaller institutions had more difficulty staying abreast of relevant regulations—that they were too disconnected from vital national IRB discussions. Cynthia was surprised at the naïveté of questions that she felt small IRBs asked at large conferences:

> It's difficult to stay on top of IRB regulations. But at national meetings it always amazes me that people from IRBs in *smaller* hospitals or communities will ask questions that to me are really obvious—about IRB composition, how many people they have to have, the difference between the majority vote and a quorum.

Whether the "obvious" questions do indeed all come from individuals at smaller institutions is unclear, but her perception is important.

TYPE AND VOLUME OF RESEARCH CONDUCTED

An institution's size can shape the types of research funding it attracts, and by extension, the type of ethical problems that occur. Jack, a physician, researcher, and IRB chair at a rural medical center, does not have big drug development programs that can in turn generate problems:

> We don't have the capabilities of coming up with a molecule in a test tube, and then scaling it up, putting it into humans for the first time, and then pushing for FDA approval. We just don't have the scientific enterprise capacity to do that—investigators with the laboratory backup to develop gene therapy. Doing that has more opportunities for an ethical misstep. Jesse Gelsinger never could have happened here.

At the same time, Jack expresses regret about his school's limitations: "We don't have big drug development programs, but *wish* we did." The larger institutions are "doing great stuff, and move things forward—when these ethical glitches don't get in the way." He continued:

> So, that's the good news and the bad news about us: we are still a small sleepy place. We do some good science, but are not breaking new ground here. So we don't have the stresses and strains that allow those lapses to happen.

He suggests ambivalence but also the present financial value of industry funding at academic medical centers.

Such a "small town" culture can in turn be self-perpetuating—because it attracts fewer relatively "high profile" players. Within the culture of the institution, mutual selection and implicit social feedback loops naturally ensue. Jack continued:

> People here know each other. It's much more of a small-town, interpersonal ecology. You can't make enemies here. If you tick off the orthopedic surgeon today, if his daughter's on the field when your daughter's playing field hockey, and your daughter breaks her leg, he's going to be the first one there. So, we are much more interdependent in this small community off the hospital grounds. That reverberates: we don't have the big institutional scale to attract high-power go-getters. We mostly tend to be here because we like the quality of life. If we wanted to make our jobs the absolutely number-one thing in our lives, we'd probably go elsewhere. So, we don't have those strains—because of both the interpersonal politics and the drive that people don't have here.

He feels that the opportunity for financial conflicts of interest may hence be less as well. "Nobody says, 'I'm going to develop a new drug, and retire with huge stock options.'"

Conversely, research-intensive institutions typically depend heavily on large research grants—not simply for research itself but also for operating costs. The NIH adds about 65 percent to every grant to cover institutional overhead. Joe, the researcher and chair, said, "The institution wants to make sure studies get funded, because, frankly, the institution relies on the indirect costs—a lot of money here."

As we saw earlier, a small institution's committee may also be more agile because the IRB staff knows the investigators and can rely on ongoing relationships and trust rather than bureaucratization, while large institutions lack such knowledge and intimacy.

Assigning Studies to IRBs Randomly

Some institutions seek to eschew the advantages and dangers of a "cozy" relationship between researchers and particularly IRBs by assigning protocols to committees randomly. This also prevents researchers from "IRB shopping" to increase the likelihood of approval. Christopher, the chair, explained:

> We have four IRBs, and some have reputations as being harder, so researchers game the system, submitting at different times of the month to try to get an "easy" IRB. If investigators don't like the issues our committee raises, they just don't submit to us anymore.

"We don't allow investigators to 'IRB shop', Jeremy, the physician and chair, said. "They can't stipulate where their protocol ends up." Yet such random rotation of submissions between IRBs has disadvantages in that one committee, but not another, may then know of a problematic PI. Jeremy continued,

> Our IRB had a long track record of lots of problems with this guy, but the other IRBs weren't aware of it. And we weren't aware he was submitting protocols to all the other IRBs, because they don't come to us. When there is a problem investigator, we should *all* be aware of it.

WHO IS IN CHARGE OF WHAT? COMMUNICATION BETWEEN REGULATORY OFFICES

Jeremy's complaint is that within the ecology of many institutions, IRBs are now set up so that one committee does not know what the others are handling, and vice versa, and different boards may therefore be unintentionally working at cross purposes, or with incomplete background information. *And IRBs are only one type of regulatory committee;* institutions may also have separate offices for compliance, COI, and their general counsel. These entities may differ, but have overlapping and potentially synergistic roles, shaped by complex institutional histories and cultures; interactions among them range from close and collaborative to very distant, with little to no communication. Institutions have officials higher in the organizational structure who are administratively responsible for the IRB—often a VP of research or of compliance. Compliance offices usually oversee a university's adherence to a broad array of financial, safety, quality control, and other federal and state regulations. Many IRBs attempt to take on some of these additional roles—such as addressing researchers' scientific misconduct and conflicts of interest related in some way to research. Yet the nature and boundaries of these broader possible scopes are not always clear.

For instance, Jeff, the chair, related that his IRB had suspended a study because the PI had kept unidentified information on samples. At his institution, Jeff reported the problem to this official, but received no follow-up. Was this PI still conducting any research?

> We've shut down several protocols. But it isn't clear to me: maybe the PI's still doing research. I don't know if he's doing nonhuman research, or working on those samples properly.

On the one hand, chairs generally thought that their IRB was already overworked and underresourced, and hence neither could, nor should, do more. On the other hand, chairs often felt that they had only incomplete information on PIs, and lacked the whole picture. Jeff continued,

> There should be a way to find out what this faculty member is doing. That is in the Compliance Officer's domain. The IRB forwarded to him a list of what he needs to do to reactivate his studies. He didn't do those. His department chair and dean are aware, from being copied on the correspondence. So, the IRB met its obligations. I didn't think that we needed to be *police* and put yellow tape across his lab doors.

Such incomplete interoffice communication raises concerns at many institutions.

OTHER CULTURAL VARIATIONS

Other aspects of medical centers can mold IRB issues as well, such as areas of specialty within an institution. A cancer hospital will face different ethical issues than an orthopedic center. Liza said,

> The culture here is due to the fact that we're *pediatrics*. The type of people that work with children just have a different attitude. They can explain things. There's a different ethics. It shows in a culture of an institution, too. Maybe that's why we don't have so many problems.

Anecdotally, pediatricians have usually struck me, personally, as being the nicest group of physicians. Institutions may specialize in areas from eyes and ears to diabetes, obstetrics and gynecology, psychiatry, drug abuse, or social science. The types of protocols that IRBs see range accordingly.

Institutional Support for IRBs

POLITICAL SUPPORT

Institutional leaders vary greatly in how much they understand or back the IRB. Chairs felt that institutions need to "buy into" and "be committed to the culture of compliance," but conceded that they differ considerably in doing so. Within each institution, the standing of the board may vary, whether due to particular leaders or recent scandals.

Occasionally, a research ethicist holds a high position in the university administration, thereby buttressing the IRB's value. "Our university is very supportive of our IRB," Dana, a social scientist and chair, said, "One of the vice presidents is an ethicist, and brings status to our IRB and what we do. So the institution allots money." In this particular case, it is unclear which came first—the ethicist being high up in the university, or the university valuing ethics.

Having an ethicist or IRB leader in a powerful administrative position in the institution is not the norm but not entirely unique either, and can provide many direct and indirect benefits to a committee. Scott, an IRB director, said,

> At my previous institution, the IRB ruled the roost. Here, it's the exact opposite—it's an uphill battle. There, an associate dean for research who had an iron fist oversaw the IRB, and never really faced any resistance or noise from PIs. He was in a position of authority *outside* of the IRB, so we got less flak from PIs. If the dean is a huge advocate and supporter, and gets involved as a buffer for IRB chairs, the IRB gets respect.

Friends in high places are particularly valuable for IRBs, since much of their work takes place against the backdrop of widespread criticism from disgruntled researchers.

Some IRBs attempt to enhance attitudes toward them through "PR work"—distributing newsletters about their activities, and sending out "helpful hints" to PIs.

Still, these relationships may remain ambivalent. Many institutions consist of both a medical school and a separate hospital, and these two entities can themselves clash, having different cultures and priorities. IRBs may thus be interacting with competing organizations. Christopher, the chair, said,

> The institution is and is not supportive of the IRB. We're about to have a potential blow up. Our hospital system is independent of the medical school. The IRB is now joint, so all the hospital research has to go through the university IRB, but there's a conflict.

An IRB may be forced to straddle these tensions, reviewing research for both institutions without necessarily knowing the researchers equally at both.

FINANCIAL SUPPORT

Institutions vary in the amounts of money they spend on their IRBs, which also causes strains. Compensation, Scott pointed out, is a very tangible form of support that also signals to the wider community that the work of IRBs is valued:

> A few years back, no members were paid. Now, we compensate our members. They spend time, and put themselves in positions that may not be favorable with some of their colleagues. The support IRBs get from institutions highlights the differences in how [IRBs] are viewed in different locations. It's a matter of perception and support, which pretty much determines the IRB's standing from institution to institution.

Almost all of these men and women felt that their IRB received insufficient resources, yet obtaining additional funds was difficult. Individual compensation was only a small part of the issue. As Jaime said, "there are never enough staff." Chairs usually request more resources, but compete against other institutional priorities. Several interviewees felt that a limited budget, exacerbated by the recent economic downturn, was the major obstacle facing their board. Scott, the IRB director, said,

> Losing a few million in research funds decreases staffing throughout the institution. There's a hiring freeze. That's the biggest challenge—the lack of resources to support the traditional expectation of growth.

Additional resources can expand a committee's capabilities, providing extra staff to conduct better and more frequent audits, orient new members, assist community members, or help with student research or consent forms. Conversely, at small institutions, a board may have fewer resources and meet less regularly—only nine times a year—slowing approval.

Limited resources can demoralize staff, and engender perceptions that institutions are unsupportive. Scott said,

> Additional resources haven't come in to make up for the additional workload. That demoralizes people who want to work. Chairs are demoralized, because they see the same pattern going forward.

Long hours can erode IRB staff morale further. "We're all overworked," Scott continued. "The staff take on a larger chunk of the workload. It doesn't help their morale."

IRB STRATEGIES TO GET MORE RESOURCES

While recognizing that universities have numerous other competing demands, many chairs nonetheless try to obtain additional funding. Since his school has a new incoming dean, Scott is planning to ask for more money.

> We are taking advantage of that. We are hoping to negotiate to revert back to the good old days where we had discretionary spending—not one hand tied behind our backs.

Frequently, IRB chairs argue that support to IRBs is not only crucial morally, but is also pragmatic—to avoid potential mishaps and/or scandals. Jeremy, the physician and chair, said,

The institution has less money than it needs for all the things everybody's asking it to do. But clearly, *this* is crucial. And it's the right thing to do. If things go badly, much is at stake for the institution. It's a time bomb—if you don't have the resources, you can almost predict [what's] eventually going to happen.

Unfortunately, legal trouble and "bad press" that could hurt financially generally carry more weight than do ethical principles by themselves. Often, institutional leaders feel compelled to support IRBs more only after scandals at their own institutions. Absent such a violation, several chairs have tried informing their institutions about scandals *elsewhere* to get more resources. Liza said,

> I advise other IRB chairs about what I call the *raindrop effect*—they need to keep their institutional officials informed when things happen elsewhere—not telling these officials, "This means we need more resources," but just sort of *raindrop them* throughout: "Geez, this went on at that institution. We're trying to figure out how to prevent this here."

Ultimately, however, interviewees felt that institutions may be wary of additional expenditures, and appear more interested in meeting their own needs than bolstering subjects. As Greg, a chair, said,

> Most institutions don't want to spend a lot of money if they don't have to. They tend to do what they *have* to do—based on regulations or needs to get accredited and maintain accreditation. Accreditation seems to be one of the main drivers—not necessarily the ethics.

Fears of lawsuits can also impel changes and increased support, but have disadvantages as well as advantages. "Liability," Greg added, "drives a lot of issues":

> Our institution has restructured to become more...bureaucratized and centralized...to handle issues in more of a lawyer fashion.

The institution's direct aim then, arguably, may be protecting itself more than subjects. The former may lead to the second, but not necessarily or efficiently.

Greg wanted his office to emphasize ethics, not merely compliance per se, and to include more education; but he only partly succeeded. Limited resources can significantly restrict an IRB's ability to broaden its scope.

CHARGING FEES?

Increasingly, to obtain additional resources, many committees charge fees to industry-funded studies, raising questions, in turn, of how much to charge, and where the money should go. Free-standing for-profit IRBs, which charge researchers fees, have grown in recent years. Recently, some university IRBs have also started to charge industry sponsors for evaluating protocols—around $2,500 for initial reviews, and $500 for continuing reviews. But requiring such payment for reviews poses problems.

These institutional IRBs may then be competing, either intentionally or unintentionally, with these private boards. University committees that charge fees generally appear to request less than these for-profit businesses, so they see themselves as offering a relative advantage. Christopher thought,

> As more companies are going to central IRBs, which charge even more, they're realizing that universities are a good bargain—not faster, but at least not more expensive.

Unaffiliated with any university or hospital, such for-profit committees review studies simply for the money. Critics contend that such companies consequently have inherent COIs, getting paid to approve protocols. Questions arise of whether collection of such fees by IRBs might then pose conflicts of interest as well—the temptation to approve such protocols more readily.

University IRBs that charge fees face problems, too, because some of these larger institutions have started taking these funds from the IRBs. Scott said,

> It used to be collected as a discretionary fund, used as IRBs chose. Now, it's been expropriated by senior officials and absorbed as part of the whole school revenue stream, which has affected our turnaround time. There is less of an incentive for IRBs to decrease their turnaround time if they know they are not going to reap the rewards.

This expropriation of funds earned by the IRBs may hence lower their incentive to improve.

Yesterday's Scandal/Tomorrow's Cash Flow

Almost every year, well-publicized research controversies shake IRBs nationwide. Ethics violations can challenge prior assumptions about what is permissible or not, highlighting complexities posed by new permutations of research studies, and thereby changing IRBs' views. "An event calls into question the way you view the world," Martin said. "You think: maybe I shouldn't have taken for granted something that I did."

Institutions also dread "bad press." As Kevin, a health care provider and chair, described,

> After wrongdoing at another institution, *soul searching* always goes on. You always look at yourself and say: "Could that happen here?" Sometimes the answer is difficult.

Generally, though, institutional leaders pay more attention to crises at home. Interviewees thought that variations between IRBs can stem in part from the fact that some institutions have had "scandals," or been cited or investigated, increasing attention and resources to these areas. Indeed, the few IRBs here that felt relatively well supported had all had major breaches in recent years.

Jeremy, a physician and chair, explained that his institution's IRB process was transformed after being investigated:

> We went from two committees to five, and regular members are now paid 10 percent salary support. Before, nobody was. Now, there's a huge IRB central office with consent form specialists, a regulatory person who's a lawyer, and administrative support. A whole leadership structure was put in place that didn't exist: a dean for clinical research, retreats once or twice a year. The institution takes it extremely seriously now—making resources available.

Yet unfortunately it took the shutdown to produce these beneficial changes. Crises alone may generate funds. He continued,

> Getting shut down had an absolutely seismic effect on this institution—all for the positive, I think. After our tragedy, everything got upgraded. *Unless there's a crisis, it's very hard to get resources.* Trying to get money and support for ethics has not been easy....I asked the former dean for money, and was told, "You're doing great work. Keep it up." No money. Then there was a disaster, and suddenly the coffers opened. Unfortunately, that's the way institutions work. It takes exceptionally strong, smart leadership to identify these things ahead of time.

Federal audits can take years, and make institutions, IRBs, and researchers anxious; but ultimately these probes can compel institutions to provide their boards with additional support. Laura, the lawyer, said,

> I came in the middle of a big federal investigation, and the school was desperate for help in getting out of it. It was pretty bad, but a blessing for me. It gave me leverage to get resources, hire staff, and make changes.

Such exigencies can galvanize IRB reorganization and improvement. Dana, the social scientist and chair, reported, "With restructuring, we decreased our turn-around time for reviews from six months to six weeks. Before, the IRB wasn't functioning—we would just sit on studies."

An institutional audit by the federal government for purported ethics vio-lations can create stresses for IRBs and therefore PIs. Joe felt that differences between IRBs depend on the institution's experience with OHRP—how much federal audits have made institutions and IRBs *risk averse*. Elaine, an administra-tor and member, continued:

> We've had three audits, two from the OHRP and one from the FDA—not about major things—they aren't going to shut us down—but we're on their radar. They could come back. The IRB is really trying, because they'll find stuff. But researchers are complaining.... It's uncomfortable.

Ironically, however, with fewer federal shutdowns of research in the past few years, less money may now go to IRBs and compliance, given other competing needs. As Scott, an IRB director, said,

> It's not that deans don't respect IRBs, but the government is taking money away from NIH to fund the Iraq War, and expects that institutions will come to bat for their IRBs. But I haven't seen that. Institutions look at us as a regular department, like the clinical trials or technology transfer office. Money speaks loudly here, and is more important than compli-ance these days.... Support is going more towards offices that bring in revenue: the grants office. The IRB is simply *compliance*. These days, we don't have much noncompliance, because everyone pretty much knows what they should and shouldn't do. As a result, there are fewer shutdowns, and attention goes to the money-making, revenue-generating groups.

Interviewees often felt that medical centers aim implicitly to determine how little they can give the IRB while avoiding federal audits and/or shutdowns. Scott continued,

> Whether or not we have the funds to hire another two people largely depends on the *good graces of the school*, instead of how much revenue we generate, and whether we can afford it. But we need expansion.

Unfortunately, tensions and potentially COIs can ensue. IRBs may feel the need to obtain support from their institutions, and thus lean more toward supporting their institutions and colleagues seeking to obtain grants.

Moreover, interviewees felt that even at institutions where scandals have occurred, IRBs may initially receive more resources, but over time see these added funds then decline. Stephen, a chair and health care provider, said,

> Initially, there was a lot of support...Now, it's not in the forefront. We're certainly, at our institution, light years ahead of what we were in the late '90s. But to a degree, we may have lost some of that edge that we had right after the government shutdown.

Apart yet a Part: How IRBs Manage their own Conflicts of Interest

Even after Ellen Roche's death, the Johns Hopkins internal review committee assessed the institution's IRB performance far less critically than did the three external review committees—including one each from OHRP and the FDA. This discrepancy highlights how an institution's employees may seek to protect the organization. Committees may be more inclined to help compatriots, however defined, over strangers. Although IRBs are *set apart* from the normal workings of their institutions in various respects, in other regards they are also very much *an integral part* of them; and as a consequence all sorts of biases, both for and against certain protocols, can come into play. In addition, some chairs, despite their ethical role, still feel implicit pressure to help their institutions by encouraging research and researchers. Identifying, monitoring, and responding to these conflicts can be challenging.

POSITIVE BIAS: WHEN IRBS GET TOO COZY WITH RESEARCHERS

One danger is that committee members will judge some researchers less rigorously than others. A few chairs spoke of trying to *avoid* giving help to friends who were investigators. Aaron, a chair, said:

> When somebody from my department comes through with a protocol, I probably *bend over backwards* to try not to forgive things—for just that reason. They are friends, but I'm not there to help my friends—I'm there to do a job.

But these strains can be subtle, especially when the institution stands to gain large amounts of financial support, and IRBs and faculty may in fact have close bonds. Jeremy, the physician and chair, invoked the metaphor of a sports team:

We are all part of the same club. When a PI came in to explain his study, it was like a *locker room*. The guys were very friendly, chumming around.... The IRB is supposed to be objective, professional. But on a personal level, it may not be as strict or stringent with friends or long-standing colleagues than a regional IRB, with no personal relationships, just dealing with the facts, regulations, and principles.... To what extent do the facts that we are all colleagues, and know the investigators, affect our performance—our ability to protect subjects?

This last question remained unanswered in his mind.

"There's still a good-old-boy, nepotistic kind of atmosphere here," Louis, a chair at an institution in a relatively conservative state, said. "I'm one of the outsiders, from a different part of the country."

There can also be strong unwritten rules against criticizing colleagues, especially more senior ones. Charlotte added,

One scientist quit the IRB because he was unwilling to confront another scientist. He said, "This is bad science." But rather than confront the guy, he quit, because it's taboo professionally to criticize a colleague. He was new to the institution, and didn't want to be in the position of The New Guy sitting there judging all these esteemed colleagues.

This sort of indirect conflict of interest can be difficult to detect or prevent. In such an environment, many feel limited in their ability to "stand up" to certain researchers. Aaron, a chair who does not yet have tenure in his academic department, faced a researcher who was "a real jerk." Aaron wanted to confront this researcher, but was advised by his superior, the university's vice president, to delay doing so: "I'm going to be tenured this year. The VP of Research said I should wait until I get tenured. So I'm making nice."

NEGATIVE BIAS: WHEN IRBS COMPETE WITH RESEARCHERS

Sometimes committee members can feel competitive with PIs, and not want to approve certain protocols. Consciously or unconsciously, members may resent or feel jealous toward colleagues proceeding readily with an important study. Members walk a fine line between criticizing investigations when they feel that it is indicated, while not being overly critical and disparaging colleagues' protocols due to competitive feelings. A good chair can potentially detect and limit such discussion.

At the same time these researchers and their colleagues may have helpful expertise in an area, justifying their inclusion in discussions: if they are forced to recuse themselves entirely, much valuable information can be lost. Nonetheless, their presence can be awkward. If they criticize a colleague's study, their disparaging remarks must be kept confidential.

To stymie such discomfort, Kevin starts every meeting with a blessing.

> We start every meeting with a benediction of sorts, saying, "The things that we talk about in this room can affect the careers of the individuals involved. *What goes on in this room stays in this room.* Consider it like Las Vegas: we don't discuss anything outside of these doors." We really do let our hair down, take down our defense shields, and call a spade a spade.

His practice of a "benediction" also suggests how IRBs may to a degree engage in *rituals*—established systematic means of addressing difficult emotions.

Should I Vote or Go? The Complexities of Recusal

Some committees may try simply to be "above" financial considerations involved in research, unaffected by these issues. "We try consciously to be *purer* than money," Troy, the urban researcher and chair, said. But how to achieve that goal is not always obvious; and sometimes a committee member's bias may either have nothing to do with money, or tie into financial considerations only in some very subtle and indirect way.

Often, chairs either request or demand that members with actual or potential COIs identify and recuse themselves. But the definition of such conflicts (e.g., whether these include nonfinancial strains) may not be clear. A chair's position may also vary, depending on the details of the conflict or other, subjective factors. As Laura, the lawyer, said,

> At meetings, the chair reminds everybody: if you have a conflict, identify and disclose it, and if you need to, recuse yourself. They then leave the room before the vote. They might stay for *some* of the discussion, and answer questions.

Other IRBs may bar the member from the discussion entirely, or leave these decisions up to the individual conflicted member. Kevin said that a member "could be doing research for the company that makes a drug or a competitor, and be conflicted. We allow them to take part in discussion, but not vote."

ALLOWING "BIASED" IRB MEMBERS
TO JOIN THE DISCUSSION

Having on the IRB a member of a research team whose work is being reviewed can be both good and bad. Jeremy said,

> I think we've been pretty good about not being too cozy. One member is part of a research group, but that has not been an issue. We were pretty tough on protocols from his group....He tried to defend or explain what the researcher was doing, and the discussion didn't go his way. On balance, it's been helpful to have him to explain the research, because on the face of it, the research seems a little crazy. Why are we exposing healthy research subjects to this particular drug? He can explain it.

In this instance, the committee was able to achieve a greater understanding of the protocol from the researcher, while maintaining sufficient independence in the face of his opinions. Kevin permits conflicted or potentially conflicted members to join the discussion, but other IRBs ban such participation, and make such members leave the room during the deliberations. The logic behind this stance is that allowing conflicted members to remain in the room, and/or participate in the conversation—even if they can't vote—could still potentially sway the board's conclusion.

Andrew felt that recusing members may be particularly hard at smaller institutions. "Usually, the researchers doing the studies are sitting on the IRBs! They're not supposed to be voting on their own studies, but they are present. Even if they go out of the room, everybody knows." The PI may deduce their views and members may still hesitate to criticize a fellow member's study too harshly.

Even within the same institution, IRBs vary in decisions about *recusing* department members. Christopher explained,

> A PI on the committee has to leave. But we don't change the *chair* if *he* happens to be in the same department as the PI. One of our other IRBs does that: the chair is a pediatrician, and any time the PI is a pediatrician, the chair leaves that discussion.

Questions also surface of *when* exactly members should recuse themselves—whether it is when *any* protocol from a department is discussed, or only for those in which they are closely involved. Some committees are very cautious. As Stephen, the chair, said,

> Our department is receiving payment for services that we're providing in a study. Generally, I'm pretty upfront about that, and declaring that

as a conflict of interest. So I would not take part in discussions, deliberation, voting, assessing amendments, updates, and safety reporting. Is that *really* a conflict of interest? I look at it: we're published as a headline in the newspaper, "The IRB chair gets salary support for working on this, and he's doing this." How would that look?

Other chairs in similar positions might be less conservative, however, and choose to stay in the room if they have the authority to do so.

Recusal may also be used to protect an IRB member. For instance, fellow committee members may suggest that a colleague recuse him or herself to prevent possible recrimination from reviewing a protocol negatively. Still, in these instances, the member may decide to participate nonetheless. Kurt, the researcher and chair, said,

> A resident on the IRB reviews protocols, and tells his faculty what he thinks is wrong. We've told him he can recuse himself—that he needs to worry that his department may not like him rattling cages, if he's only a resident.... But he feels OK.

The specifics of the department and the individuals involved can therefore differ substantially.

POTENTIAL COSTS OF RECUSALS

When people *do* recuse themselves, their absence can make a *quorum* of expertise difficult to obtain. Senior faculty on an IRB may be involved in many studies, and therefore have to excuse themselves relatively frequently. Unconflicted experts in a field can be hard to obtain, as well; chairs may have to find outsiders to review certain studies. As Christopher said,

> We have a limited pool of experts. One cardiologist consults for all the companies, so can't review for us.... But then no one on the committee has the expertise. In some ways, it's better to have someone involved who knows the field.

Pressure from Above? Indirect Institutional Influences

Some interviewees thought that, generally, their institution did not try to influence the IRB. "I'm amazed," Judy, the physician and chair, said, "at how little institutions pressure IRBs to approve studies." But other interviewees thought that such influence did exist, though implicit and subtle. As Stephen said,

The IRB is supposed to be very free from all those pressures. But subliminally, they are still there. Investigators are unhappy about review turnaround times, and complain up the chain. Then the institution says: "You guys have to do better at review times," or this and that.

INSTITUTIONS MONITORING IRBS

While the regulations dictate that institutions designate an official to be responsible for the IRB, questions surface about that person's role. As Elaine said,

> Our institutional official is a researcher. In the past, he came to the meetings. The committee then voted to make them closed, because they felt that he was swaying the vote.

Yet, at other institutions, such pressures persist.

IRBs may debate whether to allow other institutional representatives, too, to sit in on committee meetings or participate, which may allow the institution to influence the board's deliberations. IRBs varied on this; sometimes a hospital's lawyer observed and/or spoke at committee meetings. Louis permitted an institutional official to be involved, yet members and chairs can disagree about these decisions.

> The old-timers on the board say that the IRB is a faculty committee, and that the administration *shouldn't* have any input—that the administration's always the dark side. . . . I don't see the harm in getting input. I make sure the [larger] institution's protected.

COMMITTEE CHAIR AS HOT SEAT

Medical center CEOs or other officials may seek to influence committees in other, bolder ways as well—even to pressure IRBs to approve particular protocols, although this practice appeared rare and to have occurred more in the past. Ultimately in these instances, institutions appeared to demur, and IRBs prevailed. As Christopher said,

> I've gotten calls from the Dean and the hospital president, who say, "We need to approve this right away: we have 25 people lined up for this surgery, and it needs to be approved." I say, "Well, the PI didn't fill out the forms," or, "We can't approve it. I'm happy to work with them, but they need to go through the process. I'm not going to speak for the whole committee." So, there has been pressure to circumvent things.

Generally we resist.... They eventually understand. It can take a bit of time. The hospital administrators "get it" the least—because they're just interested in getting the money, and don't understand the whole process and the issues. But they understand administrative process: it's no different from trying to cut a check. It's just new to them as a bureaucratic hurdle. They view it as a barrier.

In recent years, the growing prominence and importance of IRBs have also often counterbalanced and diminished these forces. Kevin said,

Ten or 12 years ago, the regime was different here, and there were attempts to force things down the throats of the IRB. But that's long gone. The regulatory issues have gotten much stricter.

When researchers complain about their IRBs, however, institutional leaders may nonetheless side with investigators.

Chairs can react to these pressures in several ways—ordinarily not succumbing to such forces, but resisting, or in some cases resigning. Elaine, the administrator, added,

I'm trying to do what I think is right—which is going to upset some people.... Most of it runs quite fine. But chairs are going to still get pressured to approve studies. Unfortunately, politics are everywhere. In these situations, chairs may cave in, and change what they do, or get frustrated, or nervous, or say, "I've had enough."

Institutional officials cannot directly dictate IRB decisions, but they can and do exert influence by replacing chairs—sometimes in response to researchers' grievances. The degrees to which these measures are justified can vary widely. A chair might be removed because he is raising too many inconvenient ethical questions about potentially lucrative protocols the university is afraid of losing. Or he or she might be removed for being inefficient or overbearing. A new chair can improve communication and efficiency, which can be good not just for researchers, but for other IRB personnel and broader institutions. "The new chair is much more conducive to researchers," Dana said, praising a new chair who had replaced an older, less effective one.

AVERSION TO RISK

In clinical care and research, risks are inevitable. But institutions range in the degrees to which they are risk avoidant, related in part to other institutional events—past and present. An institution or close affiliate may have recently been investigated, or gone bankrupt. One medical center became far more cautious because of an affiliated institution's financial woes. The IRB has asked the medical center to get an insurance policy, but without success. Jeff said,

> Since the bankruptcy of an affiliate hospital, our institution has been immensely risk averse. An IRB does its best to protect human subjects, but risks are intrinsic to research. The university ought to live with that, and get an insurance policy.

Financial risk may affect multiple aspects of IRB processes, including consent forms. These documents must state whether treatment or compensation will be provided in case of injury, and if so, of what it will consist. However, the federal regulations do not specify how institutions must *answer* these questions—whether participants will in fact receive treatment or compensation in these cases, and if so, what. Some institutions, concerned with expenses, have said that they will not provide any care to research participants injured during a study. The subjects' insurance will have to cover such costs. The IRB may object—in part because poor subjects without insurance will be excluded—but the committee may then have to fight institutional leaders, which can be difficult, and ultimately fruitless. Jeff continued,

> Our "in case of injury" clause changed from one that [said the institution] would cover the cost of care for injury, to one that would not....It used to say that in case of injury, they'll cover it....That's appropriate. We've appealed to the administration to change that, and have never even gotten a formal answer.

These financial pressures can impede research in other ways, too. For example, investigators often know the areas in which IRBs or institutions are risk averse, and as a result choose not to pursue certain studies. Jeff, the chair, added, "Investigators in cardiology and oncology knew: if a study looked high risk, [these researchers] didn't want to do it."

Other Institutional Conflicts of Interest

IRB members must struggle with not only their own conflicts of interest but also, potentially, those involving their departments or the institution itself. For instance, a drug company might fund an oncology department, but not directly the salary of a researcher in that department. However, that investigator might benefit inadvertently from the funds and thus have a conflict. Yet such strains can be less obvious, and hence overlooked, and IRBs may avoid discussing them. Martin, the researcher and chair, feels that such tensions "can be far more subtle. And there aren't any guidelines on that. People are reluctant to open up that box."

Such conflicts often involve finances, but not always; sometimes, for example, administrative officials might try to block research that may question the institution's own practices or policy. Martin said,

> Our institution has very specific guidelines for regulating faculty members' COIs, but not the *institution's* COI—those of the hospital or medical school. The IRB has to regulate those. One incident made the hair stand up on the back of my neck: Health policy faculty wanted to look at the health records of university employees to determine if lower paid employees had the same access to health care as higher paid employees.

The IRB approved it, but when the researchers attempted to get the health records from HR, they were denied access. Martin continued,

> The university administration and president disallowed the protocol, saying they were afraid about loss of confidentiality of employees' health records. But, in fact, *they have a COI*: what if these researchers find that access to healthcare is not equitable? The university is at risk, and is judging whether the research can be done. That's a COI. In other research, the hospital itself stands to gain, which can affect the review of protocols. From time to time, the fact that the hospital stands to gain filters into the review of protocols.

AVOIDING THE MIRROR: IRBS MAY NOT ENCOURAGE RESEARCH ON THEMSELVES

My own institution's IRB reviewed this study on IRBs. For the first and only time in my 25 years of research, they asked me to appear and defend my protocol at a meeting of the full board. Most of my prior research had been considered minimal risk, and therefore received expedited review. When the full board or a subcommittee reviewed it, I was told simply to be available if members happened to have any questions for me to answer immediately (rather than via memo), which they never did.

This request to appear before the full committee was unusual and somewhat intimidating. "What are you going to do with all of this sensitive data?" they asked me. "How are you going to analyze it?" I explained that I would do so as I had analyzed all my prior qualitative data in my previous studies on subjects that I considered "more sensitive"—exploring individuals' HIV sexual risk behaviors, illicit drug use, et cetera.

The IRB was questioning me more than they ever had before. Yet there was an obvious COI at play, in light of my subject matter, which was never acknowledged. For me, this experience exemplified both the complexities of the issues I am examining here, and the blind spots inherent in this work.

Conclusions

These interviews, the first to explore how IRBs operate in the contexts of dynamic local institutional relationships and systems, illustrate how these settings can exert both direct and indirect effects. Although these forces may be ineluctable, they fuel inconsistencies between IRBs, impeding studies and frustrating researchers. Implicitly or explicitly, subtly or directly, committees may feel pressured by their institutions, producing and exacerbating conflicts. These boards usually try to fight these forces, but doing so can be hard—especially since institutions determine how much support their IRBs receive.

These institutional relationships and processes can also shape how any new regulations get implemented in an institution. Despite proposals for more uniformity through centralized review, interinstitutional variations may well continue, underscoring the needs for other improvements. IRBs, policymakers and, in the end, all of us should thus be more aware of these phenomena.

Complex feedback loops exist. Investigators complain about IRBs to institutions that may consequently pressure and/or alter IRBs. Institutional leaders may decide to replace IRB chairs, significantly altering a committee. As we saw, over time PI complaints can also prompt federal agencies to consider altering regulations governing IRBs, as seen with the ANPRM.[7,8] Subjects seemed rarely to complain to an institution, in part since they may feel disempowered to do so. Yet the death of a subject can trigger media and federal government attention, forcing a major investigation and shutdown of an institution's IRB or research. Overall, these feedback loops are not very efficient or effective, and should be improved.

Though a few aspects of financial COIs among IRBs have been probed,[9] the men and women here highlight other areas, such as how IRB members confront *non*financial conflicts and respond to both types of strains—whether members should vote and/or leave the room in the presence of such *non*financial binds as well. Members can potentially either aid or hamper researchers—"helping their buddies" or impeding rivals—and IRB meetings can be "like a locker room," involving informal as well as formal interactions and relationships between members and researchers. These impediments can be subtle, subjective, and invisible, and therefore hard to detect, monitor, regulate, or prevent. IRBs' responses to their own potential COI range considerably, and conflicted members may still be allowed to observe, participate, and/or vote in discussions. Mechanisms for handling these COI often appear informal, ad hoc, and case by case.

Definitions of COI can be blurry—for instance, if researchers are developing a device that they might sell and hence have financial interest in, not now but in the future. Questions arise, too, of whether IRBs should use, as a standard, not having even the *appearance* of a COI, and whether these conflicts are less important in minimal-risk studies.

While prior discussions distinguish between financial and nonfinancial COI, distinctions more commonly arise here between *direct* and *indirect* financial COIs. Nonfinancial biases have been described, based on political or other commitments,[10] allegiance to a particular theoretical framework,[11] or career advancement and ambition.[12,13] A researcher might be biased in interpreting data because he or she is a Marxist or a strict Freudian or thinks certain drugs should be legalized, thus slanting studies to support that position. But the men and women here reveal *indirect* financial COIs that are based on gain or loss not to themselves, but to their colleagues or larger institution.

Importantly, IRBs themselves wrestle with competing priorities—such as managing COIs *vs.* having a quorum, and/or expertise to review a protocol; and avoiding these conflicts *vs.* wanting to help their institution to obtain industry funds. To gauge these tensions, IRBs also rely on trust of each other and of researchers. Committee approaches to these strains may be suboptimal because of perceived "knowledge" of local PIs—faith that these PIs would not have COIs, and/or would readily report it. But such beliefs may not always be fully justified. Just as researchers and clinicians may be unconscious of their COIs, so, too, may many IRB members.

One could argue that IRB conflicts of interest with PIs can cut both ways—helping or hindering investigators—and that these phenomena in effect cancel each other out. But such "balancing" may not always occur. Rather, at any one time, an IRB may tilt more one way or the other, raising concerns.

These interviewees highlight, too, inefficiencies in current bureaucratic structures for overseeing these tensions. Separate institutional COI offices, other than IRBs, may know of and manage investigators' financial conflicts. But many IRBs then do not learn of these other offices' decisions, though IRBs would often like to, in order to review protocols appropriately and determine what the consent form should include. Thus, institutional relationships and structures may need to be altered and improved to facilitate increased sharing of relevant information.

Some critics have advocated disclosure to study subjects of both financial and nonfinancial COIs,[14] but doing so may not be feasible or realistic for *indirect* financial conflicts. In part, IRBs, not researchers themselves, may be conflicted. It may not make sense for informed consent forms to state, in essence, "The IRB may also have been trying to help the PI by approving this study, in order to maintain his lab." Just as needs for career advancement pose intrinsic nonfinancial conflicts, so, too, indirect financial strains may be inherent in academic institutions. Consequently, efforts to enhance awareness and education about these tensions are vital.

These men and women also underscore the need to consider guidelines and clarifications concerning when and how IRB members should recuse themselves from discussing, reviewing, and/or voting on protocols. IRB members are familiar with many faculty members, posing potential conflicts. Hence, the criteria for COIs should not be whether members know the researcher, but rather to what degree that knowledge may influence deliberations one way or the other. Still, these determinations, potentially shaped by these long-standing, but possibly weak influences, can be highly subjective and hard. Guidance can, however, help these committees.

While the Obama Administration has proposed "excusing" certain studies from IRB review, the onus of review might then fall on academic departments to assess studies internally. But such departments may be conflicted, wanting to advance its faculty's research. The current system of having two parties involved—researchers pursuing science, and IRBs protecting subjects—may have certain advantages. How departments would approach and resolve these conflicts of interest is unclear.

Though increasingly proposed, centralized IRBs (CIRBs) may have inherent COIs as well. For-profit IRBs, for instance, get paid to approve protocols.[15] CIRB members, too, may know and potentially want to aid or hinder PIs. Hence *both* local and centralized IRBs may have COIs, which need to be weighed in discussions about changing the status quo.

The fact that institutional support of committees may increase after a scandal, but subsequently diminish over time, is troubling. Unfortunately, human nature is such that at times, only avoidance of crisis, not appeal to ethics will impel such improvements. But for getting more resources, other means besides scandals would be best. Some institutions respond to scandals elsewhere, and preventively bolster their IRBs; but especially as broader financial constraints continue, such additional funding may decrease, potentially constraining IRBs and prompting added problems. IRBs may try to charge fees, but doing so can trigger difficult negotiations and tensions concerning when and how much academic boards should charge for reviewing protocols, and who should keep the money.

Though IRBs now minimize or dismiss complaints they receive from researchers (e.g., that IRBs are interpreting the regulations in ways that PIs feel are overly stringent and impede research), researchers also complain to institutional leaders and national policymakers. Committees might therefore benefit from being more responsive to researcher feedback. Still, IRBs should obviously not necessarily simply comply with all PI requests.

Questions arise of how much support IRBs do and should receive. Future research can explore more fully whether and to what degree more resources enhance the quality of reviews—for instance, whether relatively higher IRB budgets reduce PI frustrations and tensions or violations of research ethics. Ethical questions emerge, too, of how institutions should split limited resources between IRBs *vs.* other competing needs. Institutions should also be more aware of the costs of *not* providing more resources to IRBs. To persuade funders and institutions to "pay" for ethics is often difficult. Institutional leaders may find it hard to justify such expenses, given competing needs. Hence, standards and expectations are needed for approximately how much funding IRBs need to protect human subjects appropriately.

Many IRBs struggle with institutional contexts that can affect committee decisions. But, anecdotally, PIs generally appear unaware of these restraints. More explicit awareness of these institutional constraints among IRBs, PIs, and institutional officials can potentially help ameliorate IRB relationships with researchers. In sum, these institutional contexts can generate COIs that affect IRBs in several ways. CIRBs eliminate some of these tensions, but could potentially foster others. In both cases, ever-vigilant management of such moral challenges is key.

IRBs *VS.* RESEARCHERS

CHAPTER 10

Trusting *vs.* Policing Researchers

As we saw in Chapters 4 and 6, some IRBs demanded that Kathleen Dziak alter her study, with one board requiring that subjects explicitly send in a card and opt in to receive a questionnaire. Other committees allowed her to mail her survey to *all* subjects, and have those who wished to opt out do so simply by not completing it. The response rates and types of respondents then differed, such that she could no longer compare the data from the different sites. Still, she felt that she had no choice except to comply with these IRB decisions.

"IRBs have tremendous power," researchers have repeatedly told me in focus groups and conversations. "They can stop or change studies." Given these problems, in recent decades tensions between IRBs and researchers have mounted, with many investigators decrying these boards as "the Ethics Police."[1] Yet little systematic attention has been given to whether IRBs recognize or respond to these grievances, and if so, how, and with what results.

Researchers may cooperate fully with IRBs, or remain wary; and committees must decide how much to trust and monitor investigators. But these two groups disagree even over whether these boards have power, and if so, how much. How then should we understand these dramatically differing perspectives?

Researchers complain of IRB overreach, delays, and adversarial stances.[2] For instance, 84 percent of IRB members, *vs.* only 64 percent of investigators, felt their IRB "runs with reasonable efficiency."[3] Scientists protest the extension of these boards beyond their original intent and mission. But surprisingly, little if any research has examined how committees view these issues, whether they try to address these tensions, and if so, how; and what else, if anything, can be done to ameliorate these animosities.

IRBs generally feel good about their work and that they have relatively little power; researchers feel the opposite. Yet these two groups must be able to achieve some measure of common ground to do their respective jobs properly. As seen in Figure 10.1, I discovered that IRBs typically feel they have no power, or only very little—because they are "merely following the regulations," have an "open,"

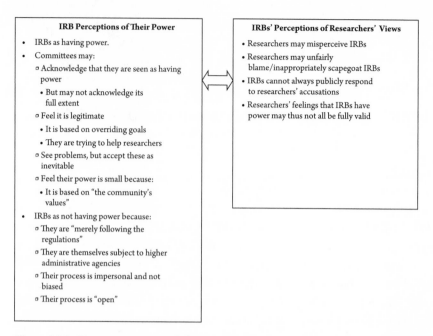

Figure 10.1 Themes concerning differing views of power and PI complaints among IRBs

impersonal, and unbiased process, and are themselves beholden to higher administrative agencies. How can these views conflict so markedly?

Differing Views of the Nature and Causes of Researcher Complaints

DO IRBS THINK THEY HAVE POWER?

IRBs often recognize friction between themselves and investigators, but tend to view the nature and causes of these conflicts very differently than researchers do. Several interviewees acknowledged that their IRB had considerable authority, but they then focused only on particular aspects of it. "My IRB is pretty darn powerful," Patrick said. "I've been amazed at how many consent forms they will actually send back. We're really hard on the informed consent form." But the basis of this statement—that the IRB can force changes in consent forms—refers to only one relatively small manifestation of IRBs' authority.

Some interviewees saw their IRBs as powerful, but felt that that this power was legitimate and deserved, even if tensions ensued. "We respect the PIs as scientists, but they are going to have to do things *our* way," Jeff reported. "In two or three instances, they thought, 'Who the hell are you . . . to tell me that?' "

Other interviewees agree they have power, but feel it is warranted because of their overriding goals—protecting subjects and optimizing the quality of protocols. As Dwayne, the rural researcher and chair, said,

> PIs think the IRB has a lot of power because they can't proceed without approval. But we're there to *help you* get your protocol up to snuff. And the consent form and all the elements of the consent are now templated on the website. PIs just have to fill things out.

But definitions of "up to snuff," and whether this term refers to the science or the ethics involved, can vary. Dwayne also suggests that the straightforward nature of these forms means that the IRB approval is easy to acquire if one simply follows directions—again seeming to minimize researcher concerns.

IRBs may dismiss the notion that they have power, too, because they see themselves as simply aiding researchers follow the regulations. Robin reflected,

> The IRB has power in the sense that we can tell someone they can't do a study, but we've never done that. We can certainly tell them that they need to do it in a certain way. So the IRB has certain power. *But we're just trying to help the PI navigate through*—to do good research, but to do it in a way that navigates the federal rules appropriately.

Robin's comment, like Dwayne's, suggests both an ethical and an intellectual dimension. Her IRB is helping the PIs "do good research," which, she says, is being consistent with following the regulations.

Robin states that her IRB has not entirely rejected studies but, as we have seen, interpretations of the regulations can vary. This may be because, as a social science IRB chair, she primarily reviews minimal-risk research. In contrast, IRBs that review more invasive biomedical research may be likelier to block or fundamentally alter studies.

Some IRB members feel that their power is legitimate because it is based on "community standards"—they see themselves as representatives of a much larger group. However, as mentioned earlier, discrepancies between IRBs very often reflect other factors—having been recently "shut down" by OHRP, or having a "user-friendly" ethos—more than variations in community values.[4] Moreover, the absence of an external appeals process can bolster an IRB's position, impeding any challenges to its idiosyncrasies or subjectivity.

Others feel that researchers have an exaggerated sense of IRBs' authority. "I believe the IRB has power, but not too much," Maggie said. "But scientists would probably disagree with that. We have the power to stop a protocol."

Within an institution, several factors may affect the extent of a committee's power. For instance, the IRB chair may also head an academic department, and thus have additional weight. Such institutional authority appears very important in backing the IRB. Scott, the director at an institution with a CRO, explained that his IRB chair was also a department chair, and the administration strongly supported the iRB. Hence, as mentioned earlier, he got less resistance from PIs."

IRBs also vary significantly in how they *express* their power, how much they draw attention to it in interactions with researchers, and whether it thus proves productive or corrosive. Committees may rigorously challenge researchers, instilling apprehension; and researchers may see then these boards as harsh or insensitive. Nonetheless, these committees may justify these approaches. Gwen said,

> We have a little bit of a reputation of *grilling* investigators when they come in, and I think they're a little bit nervous when they walk in. But I don't think that's necessarily bad, because I don't think everybody should feel like it's a cake walk—that everything's going to get passed.

She suggests that fear of the IRB is good, because it encourages researchers to be more responsible and prepared. But presumably some happy medium exists between a "cake walk" and being interrogated under intense pressure.

Some interviewees recognized that perceptions of an IRB can influence in unfortunate ways what studies PIs choose or avoid. A researcher may decide not to pursue certain studies because of fears of rejection from the IRB. Phil, a social scientist and chair, reflected,

> Some faculty have learned to become strategic about projects, to avoid IRB review, and don't study vulnerable populations. But then [researchers] don't study children. For instance, one couldn't do a naturalistic study of bullying in the schoolyard.

Several interviewees do not see themselves as having power, and said they do not even understand these assertions. As Cynthia, an administrator, reflected,

> I don't really get it when the FDA says the IRB has so much power. It's only through regulations. And if things are designed according to the regulations, then it's not a matter of power.

A mandate to follow regulations does not, however, necessarily preclude the existence of power—nor does it guarantee that that power is correctly used. Police officers have also said that they don't feel they have power because they are simply following the law. Yet police have been accused of racial profiling—not enforcing the law equally with all citizens. Since the police can decide when and how to employ their authority, they have been described as having "discretionary power."[5] Given the discrepancies in how IRBs choose to interpret and apply regulations, these committees appear to have discretionary power as well.

Interviewees may not feel powerful because they are vulnerable to criticism from all sides: the researchers, the administration, and the federal government. They may also feel they lack potency because they are often disrespected. "Where are IRBs very powerful, and not the objects of scorn?" Cynthia asked.

Cynthia suggests that her IRB isn't powerful because it isn't vindictive. She continued,

> We don't have the power to say, "That doctor was really rude to us last year: he complained at the faculty meeting about how the IRB was slow, and lost studies. OK, we'll fix him! We'll put him on the July agenda."

But in minimizing her committee's authority because it does not abuse its mandate to pursue personal vendettas, she may in fact be creating a "straw dog," unfairly characterizing researcher criticisms of IRBs.

Committees may also dismiss claims that they have power because their processes are transparent and "open." As Cynthia elaborated,

> We're real visible here. At some hospitals, researchers submit stuff to the IRBs, and it's a closed door. They can't enter the sanctum. At our IRB, all the staff are available all of the time without appointment. You just come in. PIs know me.

Cynthia's statements all suggest that she sees the *expression* of the committee's power as key to its reception: the committee is objective, fair, and open. But that does not mean that her IRB lacks power.

"HOW THEY SEE US": RESPONDING TO RESEARCHERS' PERCEPTIONS

Committees often see themselves as misunderstood by researchers. Investigators may unfairly hold the IRB responsible for setbacks in their research. PIs may turn in late, incomplete, or sloppy forms, and then unjustifiably fault a committee, exacerbating tensions. As Cynthia said:

> If a PI can't start a study—a sponsor was unable to, or decided not to use the site—the IRB is always a good place to blame: "If it hadn't been for the IRB!...We lost that study because the IRB didn't act quickly

enough." OK, well, let's see the protocol: it says it was issued last July, and it's coming over here in February...We can be the source of all joy or all sorrow, depending on how their grant funding worked out.

Again, PIs may "blame the messenger"—i.e., the IRB—simply for needing to follow federal regulations.

Researchers may have practical complaints about their IRB—the long time it takes to get a protocol reviewed, for example, or the wording on a consent form that might discourage patients from signing it—or PIs may have broader concerns, such as perceived infringements on intellectual liberty. "The IRB became the *villain*," Phil, the social scientist, said, "for all the other incursions on academic freedom."

Much of this blame appears inappropriately placed, but the ability to thwart another's desires can be seen as an expression of power, which may thus be partly in the eyes of the beholder. Nonetheless, IRBs emerge here as, in effect, "caught in the middle" between federal regulations and agencies on the one hand (serving as their local interpreter, enforcer, and "face") and local PIs on the other.

Some felt that the IRB was simply an easy target. Researchers may complain to institutional leaders who may then either pressure IRBs or send protocols instead to for-profit CIRBs. Stephen, a chair at an institution that recently began using such a CIRB, said,

> A lot of the political pressure, or frustration with our whole review system was directed at the IRB when, in reality, I think we were doing pretty good with our turnarounds. *Other* reviews—the scientific advisory committee, and the grants and contracts office—were becoming problematic. Maybe we can turn it around a little quicker. But I don't think studies are necessarily starting any quicker—because of budget issues, or the hospital representative has a problem with an injury compensation statement that we're just fine with. It was a PR problem. Many times the IRB was the fall guy. It's easy and quick to say, "It's *their* fault." Rather than...figuring out where all the other delays are. It was easier to say, "Let's take this to the Western IRB and get our turnaround times improved."

An IRB's position may be complicated by the fact that it cannot publicly respond if scientists loudly criticize it within an institution. Phil observed that such constrained communication can aggravate strains.

> People assume the IRB is the big-evil-regulating-snooty-bureaucracy, and that the researcher did everything right. But we can't say, "The PI might have said this, but here's the truth."

Still, committees may also misperceive or dismiss researcher complaints. "There are always going to be complaints," Troy said, "if you don't give people exactly what they want when they want it." As he suggests, criticism may inevitably persist. Yet boards may also fail to appreciate underlying tensions and potential solutions. "PIs are primarily concerned with how quickly a project can be approved with minimal comments," Scott said. "So, IRBs need additional staff to absorb the workload." In some cases, however, not only a paucity of resources, but also IRB members' attitudes, may need to be addressed.

PI Oversight: How much should they be trusted?

IRBs faced quandaries of how much to monitor investigators—whether to police researchers more closely or to adopt the honor system. "How can we be sure we're compliant with regs, other than *the honor system*, and some audit of larger, complicated studies?" Greg, a social scientist and chair, asked.

THE NEED FOR OTHER POLICE

Some IRBs feel that they should not be the police, but that *someone* needs to be. IRBs may consciously try not to fill this role because their institution has created another office to do so. A compliance office, not the IRB, may be the enforcer. Scott did not feel that policing PIs was the IRB's job:

> The Compliance Office was created for that—on conflict of interest, scientific misconduct, and time and effort reporting. They are the *enforcement arm* of the institution.

As we saw earlier, however, the relationship between these two sets of offices can vary between institutions. Compliance offices receive information reported by PIs, but are often seen as having less power than IRBs because the guidelines they interpret (e.g., whether a researcher has more than $5,000 of financial interest in a company related to his/her research) are generally more straightforward, with little if any latitude, rather than dealing with abstract ethical principles.

When Researchers Compete with Subjects as the Principal IRB "Clients"
IRBs may differ, too, in perceiving their overall mission. Several committees see themselves as "adopting a business model," "serving" rather than "policing" researchers, and having "clients" whose cooperation they actively have to enlist. But these committees vary as to whether they see their primary clients as

investigators, subjects, funders, or the institution. Some IRBs say they are also involved in protecting themselves.

These various aims may all be correct to some degree, but collide. Many IRBs perceive their main goal as protecting subjects, and researchers' main task as conducting research. As Stephen said,

> I see our customers as subjects, investigators, the institution, and regulators. Many of them have different priorities. Investigators' highest priority is to get their research approved very quickly, and they see the IRB as more of an impediment. The institution has big grants: "We've got to get this going, and can't make any changes."

IRBs generally say their goal is shielding subjects, not institutions, but in fact these boards often seem to be protecting both. When an institution's lawyers attend IRB meetings, the board can face heightened disagreements over how much to weigh each of these client's needs.

Interviewees may admit multiple goals but then struggle to prioritize them. While some chairs see their mission as merely "protecting subjects," others acknowledge these additional aims as well. Louis listed three sets of priorities in order. "My first clients are the subjects. Second is protecting the interests of the university. Third is the faculty."

Committees usually strive to *focus* on protecting subjects, yet occasionally need to remind themselves of that goal. "We do a good job," Charlotte said, "of not getting locked into protecting the institution, but staying focused on the *subject*." Other committees, however, may not do as well.

Assessing the Trustworthiness of Strangers

Every university may have a certain small proportion of difficult researchers. "As good as the institution is," Jeremy said, "there are problem players." Most scientists are, as Andrea said, "pretty ethical," but "bad apples" exist. The frequency of "lapses" is unknown—many go undetected, and they can be defined in different ways. Violations can represent minor oversights or major cheating. IRBs therefore have to decide when and to what degree to trust each researcher, and how much, if at all, to "police" him or her.

IRBs' work becomes more arduous as they review more protocols from researchers whom they do not personally know. Bureaucracy can *both result from, and generate,* diminished trust. Indeed, heightened IRB regulation may reflect the fact that more researchers are conducting research without other formal or informal monitoring.

While in the past, IRB members may have interacted personally with researchers, that is no longer the case at many institutions—especially large ones. "The biggest issue we have is: who's qualified to do research," Christopher said. "We have a lot of turnover. When we don't know the PIs, it's hard to evaluate the protocols." He highlights the importance, emotionally, of knowing the PI personally outside of the protocol alone. In the past, before research burgeoned, "We knew all the scientists," he said; thus reviews may have been less difficult.

Boards thus must choose how much faith to have in each PI and how to decide. Such confidence may be based on reputation.[6] But to assess reputation regarding ethical behavior can be difficult. As the sociologist Max Weber wrote, bureaucratization results from needs for efficiency,[7] but emphasizes formality and inflexibility rather than flexibility or interpersonal relationships, or the need to take into account the details of specific cases.[8] In running any complex organization smoothly, however, flexibility can be critical; but requires trust. IRBs need confidence that researchers will do what they say, and report any adverse events that occur. Such faith in PIs is crucial. Confidence can be mutually reinforced—if I trust you more, you may then trust me more as well[9]—but can be fragile. "At times, trust breaks down," Stephen reflected. These interviewees describe challenges in assessing and building such mutual faith. Tensions exist, and adverse events and problems cannot always be predicted.

Economic constraints aggravate these problems. Junior faculty may be doing more research and, due to tightened budgets, departments may supervise it less. As Christopher said,

> Our state's financial turmoil has led to a huge turnover. A lot of the experienced, seasoned investigators have left. So Fellows are made PIs on protocols. We don't know their names. We've not been on committees with them for 10 years. Just because they did online IRB training doesn't mean they're qualified to lead a clinical trial.

Moreover, some hospitals have started to conduct research—partly after pharmaceutical companies persuade them—without having their own IRB. Committees at other institutions must then review these protocols. Christopher added,

> The hospital is hiring its own researchers who aren't faculty members. Certain departments aren't based here anymore. So who's vetting the science and the PI's qualifications?

To compensate for the lack of knowledge, he thought it would be helpful to collect information on unknown investigators' prior research experiences in supervising staff and writing protocols and consent forms. Committees often feel that online ethics training of PIs is necessary, but insufficient.

Conversely, especially at smaller institutions, IRBs may know, or meet with, all investigators. Charlotte said, "Because we're small, we can easily call a special meeting, bring in all the investigators, and try to find a middle ground." Such communication can enhance collaboration and cooperation.

Having a well-respected faculty member as a chair can strengthen relationships with not just institutional officials but PIs. As Troy said,

> The head of the IRB office is a long-term faculty member, here many years. So he knows almost everybody. Researchers are very responsive to him. He's also very good-natured. The guy who preceded him was tough as nails—hard to deal with.

Given expanded research enterprises with multimillion budgets, institutions cannot rely wholly on informal collaborations and relationships; yet overly bureaucratic approaches can burden both investigators and boards.

Researchers' Responses to IRBs

Most investigators attempt to collaborate with IRBs—after all, collaboration is mandated and in their best interests—but failures occur, and range from minor and inadvertent to more serious and obstructionistic. Researchers' ignorance or nonchalance about federal regulations can frustrate committees. Investigators may rail against IRBs rather than try to understand their larger rationale and purpose. As Troy said,

> Some PIs are extremely frustrating, and do it "their way." Their protocols keep coming back, and we try to work with them. Other PIs are a pleasure to deal with.

At times, researchers get annoyed and dismiss or fail to meet IRB requirements, or err in completing forms. A PI's repeated deficiencies in paperwork can anger IRBs. Dwayne, the rural researcher, said,

> Certain researchers have reputations—minor offenses, like using outdated consent forms. Sometimes that's a repeated offense. The IRB then has to watch them more closely. If someone fails an audit, we keep a close eye on them. The failure might not put a subject at any more risk, but goes against the rules. Occasionally, a researcher has done that more than once.

Yet committees must judge how severely to view an "offense" if it does not harm subjects. At times, the IRB may adopt more of a bureaucratic than a purely "ethical" perspective. These two roles blur, but the logistic one (e.g., regarding largely paperwork) may be harder to justify on moral grounds alone. On the other hand, repeated failures to comply with bureaucratic requirements might also signal a carelessness about ethical standards as well.

Interviewees often felt that relationships with PIs at their institutions were gradually improving, though certain problems can persist. Efforts on both sides can be mutually reinforcing. "We've had less outright resistance," Troy said, "but have also decreased our turnaround time." Many PIs and IRBs are now working together to reduce these strains.

Still, difficulties can remain; IRBs can be bothered by researchers' inadequate advance planning and anticipation of obstacles and protocol changes. Jeff, the social scientist and chair, complained of a PI who sent *too many* separate amendments to the IRB, submitting two in one week, rather than foreseeing and coordinating these.

> It goes on and on: he wants to change recruitment procedures, or tack on extra instruments and another procedure. It's just a blizzard of paperwork.... He should think ahead a bit more.

Researchers and IRBs may thus see each other as not fully respectful.

SLOPPINESS AND INATTENTION

Investigators exacerbate frictions by repeatedly neglecting or delaying forms. These behaviors may be prompted by frustration with the IRB, but in the end they prove counterproductive, eliciting reprimands and further postponements. Still, researchers may not recognize the detrimental effects of such behavior. "I've only seen IRBs really frustrated with a PI because he has continuously turned in sloppy work," Laura, the lawyer, said, "and refused to respond to our requests for information."

Protocols are sometimes incomplete or insufficiently detailed, creating a vicious cycle. As Jack, the rural physician and chair, described,

> One junior investigator wrote a pretty bad protocol—very open-ended: "We're going to do this, and see how it goes." What are your measures and statistical analyses? What's the dose exactly? He got really ticked off: "Well, it looks like you want me to have the paper written before I even do the clinical trial!" We tend to have better relations when we get *better protocols*!

In this instance, the PI was clearly insulted, but Jack felt rebuffed as well.

Proposals from senior PIs with more experience may be deficient for other reasons. As Olivia, the health care provider and chair, said, "Research associates may fill out the forms, and simply cut and paste old information, creating inconsistencies." Investigators with grants usually have research assistants who fill out all of the IRB paperwork. Some IRBs observed PI inattentiveness from entire academic departments.

An investigator may not allow enough time for the IRB to approve a study. PIs may want quick approval because of the timeframes of funders and/or collaborating institutions. As Louis said,

> The hardest issues we get are, "I got an NIH grant from another university, which approved it. I have until this date to send it back. Is there any way we can get this through?" I'm learning to tell them, "No," but with a smile. "I'm sorry. There's just nothing we can do. We'll do the best we can."

Researchers may also submit poorly written protocols because they are "too busy," and may not even fully read the protocol. As Christopher described,

> What drives me nuts as an IRB chair is when it's clear that the PI hasn't even *read* the consent form or the submission. There are typos that you know the PI would've caught if he or she had read it. So, it's just sloppiness.

In part, competing demands and involvement in numerous studies may spread investigators too thin. "Some PIs are on 40 or 50 different protocols," Christopher added. "How closely could they really monitor what's going on?...A lot of PIs don't take responsibility for what happens." Yet in undervaluing IRB protocols, and relegating these to junior staff, researchers may also "gloss over" risks, underestimating the potential harms they pose, and becoming insufficiently sensitive to subjects' rights.

In response, IRBs may demand that PIs engage in fewer studies. "Some we restrict: 'You can only do X number of protocols,'" Christopher continued. A researcher may be able to oversee only a few studies effectively, and play smaller roles in a handful of others. But an investigator may be involved in 10–20 different grants, if not more, partly because of the need to raise his or her own salary. Still, it is not clear what the maximum number allowed is or should be, and whether IRBs in fact have the right to limit researchers' work in this way.

Proposals of poor quality can also obscure key issues, leading both researchers and IRBs to overlook aspects of a study that later prove problematic. A committee may not, in retrospect, have perceived or pursued potential difficulties as much as they might. As Charlotte explained,

> One PI's writing is almost impossible to understand. So instead of picking it apart, and trying to paraphrase it, *the IRB just got burnt out,* and didn't pursue a lot of it. Because, "in the end it's just a behavioral study. How could you possibly harm anybody in a behavioral study?" She was getting child welfare records from county welfare offices. But they were *Indian* children. The county owns the records, and is the ward of the state for these foster children. But the Indians want a say in who gets access to their children's data—highly sensitive. We weren't savvy to that. Neither was the investigator. We just thought she was doing some sort of records check. But she was really going after sensitive data—with the permission of the county, but *not* of the Indians. Had we been able to understand where she was getting some of these data, we would have insisted that she get *tribal consent.* But we didn't really understand, because it was so poorly described.

How the IRB missed these issues—and how the PI had managed to get some information when the county said she needed Indian consent as well—is not apparent.

"PROTOCOL CREEP"

At times, PIs change protocols without first notifying the IRB, creating problems. Understandably, researchers in the field need to make clinically necessary decisions quickly; in ongoing clinical care, the investigator cannot wait for IRB approval. Hence, committees must allow for some flexibility. But how much?

Researchers may cause problems by not sticking to their approved protocols, and adding procedures without informing the IRB. Greg described such "protocol creep":

> A protocol was approved five years ago, and just had continuation reviews, but may have crept from observational ethnographies into drawing blood, and collecting genetic data, and things that may not have gotten documented. The researchers didn't tell the IRB. Over five years, this creep would add up. No one necessarily saw the entire protocol, or really noticed.

Investigators can also have a protocol approved but then not follow it. Jeremy, the physician, described researchers, "slipping in an extra CT scan, without getting us to approve it. That happens at a relatively low, but pretty consistent level."

These lapses may be relatively uncommon, and time consuming to catch; IRBs must decide how much to use their limited resources to monitor all studies for such problems in lieu of pursuing other tasks.

Researchers may also fail to update their consent forms as they should, incorporating new discoveries made outside a study—for instance, new side effects or scientific advances that had not have been previously reported and now need to be communicated to participants.

PIs may also intentionally manipulate the system, not simply by IRB shopping, as we saw earlier, but by altering a study once it is approved. In yearly continuing reviews, the chair is often the only reviewer to see the protocol, and may miss these alterations. An IRB may therefore find out about such changes only when the study is published—if then. Christopher's IRB prohibited such a researcher from conducting future studies.

> PIs may try to game the system by using expedited rather than full board approval, and then *bait and switch*. They get IRB approval, and then modify things a little bit. There's not a good way to catch it, because it's never been full-board approved. So, *the only person who sees it is the chair,* and he's not a physician, so sometimes gets fooled a bit. "This is going to be a retrospective chart review," but we're starting to add a few new scales. They might not even say they're adding these forms—they're just doing it "for clinical care." We find out about it sometimes when we audit for something else, or when a publication comes out. One PI said he wasn't doing research—only treating people with spinal cord injuries, and then referring them to a researcher. But he then wanted to publish, and it turns out he had collected all these measures. So he was banned from doing research.

Whether this investigator knew about IRB regulations and had intentionally tried to circumvent them, or was in fact ignorant of his breach, is unclear.

Researchers may not grasp the importance of either the situation or the issues it raises. Dwayne, the researcher and chair, said,

> They keep coming back, arguing with us, saying, "No, this is really low risk!" We keep saying, "No, we think it is riskier than you are saying. You need to change the language." Some researchers just don't see the light.

This last metaphor suggests broader religious or political conversion. It may reflect the "rightness" that many committee members feel adheres to their opinions; it also may suggest the importance of promoting a larger ethical culture within the institution as a whole.

RESEARCHER ARROGANCE

A researcher's interpersonal deficiencies and lack of sensitivity can exacerbate these problems. As Vicki pointed out, "Some people are difficult, 'high maintenance' prima donnas, but extremely productive." She continued:

> Other people just don't think very clearly, so we get a lot of go-around, but eventually straighten it out. With other people, we have trouble for a long time, but some become our best customers.

Scientists can antagonize not only IRBs, but communities of patients— especially those already wary of research. Charlotte, the administrator, said,

> One researcher was working with a vulnerable, under-represented population, and managed to piss off most of them. [They] then wanted to get out of the study, and wanted their neighbors out, and never wanted to see us again.

Committees may thus try to prevent investigators from harming both communities and future studies.

Social Scientists and IRBs

With social scientists, many of these battles appear with particular force. As we saw earlier, in recent years the federal government has emphasized that social science research needs IRB review, yet the regulations were designed primarily for biological sciences. Social scientists often see these federal requirements as inapplicable and unnecessarily burdensome. Committee experience with social science also varies, fostering inconsistencies between boards. While some IRBs feel very comfortable reviewing social science, others have far less knowledge and familiarity, and hence are far more cautious. "The IRB approach in social sciences isn't working well," Kurt, a researcher and chair, said. "Social scientists find it's silly or restrictive. The risks are probably not great enough to justify what IRBs do." Indeed, a large part of the Obama Administration's proposals are aimed at revamping IRB approaches to social science.

Especially if they don't have much experience with social science, IRBs may not only vary, but be overly rigid, delaying studies. "IRBs may approve it," Charlotte said, "but take a *really long time*, taking it to the full board for review when it really doesn't need to be." The boards may not have major concerns, but the process can nevertheless be lengthy and onerous. She continued,

> When our social science studies finally get to the IRB at another institution—say, a medical IRB—they are generally approved without too much flutter or comment. But just getting there is *painful*.

Social scientists may also strongly resist IRBs' perceived mandates. Researchers may not want, for instance, to inform subjects as much as possible about a study; or may use deception, and debrief subjects afterwards. Yet committees may oppose such approaches. Dana, a social scientist and chair, said,

> One social scientist has a little *tantrum* every time she has to submit something to the IRB. She does individual interviews, and is going to generalize about these people's lives. I say, "Then you have to consent them. They have to know what's going on." To me it seems an honesty issue: telling people what they're getting in to. I don't think she would necessarily *not* tell people. But she might not *fully* tell people what's going to happen.

Still, questions arise of exactly how much information is needed.

Some IRBs worked more successfully with social scientists after having enticed leaders from social science departments to join the committee. Joe's IRB put together a psychosocial advisory board, including fairly senior leaders in the departments that had had many protocols with problems—"a group of strong, highly visible faculty to be the leaders, who had credibility—mid-level or senior researchers, who have some clout." Such a mechanism may aid other IRBs as well, assisting researchers and decreasing the number of complaints.

Some institutions have also established a separate social science IRB, which can have expertise in these methods. As Joe reported,

> Researchers know these various boards' members and can go to them.... Since we've given social science investigators a voice, by taking their concerns seriously, we've had fewer unhappy campers.

Open *vs.* Closed Doors: Responses to Conflicts with Researchers

In response to investigator complaints, several committees try to improve relationships and "not be the Ethics Police," but range in how and to what degree. Much attention has been given to researchers' complaints,[10,11,12,13] but little if any to IRB responses to these. IRBs may know that they are seen as "obstructionistic," but try either to address these perceptions or not to be troubled by them. IRBs tend to feel they aid PIs, but may differ widely in how and to what degree. Given their respective conflicting primary mandates to do research *vs.* protect subjects, tensions between IRBs and PIs may be inherent. Nonetheless, both sides can potentially reduce these strains. In both formal social structures and the content and tone of interactions with researchers, committees vary considerably.

FROM ANONYMITY TO "OPEN DOORS"

As shown in Figure 10.2, IRBs range from being open and accessible to distant and anonymous. Chairs generally say that they are supportive of PIs, but differ in how and to what degree.

IRB Anonymity

Much of IRBs' work occurs behind closed doors, yet this lack of transparency may contribute to researchers' frustration and demonization of boards. Chairs range in how much they keep committee members anonymous to shield these reviewers from researchers' criticism. Board membership may be automatically secret, optionally secret, or wholly public.

To avoid friction with PIs, reviewers assigned to specific protocols are usually unknown to the researcher. But this lack of identifiability can fuel acrimony by potentially delaying or hampering personal interactions and the facilitation of reviews. Scott, the director at an institution with a CRO, gave reviewers a choice:

> The cancer researchers know who the cancer reviewers are.... However, friction from that confrontation is held to a minimum. We give members

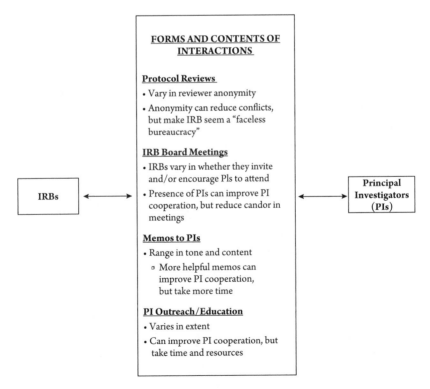

Figure 10.2 Reponses of IRBs to tensions with PIs

an option of whether to reveal themselves or not when communicating to PIs prior to committee meetings. We respect reviewers' desire for anonymity and confidentiality. If members have questions for a PI, they can go through IRB staff instead.

IRBs may have developed their own group processes and culture regarding openness to researchers, which can be difficult to change. A new chair may want members to "reach out" to investigators, and add reviewers, or dismiss members who always want anonymity. Scott continued,

> I've removed any member from the IRB who wants to remain perma-nently anonymous... That's just pure old marketing, and good will with our researchers. That's how we change the perception here of the IRB.

Hence, some IRBs may see themselves as having to "market" their services to actively engender support from PIs. When Scott revamped the IRB to improve relationships with researchers, he asked a dozen members to leave:

> ... because most of them had no desire to communicate with investi-gators prior to meetings. One of the prerequisites to then becoming a member was willingness to reach out and contact PIs prior to committee meetings. At times, they kept confidentiality when it was a personal col-league, or friend, or someone they work with closely. That's OK.

Members can therefore vary in their interest and willingness to communicate with PIs—how much they "reach out."

Similarly, although at present committees keep all minutes and correspon-dence private, heightened transparency could potentially improve investigators' perceptions of IRBs. "Minutes are not now publicly available, but *should* be," Phil said. "I guess researchers may feel it's embarrassing to have your stuff rejected." But that reason may not sufficiently offset the countervailing advantages of open-ness. Proprietary information (e.g., that companies are hoping to use to obtain a patent) could be removed, as could certain other details. Researchers, if they knew that IRB feedback about their studies might be seen by others, may be moti-vated, too, to submit higher quality protocols.

"Open Door" Policies

Many chairs also seek to improve relationships with PIs through the structure and quality of other kinds of interactions, striving to maintain "open doors" by making themselves directly and highly accessible to PIs via e-mail, phone, or cell phone. These types of physical and logistical *structures* of interaction can shape psychological and social attitudes and vice versa. As Charlotte, the small-institution administrator, said,

> Our approach here is: "Please call." Not: "We're out to get you." With a lot of IRBs, the relationship and rapport they have with the faculty causes the problem. PIs don't want to deal with them, as opposed to picking up the phone and trying to get some information. That's just a general philosophy, tone, and culture.

Both implicit and explicit IRB attitudes and practices can range.

As mentioned earlier, in response to criticisms from researchers, institutions and/or IRB chairs may even reorganize committees. Institutional leaders and chairs may thus revamp these boards due not only to their own observations but also investigators' feedback. As Scott said,

> The reorganization happened because of the usual complaints from PIs—lack of communication, board members being secretive. There was a general sense of unease, discomfort, and lack of credibility. It took two years.

In response to a researcher's opposition and angry calls, a few IRBs may reconsider their decision, but most appeared hesitant to do so—in part for fear of being perceived as susceptible to intimidation. As Jeremy said,

> We make decisions based on what we think is right. *Even if we end up being wrong, we're not changing what we do because somebody's yelling at us.* If we feel somebody has a legitimate complaint, we're always open to the idea—we realize we're not perfect—we're all ears, and we'll try to fix it, and make it right.... If somebody's unhappy, we absolutely want to understand why. Some of the time, it's at our end. Sometimes it's their misunderstanding. We try to gather data and sort it out.

Yet other IRBs are far more reluctant to alter their decisions.

Outreach and PR Work

Boards vary, too, in the amount and type of public relations ("PR work") and outreach they do with PIs. Some committees strive hard to convey the message that "we're not the enemy." As Kevin, the health care provider and chair, said,

> Our open forums and educational sessions have helped because the IRB consists of human beings—not like the FDA. [We] are approachable, and will listen to reason.

Hence, IRBs can try to improve their image and dispel the notion that they are faceless bureaucrats. But as Kevin cautioned about the effects of this outreach, "it has a short half-life."

Interviewees felt that PIs may blame the IRBs for trying to make studies conform to the regulations, yet IRBs can often alter this perception by being less impersonal and anonymous, adapting their approaches over time. As Dana, a social scientist and chair, said,

> Our IRB has done years of public relations work all over campus saying, "We're not here to hurt you. We're here to help you. How can we assist?" That hasn't *always* been the case here.

Several interviewees also felt that IRBs could better publicize the useful work they do, and get more credit for it. As Dwayne added,

> We can improve our public image by portraying some of the positive sides as well. The committee should toot its horn to the research community: here's what we do. I wish [committees] would talk more about their successes—good stories about the IRB. We just went through a huge audit of a study. Maybe the IRB sent ideas to the investigator to improve the study to make it ethical.... Researchers here just published a study in the *New England Journal of Medicine*. We could say—even if just in the university newsletter—we looked at this study.

Some IRBs may go further, asking investigators directly how the IRB can improve these relationships. Committees can therefore be very strategic, by being proactive and targeting leery researchers. "We have identified departments that are particularly hard to work with," Dana continued, "and said, 'Can we come talk to you? Let us know how we can work with you.'"

Certain committees explicitly try to reverse PIs' negative perceptions by giving the message, "We're not *devils*," as Dwayne said. "We're doing a good job"—seeking to counter a metaphor of evil (i.e., "devils"). Interviewees frequently employed metaphors that evoked both criminality and theology—both social and moral wrongs. New chairs may adopt methods that the IRB had not previously used at that institution. Anthony, for instance, started calling new PIs himself:

> I just picked up the phone..."Can I come and show you what this is all about? Because I know you're not going to know."...I tell them it's going to make life a whole lot easier.

A few chairs emphasized *two-way* education. Anthony also invites researchers to educate the IRB, and he feels this message has been effective.

> If we have new methodologies, protocols—where the committee is frankly just ignorant....We usually invite that investigator to come in....Investigators feel we're willing to be taught, and reach out.

Pre-reviews by IRB Members

To facilitate assessments, many committees have established various forms of IRB "pre-review," though these range considerably in nature, extent, and effectiveness, having different costs and benefits to different stakeholders. Some IRBs have their own members or staff conduct these pre-reviews, which can be very cost effective: such a pre-review can avoid requiring a whole committee to reconsider a protocol multiple times. IRBs may in fact require or encourage reviewers, before presenting protocols at meetings, to speak in advance to PIs to try to address any questions. Such prior discussions with PIs can be very helpful. "We can head off issues," Kevin, the chair, said, "and help PIs with the IRB red tape." Such informal openness and availability can reduce the time to get approval. It is, however, by no means universal.

Pre-review also carries with it a different sort of risk: a full IRB assessment may identify problems that didn't arise in the pre-review, incensing researchers who assumed their protocol would go through. Elaine said,

> We quit corresponding with the investigators ahead of time, because they would say, "Well, they didn't catch this during the *pre*-review." That's why a committee has all these different people. I can catch some stuff, but not everything.

Inadvertently, such pre-reviews can thus generate conflicts. Some reviewers also resist contacting PIs in advance because doing so takes time, and criticizing a colleague's work can be personally and professionally awkward. Though an outsider may not be surprised that IRBs catch scientific problems that scientific pre-review committees did not, pre-review is meant to address scientific concerns so that a second review does not need to do so. Clearly, however, scientific quality and ways of enhancing it are not wholly simple, straightforward, and objective, but vary across a wide spectrum.

Several chairs have pushed hard for "open doors" due to their own personal, political, and/or bureaucratic philosophy. Joe, for instance, was "an old [West Coast] hippie in the 60s" and, consequently, wary of bureaucracies; he tries "to be accessible." Robin, as a lawyer, also tries to avoid "policing" researchers. "I hate being the enforcer.... That's not fun. That's not what I do this for." Yet at times, many committee members nevertheless seem to adopt this role.

Other factors, such as the ways that a physical office is organized, can shape IRB–researcher relationships as well. As Cynthia, an administrator, said,

> At times, it has more to do with physical office design: we don't have a receptionist. When we had someone between us and the world, PIs said that I "suddenly started screening calls," or "didn't have an 'open door' policy anymore." Now, researchers feel they can just come in and sit down, and we can talk about their protocol—what they haven't addressed, whether they can address it, and whether I can explain to the board... that it's on its way.

At many institutions, investigators are often invited by committees to meetings, but do not attend. Potentially, such attendance could improve relationships—showing that IRBs are trying to be reasonable, and that PIs are willing to cooperate with them. Frequently, chairs are surprised that researchers do not accept these invitations, but PIs probably feel they are too busy. Dwayne, the rural researcher and chair, said,

> It's an open forum meeting. We tell all researchers to come. But they won't. It's a two- or three-hour evening meeting, though they don't have to come to the whole thing. It would help if they could look around the table and see their colleagues, and people from the lay community, and clergymen: *this isn't a group of cynics and big red pens.* We really discuss the issues... [and are] all pretty reasonable.

Even if clarification of the protocol isn't needed, the PI can observe the board, and see that it has the best intentions. Yet Dwayne's language reflects his sense of the committee as judgmental, punitive teachers, ready to fail the pupil under review.

Such joint meetings can also prompt IRBs to be more sensitive to researchers. It is harder to be overly harsh and insensitive to a PI when meeting him or her in person, rather than interacting only through memos. Anthony continued:

> It's tempting, and easier, to sit around a table and be really tough and critical and blunt when we have some anonymous individual... a name there, but nobody knows them. When you have met the individual, you tend to temper those kinds of remarks. Even if ultimately, the message is the same, we've backed off on the brute force.

Some committees have the PI come and present. The board asks questions, but then decides in private. Nonetheless, some IRBs may eschew such colloquies.

"We don't give PIs an opportunity to appear at the meetings," Scott said, "because we review too much." Other IRBs feel that even that arrangement could produce awkwardness (e.g., a researcher can later grill members who were present about why they made certain decisions). But the benefits of such openness may far outweigh these costs.

Over time, committees may also change in openness one way or the other. "In the past, the IRB would have investigators go to the meeting," Elaine said. "Now they've closed them, which is helpful." Other boards still struggle over what to do.

To address investigator concerns outside of formal reviews *per se*, several IRBs have established "clinics" and other mechanisms. Greg, a social scientist and chair, said,

> We started doing clinics. Researchers can meet with a subset of the IRB, and talk about what they want to do, and how to write their protocol. That helped...[and] worked through questions that had stymied the investigator from putting the protocol in. Mostly, they were afraid their protocols wouldn't get through. Everybody really appreciated it—both the IRB members—because they got better protocols—and the investigators—because they better understood the processes, and could then write better protocols.

Such clinics enhanced transparency and communication. Greg thought that they showed researchers "what we're thinking and brought them into the process, rather than just dropping the protocol off in some box with a closed door."

The online or in-print newsletters with updates (e.g., a "tip of the week") that other IRBs established could also improve relationships. Researchers "are not in the *IRB world*," Kevin explained. "They said, 'We'd like to know ahead of time what's going on.'...It was easy to e-mail."

IRBs may also send out such "tips" in response to errors PIs may make. Such advice may forestall additional potential problems. Kevin tries "to put federal regulations into a real world environment." Many IRBs do not have such newsletters or suggestions, but easily could do so.

At the same time, these efforts can consume much of a chair or administrator's time. IRB personnel who spend a lot of time with researchers to diminish a committee's reputation of being obstructionistic generally find that these efforts take more hours than their compensation covers. Kevin said his time is billed at 20 percent, but is really 35–40 percent. He spends more time "because I am so sick and tired of hearing that the IRB is a roadblock or a stumbling block....I work very hard with our investigators to make that not the case."

The extra time required for such enhanced IRB availability can force difficult tradeoffs. Chairs and administrators can become overwhelmed, and need to balance "open doors" *vs.* limited resources.

While some chairs are highly concerned about PI complaints and try hard to reduce these, others are far less responsive or flexible, remaining more removed and interacting with researchers more indirectly. Committees may try to strive for a balance (e.g., to adopt an overall "open" policy), but also remain firm with difficult PIs. Jeremy, the physician and chair, said,

> Some people are chronically unhappy—complainers. No matter what we do, they're unhappy. So, we try to be diplomatic, gracious, and non-confrontational, but hold our ground. We're not going to cave in just because somebody is yelling at us.

Helpful Memos

IRBs also often strive to improve the quantity and quality of written communication with individual PIs, but range in how and to what degree. Both the content and the tone of communication and interactions can be critical. Some chairs write lengthy memos to researchers, responding to submitted protocols, and assisting these investigators in rewriting these studies. Jeremy, the physician and chair, said, "For a very flawed study, I am much more likely to write back a three-page letter with 20 points, basically re-writing the protocol for them, than I am to disapprove it." Yet since these efforts can take time, chairs and staff need to choose carefully when to make such efforts.

If an investigator has a track history of poorly written proposals, the IRB may simply invest much less energy. "Some people just want you to write the darn thing for them," Elaine said. "That's not my job." Jeremy recalled:

> I disapproved one from an investigator with a track record of submitting flawed protocols, and sloppy work—making us do a tremendous amount of work. Instead of doing the work for him for the fifth time, I said, "No. Here are the major problems. Fix it." Instead of a three-page letter, I write a half-page letter...and put the ball back into their court.

Researchers may not appreciate or respond to these efforts as IRBs hope. After receiving the aforementioned three-page memo, this researcher never resubmitted his proposal. "My guess is that he couldn't fix it, and was overwhelmed," Jeremy said. "He is not a good researcher. But, for 99 percent of researchers, the concerns are fixable. They fix them, respond, and move on." To enhance relationships with investigators, other IRBs might adopt such strategies as well.

Charm: Establishing the Right Tone in Communications

Several committees attempt to mitigate friction with individual PIs through not only the *content*, but the *tone* of communication. Some chairs try hard to use a respectful tenor to bolster the message that they wish to be helpful, not obstructionist. A few interviewees described the importance of having what Kurt, himself a researcher, called a "deft touch":

> I always fear that faculty feel worn down by regulations and don't have enough time for anything. I just try to get them to keep true to the IRB's mission, and not just dismiss it as a whole set of hoops they have to jump through. Sometimes that just requires *a deft touch*. I don't know if I'm even good at it—I hope I am...I'd much rather somebody get a phone call from me, since I'm also a doctor and have done research, than just hear from somebody in the office that they didn't do something.

Yet achieving this tone, while simultaneously ensuring that researchers follow the regulations, can be tricky—doing PR while policing. As Thomas added,

> The hardest part of being an IRB administrator is walking this *fine line*. We are facilitators as well as monitors, and maintain a positive PR— we're here to facilitate and help you with the process. At the same time, we're here to *make sure you comply* with the regulations!

Enforcement of compliance can make researchers wary of these PR efforts.

Establishing and maintaining appropriate tact can be hard, reflecting in part an innate ability that not everyone equally shares. IRBs may thus struggle to have their staff use "the right" manner to improve relationships. As Laura, the lawyer, said,

> It's a challenge to not only find folks who have the talent for IRB work, but to teach people to get the right tone and balance, not shaking a stick at researchers, but trying to be collegial...when and how to make exceptions, be flexible, or compromise. We don't want to be one of those IRB offices that people hate, and complain about all the time.

To strengthen relationships with PIs and defuse animosity, chairs may try to "say no with a smile." Cynthia, the administrator originally from the South, uses "Southern charm" and a sense of humor. When investigators don't turn in paperwork, she accepts the blame rather than highlighting their negligence.

> PIs will say they brought paperwork over, and I know they didn't. They are sure. So most of the time, if there was an error, or they didn't send something, I try to be first to say, "You brought that consent form to me

the other day, and I have absolutely no idea what I've done with it. Could you send me another one, please?" It doesn't really bother me anymore. PIs will backdate memos to the IRB, but we have a time clock. I'll say: "I know you intended to get that over here. I'm so sorry. Can we deal with it now? How can we help you *today*?" I say that because I'm not saying that they didn't turn it in. *I'm trying to give them an out* so that they don't have to say, "I promised that, but have no idea what happened!" It works a lot better for me to say, "I'm so sorry: it was in my hands and I must have misplaced it. Do you have another copy?" rather than, "Oh, we never received it!" They know they didn't bring it. But we say, "We have looked high and low for that, but if you bring us another copy this afternoon, we'll see if we can work it into the schedule." It just doesn't do any good to make demands. Let's just move forward and see what we need to do to get everything running again.

Many IRBs thus try to send the message that they collaborate with PIs, although they vary greatly in how and to what degrees they in fact do so. Liza tells researchers, "You recognize that you need a biostatistician...When you need help about human subject protections, that's collaborative, too." Some PIs may merely resent, rather than acknowledge or welcome, this assistance. Still, in the face of such resistance, some chairs try to remain very patient and magnanimous.

Educating PIs

Researchers and their staff vary widely in the amount and quality of education they have on ethics and IRB procedures. Institutions range in how much Responsible Conduct of Research (RCR) training they mandate for staff involved in research. Several IRBs want the federal government to require comprehensive training more fully or clearly. Research ethics training, now formally required by many medical centers, generally consists merely of relatively short online exercises. These interviewees often sensed deficits in investigators' training in these areas. Good Clinical Practices or RCR courses may not include key issues, such as how exactly to determine adverse events in uncertain situations.

As suggested earlier, students and junior PIs who conduct research may have had little if any relevant ethics teaching. At some institutions, residents and other trainees must do research but lack adequate ethical as well as methodological training—for example, concerning research design, whether the sample size is appropriate to warrant the project—thus reducing a study's intellectual benefit.

Showing PIs the Regulations

To demonstrate the legitimacy of the IRB's authority, some boards explicitly try to show researchers the regulations. Troy, the urban researcher and chair, said,

When you can tell a researcher, "The FDA says, 'No, you can't do this,' or 'You should do this,' or 'have to do this,'" they understand. If you can show them the regs, they're even happier.

Other chairs explain to PIs not just the regulations but the overarching moral principles as well. Charlotte, an administrator, said,

There's nothing worse than saying, "The regulation's required." You always have to tie it back to an ethical principle—say not only *what* they need to do, but *why*. It's not *what* you say, it's the *way* you say it.

Again, not only what, but *how* IRBs communicate can play a crucial role. Here, both IRBs and researchers need to try to advance not only the letter, but the spirit of the law—in this case, not just enforcing the regulations, but explaining the larger justifications. Yet not all IRB staff may offer investigators broader explanations for their decisions.

IRBs can face difficulties, too, in getting PIs to understand the ethics behind the regulations. Researchers may resist or lack interest in these rationales. "Getting faculty or investigator buy-in, so that they understand *the reason* behind the regulation, is a challenge," Greg, a social scientist and chair, admitted. Many PIs just fill out the necessary forms without acknowledging that these documents are related to larger ethical issues. Greg felt that many researchers don't think about "why there's compliance, or put it in an ethical context. Whether the answers are right or not may not matter to them." To encourage PIs to appreciate the ethics behind IRB concerns also requires resources that IRBs may lack. Greg saw needs for IRB staff to

spend time with each investigator to understand the ethics behind the regulation, and help them write protocols in a more informed way. The science would be better, the subjects would end up better, and the investigator would feel a lot more buy-in.

While a common adage in clinical care is that "good ethics makes good medical care," Greg extends this analogy to research as well—that good research ethics also makes good science. It is still possible, however, for a researcher to disagree with how a particular IRB interprets and applies those regulations.

Conclusions

These interviews suggest that IRBs and researchers frequently differ markedly in their views of their respective roles and relationships. While investigators commonly see IRBs as having power, IRBs themselves often disagree, and minimize, deny, or seek to justify it.

One can argue that this friction is inevitable and unavoidable, given the conflicting roles of IRBs and PIs, and may even be desirable to some degree. After all, if relationships are too cozy, human subjects may not be adequately protected. The key questions, though, are not whether such tensions should exist, but *how much*, in what way, who should decide, and what checks and balances should exist. IRBs may know that they are seen by researchers as "obstacles," but committees differ in how much they are troubled by or try to alter these perceptions.

Boards frequently appear to try to justify their power, arguing that it helps researchers and human subjects. But no clear data exist to support that claim. At times, an IRB's power may actually delay or impede research, causing harm that the committee may insufficiently recognize or acknowledge.

These conflicting views of IRB authority partly reflect larger social structures and tensions within complex, hierarchical academic medical institutions. Researchers and IRBs wrangle because of underlying conflicting primary agendas—pursuing research *vs.* protecting subjects. Yet both sides can, ideally, work to ameliorate these tensions. The strategies presented here, such as open doors, may not always wholly eliminate conflicts, but they can help.

IRBs' power may be legitimate, but discretionary. Committees' abilities to interpret and apply regulations as they think best confers an important degree of authority. These boards can follow specified processes, but still interpret regulations in varying subjective manners.

Writers from Aristotle[14] to Madison and Hamilton[15] have argued that power plays vital roles in political and social structures, but can be used well or misused and abused. So, too, IRBs will invariably have a modicum of authority that they can exercise in more or less justified and effective ways. Unlike the police and many other entities with clout, no appeals process exists for IRBs. Citizens can readily appeal, externally, police officers' and judges' decisions; researchers cannot. Yet these interviewees rarely allude to this fact—they appear to take it for granted.

IRBs and PIs should both strive to understand more clearly and be sensitive to the nature of these conflicts. IRB power varies in the degrees to which it is legitimate, discretionary, agreed upon, and understood. It operates through several mechanisms, and generates tensions.

Definitions and implications of the terms *power* and *police* also vary. While researchers think IRBs have power, these committees typically think otherwise, or minimize it. In many ways power is in the eyes of the beholder. Both PIs and IRBs have myths about it. PIs may inappropriately "blame the messenger" for the need to follow the regulations. IRBs frequently see themselves as not having power, because they are "merely following the regulations." Neither of these views appears wholly accurate.

Transparency can reduce power, but not entirely. Authority can be transparent but persist. *It can follow a process, but still be somewhat arbitrary if sufficient checks and balances are absent—as is the case here.*

Committees need to become more aware of how they are viewed by researchers. They must understand and address the underlying causes of these strains, recognizing these subjective elements more fully, and integrating this awareness more into decisions. Many IRBs try to respond to PIs' complaints, improve relationships, and "not be the ethics police," but range significantly in whether, how and to what degree they do so. In the end, *I do not think that IRBs are in fact "the ethics police," but the common use of that term reflects an important phenomenon—how researchers often view these committees.* This descriptor is inaccurate, but suggests underlying frustrations and tensions that IRBs, researchers, and others must all acknowledge, address, and reduce.

Committees can work to improve relationships with researchers—through the quality, contents, and tone of memos and communication, and "openness and transparency," rather than anonymity and distance. Boards can establish clinics, educate researchers about the underlying ethics and rationale, and help PIs as much and as proactively as possible. Pre-reviews by IRBs can potentially help as well, but require resources, and can foster other complications. Still, these efforts can counter researcher resistance.

In establishing the right balance in these relationships, committees encounter challenges. Since IRBs monitor PIs, these committees' PR efforts may be suspect. With competing demands for their time, researchers are also very busy, making IRB meeting attendance difficult. Moreover, while many chairs would like investigators educated to "understand the ethics behind the regulations," researchers may disagree with an IRB's interpretation and application of the principles involved.

The fact that much of IRB work occurs behind closed doors aggravates these tensions. Minutes are not publicly available, but should be as much as possible. Redaction of details may be hard for industry-funded studies, but not completely impossible, or as difficult for other protocols; the benefits could be considerable.

These committees should realize that the absence of an appeals process bolsters their clout. To ignore this fact aggravates these tensions. Conversely, increased acknowledgment of this perceived authority can strengthen committees' interactions with researchers, and thus help protect subjects. Chairs who see themselves as having power, but try to use it as prudently and sparingly as possible, may impel researchers to value research ethics and follow regulations more closely, and to resent IRBs and violate research integrity far less.

IRBs vary not merely in formal structures, but also in tone and attitudes, shaping communication both formally and informally. Committees face choices in how and when to interact and communicate with PIs, in turn affecting researchers' attitudes and behaviors.

Though CIRBs have been suggested as mechanisms for improving relation-ships between IRBs and PIs,[16,17,18] the *content, tone, and* formal *structure* of these interactions are crucial. Centralization alone may therefore not resolve all these tensions. Informal behaviors and attitudes of both IRBs and PIs will be key.

Some beneficial approaches to researchers outlined here require relatively little time and energy. Importantly, IRBs should realize more fully that they have a wide degree of latitude in their interactions with investigators, and strengthen these relationships through not only *what*, but *how* they communicate.

Hence, IRBs need to be improved through not just formal macro policy (altering federal regulations and establishing CIRBs), but more micro levels as well—in daily interactions.

CHAPTER 11

"Bad Behavior"

RESEARCH INTEGRITY

▪

In 1998, a British surgeon, Dr. Andrew Wakefield, claimed that the commonly used combination vaccine for measles, mumps, and rubella caused autism.[1] As a result, thousands of parents refused vaccinations for their children, some of whom later became sick and died. In 2004, a journalist discovered that Wakefield, who was trying to market his own three separate vaccines for these disorders, had completely faked the data.[2] Over the years, other instances of data fabrication have appeared in the media as well, such as Hwang Woo-Suk in South Korea Photoshopping pictures of stem cells to demonstrate that he had cloned human embryonic stem cells.[3]

Scientists occasionally falsify data, yet the extent of such falsifications and the institutional responses to them remain fairly unknown. Gross violations of research integrity (RI) may be rare, but they cannot be ignored. Moreover, as the amount and complexity of human experiments continue to expand, opportunities for lapses have increased.[4] When IRBs see or suspect scientists "behaving badly," they must decide what to do to prevent either under- *or* overregulation.

IRBs play vital roles in monitoring and responding to researcher transgressions, but often struggle with how much and in what ways to do so. Through yearly continuing reviews of renewals, IRBs monitor studies to help avoid research scandals and optimize public trust,[5,6] but little is known about how often these committees find problems, and if so, what kind. Definitions of RI themselves vary. *The Oxford English Dictionary* defines *integrity* as "freedom from moral corruption...soundness of moral principle; especially in relation to truth and fair dealing; uprightness, honesty, sincerity."[7]

But how RI becomes interpreted and applied in research differs widely. The Office of Research Integrity (ORI)[8] defines *RI* as "the use of honest and verifiable methods in proposing, performing, and evaluating research and reporting research results with particular attention to adherence to rules, regulations, guidelines, and commonly accepted professional codes or norms."

The scope of RI problems can range from obvious breaches (focused on "major falsification and fabrication and plagiarism") to broader notions that incorporate less egregious cases. Among researchers, 27.5 percent have reported keeping inadequate records, 15.3 percent dropped observations or data points from analyses based on a gut feeling that these were inaccurate, 13.5 percent used inadequate or inappropriate research design, 10.8 percent withheld details of methodology or results in papers or proposals, 6.0 percent failed to present data that contradicted their own previous research, and 7.6 percent circumvented certain minor aspects of human subject requirements.[9] However, it is unclear what some of these categories (e.g., "circumventing certain minor aspects of human-subject requirements") include, whether IRBs are ever aware of these issues, and if so, when and how.

Compliance offices are frequently charged with handling major violations, but IRBs increasingly play key roles as well. Within a medical center, IRB members may be the only detailed reviewers of protocols, and hence potentially play important roles in monitoring RI problems; but they vary considerably in their decisions.[10] For example, 17 percent of hospital IRB chairs "had dealt with scientific misconduct allegations," but 42 percent did not have a written policy regarding RI.[11]

Yet although IRBs may be involved in ensuring compliance, how they assess it, and how effectively, is uncertain. Surprisingly, very little, if any, research has probed *how* IRBs view and approach these pressing RI issues.

Social systems in general—whether government agencies, corporations, schools, or the military—establish mechanisms of social control.[12] Institutions need to determine how to counteract unacceptable behaviors that may arise. But many questions remain about in what ways and how effectively IRBs do and should respond. Medical institutions' responses to violations to RI can differ. Researchers, when they become aware of lapses in RI, have been found to be more likely to inform their colleagues, whereas administrators were more likely to notify supervisors and deans.[13]

Potentially, IRBs can promote integrity not only by discouraging deviation from ethical guidelines but also by making them easier to comply with. Patricia Keith-Spiegel and Gerald Koocher have argued that researchers may violate ethical norms and regulations because they feel that the system and IRBs are unfair—that perceived unfairness in a social system triggers unethical behavior.[14,15,16] Yet researchers' perceptions of injustice may be inaccurate, reflecting post hoc rationalizations and prompting self-justifying misbehaviors. Nevertheless, the fact that PIs may cooperate more fully with a system that they perceive to be fair highlights why IRBs should function as transparently and judiciously as possible.

As suggested in Figure 11.1, my interviewees observed and addressed integrity in varying ways, and wrestled with whether and how involved to be, given the competing demands on their resources.

Roles of IRBs Concerning PI Problems
- IRBs differ in:
  o Interacting with other institutional offices
  o Feeling they have in amounts of responsibility for RI problems

Types of Problems
- Poor informedconsent
- Non-submitting to the IRB
  o Entire protocols
  o Changes to protocols
- Altering aspects of approaches being compared in a study
  o Inclusion/exclusion criteria
  o Number of subjects

Severity of Problems
- Vary in concern, but are generally relatively minor (i.e., not involving harm to subjects)

Ways IRBs Learn of Problems
- Continuing review
- PI self-report
- Audits
  o Audits for cause (which raises questions of when to audit)
  o Random audits
- Complaints by subjects
- Complaints by staff ("whistleblowers")
- Chance

Causes of Problems
- Generally not malicious
- Poor supervision of staff or students by PI
- PI Ambition
- PI mental health problems

Responses to Problems
- Vary in degree of severity and type
  o Educating PI
  o Suspending study
  o Reporting problem to federal agencies

Figure 11.1 Aspects of research integrity problems confronted by IRBs

How to Define Research Integrity

Interviewees define RI broadly and in different ways. Louis saw it as transparency and openness: "It's like playing cards with your hand open—actually executing the study exactly the way you said you were going to." A few chairs defined RI as also *reporting* research accurately. Other interviewees viewed integrity even more widely—akin to "research ethics" itself. Phil, the social scientist and chair, spoke of designing research that works against one's own biases, "to unpack them." Such studies should therefore seek to disprove one's favorite hypothesis. He thought that RI also includes

> how you deal with your subjects afterwards... [whether you] involve them in dissemination, or give credit for their contribution. It could be about 9,000 other things, too.

Though mandated to protect human subjects, most interviewees seek to "go beyond" the narrowest possible definition of that task, to include key aspects of integrity. Many noted that although compliance offices were often involved, those offices range significantly in their scope, size, and functions; IRBs therefore can and should have important roles in RI, and may even ultimately share part of the responsibility for problems that emerge.

Others struggled to distinguish what they were *vs.* were not responsible for; they thought that they had a broad mandate, but that it did not include *all* potential aspects of compliance per se. Jeff, the social scientist and chair, felt that the committee's purview excluded:

> ... integrity in reporting data and publishing, and acknowledging contributions, sources of data, and others' "work." ... But following protocol and decency in treating human subjects... *is* the IRB's jurisdiction.

Given budget cutbacks and threats to integrity, several of these men and women thought that the IRB's role may in fact be increasing. Lack of NIH money may make research more arduous, encouraging researchers to bend or avoid rules. Constraints in funding, Troy said, "may lead to more desperation and cheating." The intense pressure of academic medical environments can contribute to integrity violations. For some scientists, the "pressure cooker" may simply get too much. As Olivia, the health care provider and chair, said,

> A lot of it is competition. Many people thrive in pressured environments like this; but many do not. What length will people go to when they feel threatened, and how do you reduce that threat?

Novel information technologies provide additional opportunities for integrity violations. Photoshop, for instance, lets researchers alter images. "The degree to which people go to the trouble of doctoring a picture," Olivia said, "is startling beyond belief."

Common Infractions

In 2001, a faculty member at Columbia Business School, interested in studying how businesses respond to consumer complaints, sent letters to the owners of leading New York restaurants, claiming he had become severely ill after dining at their restaurant, and wanting to know what they were going to do as a result. Many of the restaurateurs took the claim seriously, shut their kitchens, and interrogated and fired staff. The researcher had felt that since his study was minimal risk, he did not need to submit it to the IRB. Only when several restaurant owners found that they had no reservation or credit card record of the professor dining at their establishment did they suspect a hoax. Outraged at being deceived, they complained. Ten sued.[17]

IRBs observe integrity problems regarding not only COIs and data falsification but also other, generally less serious issues—most frequently researcher noncompliance with regulations. Mostly these instances are minor, but occasionally more significant concerns arise. Researchers do not always adhere to all aspects of their submitted protocols. Some IRBs see *only* such minor deviations—in Jeremy's words, "a PI who exceeded the number of approved subjects, or is sloppy." Investigators may use the wrong consent form or fail to follow the time frames listed in their protocol. Patient revisits supposed to occur at 60 days may not happen until 90 days. Given the exigencies of conducting studies in the field, such mistakes may be inevitable. Yet periodically IRBs wondered whether such sloppiness and inattention to details reflected deeper trouble—whether these deviations represented only minimal problems or constituted "the tip of the iceberg." Researchers' sloppy paperwork can undermine trust, making boards wonder whether their prior confidence in the investigator is unwarranted. Elaine said about a researcher whose applications are sometimes disorganized:

> There's discomfort. Is he appropriate to be doing this research? Is that the IRB's job? If that's how they're going to treat IRB staff, how are they going to treat their subjects? I worry with a lot of these people, if they're such jerks. But what do you do, deny everyone that's a bad person? You hope that they're going to do what they say. But you can't disapprove something based on a gut feeling, I guess.

She and others remained unsure. At times, IRBs suspected researcher obfuscation. "It's hard not to believe those actions were not purposeful," Kevin said. "That there wasn't some attempt at concealment."

RESEARCHERS NOT SUBMITTING PROTOCOLS OR CHANGES IN PROTOCOLS TO THE IRB

IRBs discover PIs who have not submitted studies, or not submitting changes to approved protocols. Interviewees felt that ultimately *they*, not the researchers, should determine what constitutes "research." Still, investigators may make this call on their own, and feel that their work is exempt—that it does not constitute research on humans, and thus does not need to be submitted to the IRB. Cynthia, an administrator, reported,

> Researchers argue, "I'm just writing a paper, holding a focus group, doing an anonymous survey—isn't that exempt?" Well, it may or may not be, but PIs do not self-determine that here. It has never worked in an academic situation. We want all researchers to run everything by the IRB, and get a determination letter: "Yes, it is research." Or, "No, it's just quality improvement."

Researchers have argued, for instance, that they "don't need IRB approval for chart reviews," but confidentiality can nonetheless get breached. Cynthia continued,

> Nice patients come for treatment here, thinking that only their doctors look at their records. Researchers can write things down. But don't carry them around in an open tote bag, with patients' names on the data collection sheets that you're taking to the office once you've gotten coffee at Starbucks, with all this stuff flopping around!

Some researchers get caught because IRB members spot recruitment flyers posted, or lists of research-based dissertations that the committee never saw. But how many studies researchers conduct but do not submit for review is a mystery. Nonsubmission may occur, particularly in fields where regulations are not entirely clear. As Jeremy, the physician and chair, said,

> It is hard to know how often researchers do not submit to the IRB at all. It is a black hole. I think it happens more in areas that are a little gray without clear consensus—like educational research. From the federal level down, we have not been clear about what is and isn't exempt. So

there is confusion, and researchers want to avoid the hassle of submitting a project. So they will just go ahead and do the research.

IRBs may try to identify all research, but doing so can prove elusive. "We're trying to get a foolproof method of detecting research," Nancy said, "to make sure it goes through review. But there's still an awareness problem." Committees may learn of these protocols, or key aspects of them, only indirectly through grants and contracts offices. Hence, IRBs may routinely screen lists from these other offices. Nancy continued,

> We examine the records from our contracts and grants department every month and try to pick out new ones, and publicize: "Here are the telltale signs that your research should be reviewed." But it seems like an awful lot of screening effort.

As mentioned earlier, PIs may also substantially alter their protocols without informing the IRB. Such changes are often, but not always, minor. One study abroad posed problems by adding the collection of biological samples to their protocol. This sort of breach in another country can be particularly troublesome, given cultural sensitivities. Robin said,

> A professor called a student down in Latin America and said, "Collect a couple of stool samples from kids and bring them back." The student did, and the Health Authority in that country caught wind of it and was not happy. We weren't happy either.

IRBs find other problems that involve "only" paperwork, but these, too, range in significance. Many are relatively small. For example, as Christopher explained, staff may simply be inadvertently using outdated consent forms: "One version was approved, and then a Research Assistant prints another one that's not stamped, and there are 12 versions, and no one can remember which version is right." Other IRBs found PIs "getting out of the gate before approval" or "having non-approved personnel do the consenting."

Yet at times, "record keeping" problems can have serious implications—for example, "giving medication they weren't supposed to." Poor record keeping can also extend beyond mere sloppiness, and threaten patient confidentiality. Jeff, the social scientist and chair, described how one researcher retained identifying information about biological samples:

> We made a site visit because a cell biologist was egregiously late in submitting some continuing reviews. His record-keeping was in shambles.

His protocols stated that he was getting cell samples from a couple of other, de-identified hospitals. Yet information sheets that had accompanied the samples were in his files with patients' names, addresses, and diagnoses. He had mixed records from different studies. It was very hard to figure out if he was compliant in the numbers of samples that he had taken, and when he'd taken them. That [audit] has been going on for a couple of years, and hasn't been resolved. We have disapproved him to do the research. The finance office asks us every so often if they can tell NIH to clear the flow of funds for the PI. We've said no.

The confusion caused by such carelessness can be hard to disentangle.

Researchers may also be lackadaisical regarding *both* regulations *and* cultural sensitivities. For instance, an IRB chair at an institution with a relatively high number of Native American students encountered problems with researchers who conduct studies there, but are based elsewhere. As Greg, a social scientist and chair, said,

Universities want to use our student population for their studies. Two studies came in on campus. We thought they were targeting the student population, but it turns out they were targeting the [Native American] population. That was offensive to some participants. The investigators lacked sensitivity about how to approach these people in a culturally appropriate way. Our IRB hadn't been notified that they were going to be on campus questioning students. An instructor asked them, "Do you have IRB approval?" They said, "Oh yeah, we're at the University of blah blah in the Midwest, and here's our IRB approval letter." I was a little surprised. We contacted their IRB, and said, "Do you know your group is doing this?" They said, "No. They have [our] IRB approval, but were supposed to contact *your* IRB, and get approval." It was a grad student. The advisor just wasn't paying attention.

PUBLISHING STUDIES THAT NEVER RECEIVED IRB APPROVAL

Occasionally, researchers want to publish their data without having previously sought IRB approval for the study. But, as discussed earlier, when researchers start to collect information, they may not initially know that they will eventually want to publish it, since they do not know in advance if the findings will warrant publication. Louis described a "fine line":

A study was intended just for the classroom, so is exempt from an IRB review, but later on, a professor wants to write about it. We may not see a proposal from him. He'll just publish it.

IRBs then have to decide how to respond, and will often refuse to grant approval, since subjects may not have been informed that they were participating in research.

Investigators may also dissemble about their intentions. They may have gotten approval for a study to which they then add data or sample collection without informing the IRB, and about which they then want to publish. However, IRBs generally do not have the capacity to investigate all research to prevent such lapses. "If they submitted a proposal," Louis continued, "and don't write that they had collected this data, I can't go back and think: did they do that? Were they honest?"

Once more, IRBs confront questions about the extent of their responsibilities. Given competing demands on their resources, these committees differed. Some interviewees, such as Louis, felt no need to look further than the specific information researchers gave him. "I don't think it's my job to read beyond the document in front of me." Others disagreed.

The Ambiguities of Adverse Events

I have often wondered how much of the immediate cause of my father's death was his disease and how much was the side effects of the chemo. Though the question is now of course moot for him, it remains crucial in ongoing studies of new treatments. Indeed, the deaths of Jesse Gelsinger and Ellen Roche might have been avoided if the researchers in each study had reported to their IRBs the adverse reactions that earlier participants had suffered from these same experimental drugs. Instead, both investigators pushed forward, despite evidence of problems. IRBs are mandated to monitor and report serious and unexpected adverse events (AEs)—especially in studies of new drugs. Yet while many reports of these events are straightforward, others are not, leaving IRBs to struggle.

At times, IRBs are in a unique position to detect important patterns across studies. In multisite studies, for example, chairs receive AEs from all the sites involved in the study. Committees receive numerous reports of these from both their own and other institutions, and then have to assess whether and how to respond. Christopher reported that only by viewing many protocols did his IRB recognize that an experimental drug was reactivating hepatitis. "Twenty different protocols used it, and each investigator only saw one or two cases." After his IRB discovered the trend, it "made all the PIs change their consent forms."

But discovering such patterns and establishing such clear causal links is often hard. AEs can be burdensome because of uncertainties whether an adverse event results from the research or the subject's underlying condition. "For some patients, it's very tricky," Christopher said. "If someone with terminal cancer has a problem, is it from chemotherapy or part of their illness?" Particularly with seriously ill patients in trials of new treatments, determining whether a death or serious medical event occurred because of a study remains very difficult. As Kurt explained,

> Some patients are fragile, and have a fairly high rate of complications and death. But it's often hard to tell whether the study did anything to them. In some other study, a death would be a major catastrophe, and a reason to stop the research. But fragile patients have calamitous courses, and you often can't really tell. If they had a catheter in their head, and an intracerebral hemorrhage, and the surgeons say 30 percent have hemorrhages after head surgery, I can't tell if the catheter did it, or if the subject is in the 30 percent. We're stuck.

IRBs face difficulties, too, because they may not know the rate at which a particular side effect occurs, or because they don't know how many patients are in the protocol across all sites. Kevin, the health care provider and chair, said,

> We see individual reports, but have no way to put them into perspective. If adverse events are associated with a drug, I need the number of exposures. Someone had a cerebral aneurysm at another institution while receiving a skin cream drug. We have to review it. But it just blows my mind.

IRBs struggle to proceed, with unclear success. Kevin added, "We get frustrated. Then we go out for a drink."

The degrees to which problems are due to a drug can be very uncertain, hinging on questions about the meaning and extent of causation. Jeremy, the physician and chair, said,

> A subject getting a new cholesterol drug is hospitalized with bad pneumonia. It may be unrelated to the intervention; or possible, but not likely that the drug played a role. Or it's possible, not probable, but you can't completely exclude it. Few times are you pretty sure. The vast majority of time, you get a report that a bad event happened, and there is *no* relationship.

Problems arise as well because IRBs may not know the base rate of a particular problem in the general population—how often these problems occur outside of a study. Stephen said,

> One investigational drug was for heart disease. We were concerned about occurrences of depression and suicide ideation. We wanted to make sure our local investigators screened and monitored very carefully for these

AEs....I was getting 25 or 30 incidents of suicidal ideation and anxiety attacks at a shot, but I didn't know the denominator. I was only seeing them on study-drug-assigned subjects. What's going on? The response was: They were reporting these events only in the active drug subjects, not the placebo. I was seeing the baseline rate of depression in the population!

In social science, too, AEs occur, though far more rarely. Researchers may misplace or lose laptops, flash drives, or CD-ROMs that contain confidential data. An IRB may then have to tell a researcher to notify all the subjects that their information was lost or stolen. Or a subject may indicate on a form that he or she is suicidal, but the researcher only reads the form months later. "So now we have to find the person," Phil, the social scientist and chair, explained. "*Can* we find them?"

Furthermore, AEs can be hard to assess because of difficulties differentiating these from other problems in participants' daily lives—especially in research on groups that face multiple challenges. For instance, one subject was killed while in an HIV study. The PI thought the death was unrelated to the study, but questions lingered. Judy said,

> The women were being tested for sexually transmitted diseases, and if they tested positive, were supposed to tell that partner to come in and get treated. One woman told her partner, and a few days later was murdered. Was that related to the study or not? The investigators didn't think so. But maybe it was. We asked the researchers to come up with another way to guarantee more safety for a woman disclosing her results to her partner. Perhaps a study staff member could go with them. The investigators felt that could be very intrusive.

IRBs may also suspect AEs if recruitment is very slow. For instance, in a study of a new drug, subjects may be suffering significant side effects and thus drop out of the experiment; and the researchers may hence have stopped recruiting participants, but not yet disclosed the problem to the IRB. Committees can then struggle, however, with whether it is their responsibility to seek and assess all such delays. Martin, the researcher and chair, said,

> The investigator intends to recruit 100 subjects a year, and has recruited only six. Sometimes there's an AE: Is this a doable, feasible protocol? Whether that's the IRB's responsibility is a little ambiguous.

Frequently, committees are forced to trust researchers' determinations of the causes of AEs. "The PI has a lot of latitude," Christopher said, "attesting to whether he or she thinks it's related or unrelated to the study. If researchers attest that it's not related, we leave it at that." But investigators may not report AEs quickly or completely, and may be biased in judging whether their study is at fault.

After learning of an adverse effect, some IRBs may respond by simply adding to the consent form a mention of the new side effect; but other times they wrestle with to what degree the study *caused* the event. Stephen said,

> You get items that are *possibly* related because there's a time relationship. Is this already in the consent? Is it more severe or frequent? Do we need to change the consent, or have other monitoring?

PIs, however, may resist altering the consent form. "If they make the study sound more risky," Stephen continued, "maybe fewer people will participate."

In multisite studies, chairs receive AEs from all sites participating in the study, and the volume can be inundating. Lots of uncertain information can prove confusing. "Everyone is overwhelmed," Jack confessed, "moving pounds of paper with random pieces of undigested data, and no way of making comprehensive sense out of it." IRBs may feel, as Stephen said, that they are "looking for a needle in a haystack." Committee personnel may rotate doing these reviews for a month or year at a time, but each may then take several months to develop optimal skills in making these determinations.

The current system encumbers IRBs, giving them responsibilities that no one else may want. Several interviewees thought that AEs should instead be evaluated by another board, such as the FDA or a Data and Safety Monitoring Board (DSMB). Yet no such alternative has yet been instituted. In recent years, DSMBs have been established to examine the results of studies already underway to see if these should continue. These boards unblind results (when the researchers cannot do so) to see if the experimental treatment is proving to be worse than the standard one. If this turns out to be the case, the DSMB decides whether the study should be altered or stopped. Yet IRBs' relationships with DSMBs can generate tensions, too, since the latter have more information about what is actually happening in a study than the IRB does.

DSMBs have spread, but still do not generally have primary responsibility for overseeing AEs. In the meantime, many AE reports are merely distracting for IRBs. As Jack said,

> For one AE on one drug, I get five different AE reports, with five follow-ups. Each piece of paper may change one piece of data: a patient's temperature was 37.4, not 37.5. These things just turn into distractions and noise. I'd love to see some central reporting system, someone with intelligence say: "Don't bother."

Some IRBs streamline reporting, so that researchers don't report "every little thing."

But such a systematic solution is not yet universal, in part because stakeholders want to avoid legal responsibility for these negative events. No one wants to judge an AE as minor and later be found to have been wrong. As Jack added,

> No one ever wants to say, "This is not important." They want someone else to take the blame. Investigators say, "I'll just give it to my IRB. Let *them* deal with it."

For legal and regulatory reasons, drug companies want to know all AEs for the studies they fund, which can burden committees. Christopher explained,

> The biggest issue we have is that more and more drug companies want every AE reported, whether it's serious, or changes the consent form, or not. It's a ton of work for the IRB. Drug companies usually want everything going through full board, because they want to be able to document that everyone has seen it. We've been fighting that.

Yet companies' concerns may be legal more than ethical per se.

At present, IRB chairs have the ultimate responsibility. As Jack said, "the buck stops here with me. I think: Does this event look like some horrible real new toxicity that we have to deal with? Most of the time, it's not." Luckily, most AE reports do not reflect major new problems.

These obstacles thus raise questions of whether to alter the current system of reporting, and if so, how. Several chairs saw needs for at least developing clearer categories and definitions. Cynthia, the Southern administrator, complained,

> There's no standard. Clinicians now have several choices in describing an AE, and might differ. So, AEs are difficult to pick up in a report because there's such variation. The National Library of Medicine needs to work on developing a standard thesaurus.

How IRBs Learn of Integrity Problems

IRBs learn about ethical violations in various ways—from continuing reviews and audits to complaints by staff or, occasionally, subjects.

RESEARCHER SELF-REPORTS

Researchers must submit updates annually, and occasionally IRBs learn of problems this way. Investigators may not have been trying to conceal changes to the protocol, but merely overlooked the need to report these during the year. "In reviewing one investigator's materials for his annual review," Charlotte, the administrator, said, "I happened to notice that, unbeknownst to the IRB, he had just dropped one disease, and changed it."

Researchers may also discover and report RI problems as these occur, or designate their staff to do so. The majority of these cases are minor. Kevin, the health care provider and vice chair, said,

> Most noncompliance issues are self-reported by the investigators. The number one problem—which we consider relatively minor, depending on the study—is over-enrollment.... The PI will discover inadvertently, prior to the continuing review, that they overenrolled, and will report that. We then investigate the circumstances. Depending on the study's relative risk, we may simply ask the investigator to amend the number.

When discovering their own lapses, PIs often express feelings of guilt. "I hear about occasional lapses or mistakes because an investigator will come and confess to me," Charlotte said. "Some researchers come in and say, 'Oh my God, I just did this terrible thing. I'm freaked out. What can I do to make it better?'" One PI, for instance, misplaced a study videotape of family interactions. The researcher reported the loss to the IRB only *after* it was found. The video had been at a receptionist's desk—not in a locked location, as the protocol had promised. The researcher then agreed to protect against potential breaches of confidentiality. As Charlotte described,

> The staff kept referring to them as "missing data," which the PI thought meant: missing statistically. But they were *literally* missing. The videotape was found by the receptionist's desk. The PI...came to me and confessed that this lapse had occurred, and told me what steps they were taking to make sure the staff understood....I can slap the PI's wrists, and say: you really screwed up. But they're already coming to me, telling me that, and showing me steps...to rectify it.

This metaphor of confession suggests wrongdoing and need for forgiveness. But Charlotte's story also suggests her belief that the PI now understood the spirit of the regulations—and that he therefore deserves pardon.

IRBs then face questions of how to respond to these lapses. Charlotte continued, "I always report an instance like that to the IRB chair, and he determines whether it should go to the full IRB. Generally it does. But, on something that small, as an information item." Alternatively, IRBs can order that a PI disclose the problem to all his or her subjects.

AUDITS

IRBs also conduct audits, but vary in when, and how commonly, and what these investigations find. Institutions also vary in whether boards themselves or compliance or other offices conduct audits, how these offices interact, and whether these probes are random or prompted by suspected problems.

Who Conducts Them?

Institutional structures for handling these problems differ—for example, how close administratively or geographically the IRB is to the compliance office. These offices could be on the same floor or on a different campus; sometime they interact frequently, other times almost never. Frequently, compliance offices, rather than IRBs, perform audits; and even decide when an audit should take place, bypassing the IRB altogether. Yet in the complex exigencies of institutions, other IRBs take on key functions that a compliance office might otherwise perform. "For the past year, the positions have been vacant," Scott continued. "So I've been handling it."

Many institutions also have Quality Assurance/Quality Improvement (QA/QI) offices, but the relationships between these entities and IRBs vary as well. These offices may share members, and range in what, how, and when they communicate. IRBs may also establish their own QA/QI division. Scott, the IRB director, created such a division, "which serves underneath the IRB. They perform internal and external audits." These two divisions may then try to differentiate themselves. As Olivia said, "The QI department tries to say that we are not the IRB police." Other IRBs may want to be more involved in compliance, but already feel overburdened. As Stephen said,

> I'd like to see our institution have a Compliance Office where not only IRB issues but other fraud and legal issues are brought. We would...have the investigative arm, and also be the IRB. [But] the IRB is having a difficult time keeping their heads above water.

Types of Audits

IRBs face questions about what kinds of audits to conduct, how often, and when. Audits can result from evidence or suspicions of serious or ongoing problems. Such lapses can prompt *for-cause audits*, but committees have to establish the *thresholds* of when to perform such investigations. Triggers can be major or minor. "The two major reasons we do for-cause audits," Christopher said, "are if there's a death in a study, and if there are lapses and the PI hasn't submitted continuations on time."

Other committees investigate studies because of signs or suggestions of possible complications (e.g., over-enrollment). Pam, the administrator, said,

> Seeing a lot of serious adverse events, or a greater frequency of risk
> [than] on the consent form, or an investigator over-enrolling by, say,
> 100 people, are red flags that maybe we should do an audit for-cause.
> Are the researchers ... deviating from the protocol?

Occasionally, a PI may have a history of ongoing problems, propelling an
IRB to audit his or her research—a response that is neither wholly random nor
entirely for cause. As Jeremy said,

> There are a couple of problem investigators, where the track record is
> such that we tend to go *looking* for things a little. We may have pharmacy
> staff go audit them. One PI has a track record, [so] we end up being *pro-
> active*, trying to make sure there aren't problems that we aren't being told
> about. But that is rare.

As we will see, IRBs then have to decide what to do when they have such
suspicions.

Other committees recognize the potential benefits of for-cause audits, but
rarely if ever perform them because of lack of staff. Instead, these boards often
rely only on continuing *annual renewals*. These IRBs usually wish they had the
personnel to investigate certain studies more fully, and feel constrained without
that additional support.

A few rare IRBs perform *random audits*, not triggered by problems or suspicion, though such investigations require additional resources. Relatively well-
resourced IRBs at large institutions may even have a full-time employee dedicated
exclusively to such random checks.

Other institutions may refrain from conducting any or additional audits in
part because of an implicit COI—not wanting to uncover additional problems.
"We haven't done audits," Anthony said, "because of not wanting to rock the boat
too much—not a great excuse. And being understaffed."

Audits can also foster tensions with researchers, as well as strengthen perceptions of IRBs acting like "the police." Anthony continued, "IRB staff would just
come in like a cop, and rifle through researchers' files, and we're back to the "Us
and Them" mentality, which isn't helpful."

Many IRBs believe that having effective and trusting relationships with PIs
is vital. These committees may thus try instead to facilitate PIs' self-reporting of
problems. Anthony added,

We want PIs to call us with questions, and *mea culpas,* if that happens. Obviously, if somebody's a repeat offender, we need to have higher scrutiny. But we're all human beings. On occasions, we all drop the ball.

Indeed, most researchers' errors appear unintended—"not malicious or intentional," Anthony said. "We keep an institutional memory—if PIs repeatedly have problems like this."

Invariably, random audits uncover at least a few problems. In an ongoing study, IRBs will usually discover some deficiencies. As an analogy, Joe, the chair, said that a neurologist who looks at a person "can almost always find some evidence that looks like brain damage. So when the Research Compliance people go in there, they can almost always find something not right." Generally, though, the lapses detected through random audits are small and insignificant. "They almost always find something," Judy, the physician and chair, said, "but it may be very minor."

How aggressively, then, should IRBs respond? Based on the results, IRBs may stop or substantially alter a study, or they may recommend only additional staff and/or investigator training. The *minor* lapses generally pose no real danger, and do not significantly worry IRBs. Troy, the researcher and chair, explained,

> We find things we don't know or *want* to know about—slip-ups in doing research, things done out of the time frame window, incomplete, or undated—nothing that really concerns us yet.

He sees these problems as not only minor but as better off undiscovered, because the administrative consequences are more cumbersome than the errors warrant.

Broader policy questions emerge about whether boards should conduct more such random audit, given the additional resources required. Katherine, the administrator, conducts random audits but wonders if such monitoring could get "too intrusive," since these audits can stress PIs.

IRBs that conduct random audits tend to concentrate on researcher-initiated rather than industry-initiated or large multisite studies. PI-initiated protocols have the least external oversight and thus, IRBs seem to feel, the highest risk. Judy said,

> We usually audit investigator-initiated protocols, because drug companies audit theirs pretty well. Most National Cancer Institute or pediatric AIDS clinical trial protocols get pretty good oversight. Investigator-initiated studies are highest risk, so we focus on them.

But as mentioned earlier, whether IRBs' trust of the pharmaceutical industry to oversee the studies it funds is justified is not entirely clear.

Many IRBs would like to conduct additional types of random audits but are limited by resources. As Scott, the director at an institution with a CRO, explained,

> We don't audit pharmacy logs because of time. But to come up with a *complete* picture, you *have* to...[look] at pharmacy logs—doses logged and given to subjects—[and] protocol violations or deviations, trying to catch them in research charts. We're left with a *partial*, not a complete, picture.

But the notion that problems almost always exist, unexposed unless actively sought, poses further questions: Should that phenomenon be accepted as inevitable? Or does it suggest that more auditing is appropriate (with additional governmental or other funds to support it)? Still, audits can play important roles. The threat of a possible audit—even if it never takes place—may impel better behavior. It may not scare a serial offender, but it could motivate others to follow regulations more closely.

Whistleblowers

At times, IRBs learn of problems not by audits but by complaints from subjects or concerned staff, who alert the IRB without the investigator's knowledge. However, not all such reports of problems by subjects or staff prove major or valid. Still, IRBs need to evaluate such complaints carefully—including those by whistleblowers—looking, in part, at the informant's motives. As Stephen said,

> With whistleblowing, you need to determine: Is this just a disgruntled person, or are there very legitimate subjects' concerns here? There's been some of both. We've had very clear cases where a whistleblower has made very real charges. They have done this through no personal gain or profit, and have suffered consequences. You have to look at the motivations.

Significant complaints by subjects are rare, but they occur—for example, once or twice every few years at some of these institutions, but not much more—and can stimulate federal investigations. Christopher added,

> A couple of people have called saying, "I was asked to be in a study. They said it was going to be this and that, and it turned out to be something else. I'm really pissed off."

Often, the problem turns out to stem from the fact that the PI has mishandled some aspect of acquiring or explaining the informed consent. Christopher continued,

From the patient's view, the complaint is valid. But it tends to be a failure of the informed consent process. The form said there are unknown risks. However, consent should be ongoing.

Research staff complaints to the IRB without the PI's knowledge can also trigger audits for cause. As Cynthia said,

Usually, a staff person or one of the nurses thinks that things haven't been done appropriately. Some improprieties have occurred—usually through oversight, neglect, or lack of staff. Data should have been recorded in the charts but were written on pieces of paper. Or test results should have been filed earlier. Or researchers are going back, writing and correcting things.

Yet these examples of lapses do not appear to have physically harmed subjects.

Unfortunately, however, whistleblowers can get penalized. Institutions may protect the senior researcher rather than the junior informant. Alas, such a fate may discourage other people from coming forward. Greg, the social scientist and chair, said,

Investigators were doing unapproved procedures outside of their protocol. It turned out to be a major match of wills between the whistleblower and the upper administration. The administration didn't react very well, and ended up protecting the researcher. The whistleblower eventually left, and the investigator was more or less protected.

Some interviewees would strongly warn such potential informants about the risks they may face. Dwayne reported unfortunate repercussions against individuals who made such complaints:

Whistleblowers get screwed. I see how they are treated, regardless of policy. Everyone has to hesitate before they come forward, because there are going to be negative reactions. Everywhere.

In part, long-standing financial and personal bonds can shield the investigator, and an institution may judge the reported violation to be negligible. Greg described a complaint about the treatment of lab rodents:

A federal regulator might consider procedures on lab mice that are not on the protocol to be major noncompliance. But to a local administrator, it's very minimal, and not worth sacrificing the researcher's career. A small tarnish, at the expense of a few little mice, is worthwhile.

This institution addressed the problem by devoting more resources to the animal care committee rather than censoring the PI.

IRBs may learn of RI problems unexpectedly, through happenstance. For example, one research coordinator reported to the IRB that an investigator was "making up" subjects. The IRB then pursued the allegation. Dana, the social scientist and chair, said,

> The project coordinator was answering some questions the IRB asked, and identified a researcher who claimed to have seen patients but didn't actually see them. It was one of those accidental, *serendipitous* things, and the IRB jumped right on that.... That was the most outlandish thing I've heard of. It happens once every eight years.

Dana continued,

> This PI is not evil, but has some serious mental health issues. It was surprising, because she had gotten here in the past two or three years, with magnificent letters of recommendation. Our university called around, and found that the letters of recommendation were magnificent because they needed to dump her. The recommenders said, "I realize she's now stuck at your institution, but we needed to dump her." There's no recourse.

This ethical lapse, accidentally discovered, was unusually significant. A researcher's ostensible reputation may not predict ethics violations.

Why IRBs don't Detect more Problems

IRBs have limited abilities to uncover researcher problems and deficiencies. "We're not equipped to detect the most serious kind of problem," Kurt said. "We can tell if PIs are sloppy or late, but not if they are outright defrauding us, lying, withholding, or making stuff up."

In addition, research participants or staff who observe problems may decide not to relay these to the IRB because they are intimidated. Indeed, chairs may worry that they don't receive *more* complaints—especially from subjects. Greg, the social scientist and chair, said,

> It bothers me that more problems aren't reported. Either researchers are all doing a great job or participants may not feel comfortable complaining. We've got this big university, with big fancy researchers with

big names and titles. Maybe subjects don't feel comfortable saying, "The needle prick hurt, and I've now got a big hematoma."

Similarly, a few chairs said that they *expect* a certain prevalence of protocol violations and serious, unanticipated AEs, and may be suspicious if researchers do not report any. As Olivia, the health care provider and chair, reported,

> If we expect to have adverse events from a study, and hear nothing, we get concerned. If we don't get a satisfactory answer at the continuing review, we will usually audit, and find bad record keeping.

Yet, as mentioned, not all IRBs have the resources to conduct such audits.

Unfortunately, the baseline amount of research integrity problems remains unknown. Some interviewees feel that the frequency may simply not be very high for major violations. Questions then emerge as to whether IRBs should look further for such problems, and if so, to what degree, given their limited resources. Warren reported,

> It would be very difficult to find that one investigator in a hundred or a thousand who is not very cooperative. There have been a few. But only somebody intricately involved in the research would be able to pick them out. They could easily hide that. An IRB reviewer would not see it. They're not abusing the patients, but being a little bit cavalier about how they take and manipulate the data. I don't think that's common. And the IRB's got plenty on its plate right now.

Causes of Integrity Problems

As suggested earlier, ethical lapses might result from a range of factors—occasionally from researcher or staff psychiatric problems; but more commonly from unintentional errors or defects in understanding, on the part of PIs or their staff, of the regulations or the ethical implications of their work. Interviewees felt that almost all PIs conducted research without serious ethical violations. Lapses usually resulted from ignorance, not intentional deception (i.e., "not because they are trying to play the system or get rich").

Many researchers were also overextended, with insufficient time to train or monitor staff adequately (e.g., "The PI's off in China and India doing research much of the time"). E-mail contact alone can prove insufficient for supervising and monitoring employees. Staff turnover can also pose problems—a project coordinator may leave and not be rapidly or adequately replaced.

Investigators' responsibilities for graduate student research can also be fuzzy. Senior faculty may supervise their trainees poorly, or fail to fulfill other responsibilities. Dwayne, the rural researcher and chair, said,

> Researchers who lost their privileges due to research integrity issues…weren't bad apples. It was a culmination of being overworked and overstretched, giving a lot of responsibility to a graduate student, but not overseeing or supervising appropriately. A lot of things got out of hand, which the grad student didn't realize. But the PI was ultimately responsible.

A trainee might make errors without the PI's knowledge—for example, entering subjects into a study before the IRB approved it. Dwayne described a case where some consent form issues had not yet been resolved: "The PI was not aware. He was on this campus, but the grad student was elsewhere. The PI just lost track of what was going on."

IRBs may want to hold faculty accountable in such instances, whereas researchers may resist this responsibility or fulfill it perfunctorily, thinking that they should not be solely or primarily responsible. Greg said,

> We allow a graduate student to be the PI. But we are changing that to require the faculty member be the PI, and the student be a collaborator. But the faculty feel they'd be directly accountable for the students' actions, and that the students would *not* be.

Investigator arrogance can foster not only tensions with committees, as we saw, but research integrity problems as well. Some prominent scientists may feel they simply do not need to follow the rules. Charlotte described a researcher who felt he could significantly change his study without informing the IRB:

> He's *arrogant*—one of those superstars who cuts corners and bends the rules a little. He didn't think he was harming anybody, so he didn't think the IRB needed to know. He requires more oversight from staff.

Personality traits may exacerbate PI problems. Charlotte thought that some researchers felt they were "above" the regulations, adding,

> We have to play by the rules. The rules are made by the federal government, and we have to enforce them. It's not like we're sitting around dreaming them up.

Here again, researchers may be "blaming the messenger"—in this case, the local IRB—for having to follow federal statutes. Koocher argues that researcher perceptions of unfairness cause RI lapses, but PI arrogance may in fact exist beforehand, and reflect long-standing personality flaws that then erode integrity. Still, it is important to remember that while some researchers may cut corners and act as if they are above the regulations, most do not.

Sanctions: Responding to Integrity Problems

Committees that learn of ethical lapses then have to decide what to do. As problems can range from minor to major, committee responses vary greatly, from changing the design or consent form to suspending the study or restricting privileges, and/or reporting the problem to the Feds. Attitudes of institutional leaders, competing institutional priorities, availability of research funds, and local and national scandals can influence committee responses.

When the deviation is small, an IRB may simply chastise the researcher in a letter. The PI may have simply enrolled more subjects than the board had approved. In such cases, Jeremy, the chair, could not "think of an example of where *harm* was associated. We jokingly use this little inside phrase: 'A stern letter or a slap on the hand.'"

REMEDIAL EDUCATION

IRBs may also require that a researcher undergo additional training. For minor offenses, IRBs might require merely online training. "We don't shut that person down," Dwayne said, "but make them retake an online tutorial." Yet, such responses may not be very effective. PIs may speed through an online educational module, giving it little heed. "I don't see a big impact from formal training," Dwayne confessed. "The IRB training we require is an 'online, honesty policy.' You could whisk through it, and basically not pay attention."

Ethics lectures alone don't always fix the problem. As Olivia said, "It's very easy to take an online test, and not internalize what you learn." Courses also do not teach how to interpret and apply ethical principles to one's own research. Indeed, courses usually teach these principles as objective entities—not as being open to differing interpretations in complex situations.

To make the learning process active, not passive, committees may require that investigators who undergo remedial training also have to present newly acquired knowledge to others. Kevin, the health care provider and chair, said,

"Sanctions" is not a nice word. But we have required that a PI who has significantly over-enrolled or altered protocols without informing the IRB go back to school—take an educational module, and then present the information in a lecture to their own research group. We aim at education of the culprit, if you will, and his or her staff.

The fact that researchers may still make errors even *after* taking federally mandated online training courses raises further questions about the effectiveness of this education.

SUSPENSION AND PROBATION

Occasionally, IRBs have *suspended* a study, or placed it on "administrative hold," halting enrollment until the problems were resolved. Generally, committees seemed to do so because a researcher had completed annual renewal forms late rather than because of larger integrity problems; and IRBs took these measures rarely—usually not more than once or twice every year or two.

Sometimes, IRBs placed researchers on probation for ethical lapses, but faced questions of when and in what way to do so—whether formally or informally. Elaine said,

What if the researcher has over-sampled by 200 subjects, and we didn't find out about it until afterwards? Do we take away the data, not approve any other research, or put them on probation? We have put researchers on probation. They'd over-sampled by four participants, but all their studies were sloppy—typos or cutting and pasting from other applications, just not taking the time to put together a thorough application. The researchers said, "I'm just too busy." So my IRB said, "Well if you're too busy, then we're going to put you on probation for six months."

For such flaws, however, committees may be unsure how exactly to respond. Elaine described another researcher who was continually making substantive modifications rather than taking the time to design the study properly to begin with: "The behavior was escalating, so we put the person on probation. There was a lot of debate."

IRBs may strive to avoid having past infractions affect present interactions, but doing so is not always easy. Elaine continued,

I try my best not to hold it against the person. But, I'm human, too. 90 percent of the people I deal with are great. But, in life, you don't always remember the good people—you remember the difficult ones.

A few institutions banned researchers from doing research more permanently, but that was rare. Stephen's IRB has never done so, because, as he put it, "You're talking about somebody's career!"

REPORTING PROBLEMS TO THE FEDS

IRBs must also decide whether to report problems to federal agencies, which may then choose to investigate the institution. Legally, boards must alert OHRP of serious ongoing problems, and most IRBs have done so. Yet overall, such notifications were relatively rare (one to two times every one to three years). Cynthia said that her IRB "suspended enrollment and notified OHRP" only once. Often, she said, the lapses were "more a concern than an actual problem."

Moreover, although IRBs may see the need to report problems to federal agencies, other institutional officials may hesitate to do so. The institution may be more cautious, and delay. As Elaine said,

> At my old job, my boss, the VP for Research, was in conflict because he wanted research to occur so researchers could get their grants.... There was a lapse. We had to report to the government, and he got really upset with me: "This ruined someone's grant! You should've consulted *me* first." So, people are afraid to report to the government. I worked closely with an IRB chair, but he was not my boss. He would tell me to do one thing, and the VP would tell me to do something else. What do you do? In that case, I listened to the chair, and reported it. I should've told my boss first, but didn't. I was carrying out the vote of the committee. But my boss got really upset with me!

Boards face questions of when to report, since the definitions of "serious," "continuing," and "noncompliance" can themselves be unclear. Elaine continued,

> OHRP could be better about defining non-compliance: what's "serious" and "continuing"? That's left up to the IRBs to define. What if the researcher has been doing it for years because we did not find out in the past? One researcher enrolled a 17-year-old, but said subjects would all be 18 and older. Somehow, this year, he just reported it. If an investigator over-samples by one, is that different than over-sampling by 100 in a low-risk study? I don't know if it's serious or just sloppy. For research conducted past the expiration date, what if the investigator consented subjects, but it was a real low-risk study? It doesn't seem serious to me. But the same researcher is *always* conducting [studies] past the date. I don't know if it's non-compliance or just sloppy. You see a lot of those *repeat*

offenders. Every time I see one PI's study, I know: there goes a day of work. She always messes up somehow. That's the way some people are. They don't get it. Some is sloppiness and some is stupidity.

IRBs vary in the degrees to which they consider the severity of these lapses—rather than react the same to all violations to the letter of the law. Elaine's institution was recently audited three times, but she has tried hard not to overreact to researchers' smaller glitches.

Just as IRBs may expect AEs for certain complicated and invasive studies, OHRP may anticipate a certain number of difficulties from an institution and be concerned if these are not reported. "OHRP is not going to come shut you down if a researcher over-samples or uses the wrong consent form," Elaine added. "But they are going to say, 'Why didn't you report any of this?'"

Hence, many IRBs tended to err on the side of over- rather than underreporting. Jack, the chair, described such a scenario:

> It was more of a "concern" than an actual problem. No one was hurt. But it met the requirement: it was an ongoing problem. There was a statutory requirement that we report it to OHRP. We had to shut the study down.

At times, IRBs reported lapses to OHRP swiftly in part because they have seen other institutions castigated for waiting too long. Many chairs felt that OHRP was reasonable and thankful. Jack continued,

> We hesitated and debated, but ultimately decided that it was better to report a problem before it became a real problem. We looked back at other institutions that have really gotten nailed because they let things go on too long. It's better to put the laundry out before it gets too soiled. So, we told OHRP: "We've got this problem. Here's how we are dealing with it already." They were very reasonable: "Thanks for telling us and fixing it."

Some IRBs veer to the side of overreporting to OHRP, thinking it is better to act sooner than later. As Kevin said,

> We tend to be conservative: we would rather make OHRP aware than not, and then have them discover something. So, we may be guilty of over-reporting—once or twice a year....I would invite OHRP and the FDA to come in tomorrow. The house is *that* clean. That's why we are willing to report to them.

Yet consequently, at this institution, OHRP has never done "an on-site inspection." Over time, several chairs have grown more comfortable reporting problems and concerns to these federal agencies because they feel that OHRP and the FDA are becoming more open and flexible.

Other institutions struggle far more about disclosing to the Feds, even if, in the end, they generally do so. IRBs may fear that reporting will stimulate more onerous federal audits. "We agonize over it," Troy said, "and do it on occasion—once every couple of years."

When institutions have a separate compliance office, others may make the final decisions of whether and what to report. IRB chairs may know little about these ultimate decisions—how they're made, and of what they consist. Jeremy said,

> Reporting to the FDA and OHRP is through the dean's office, not us. We're responsible for saying whether we think there may be a serious protocol violation. *They* then have to decide what to do with that. I don't know if they weigh financial or other considerations.

Yet this disconnect between offices generates questions, since the dean's office may have competing priorities and thus be reluctant to report problems that may lead to the suspension of all the institution's studies. IRB reports to federal agencies of researcher problems may also enter the PI's institutional record, and have long-lasting implications for him or her.

Occasionally, ethical lapses become nationally publicized scandals, and IRBs have to consider the potential impact of this as well. When a serious problem or "scandal" occurs, even if participants are not harmed, committees may question whether to force researchers to reveal their problems not only to subjects but to the wider public.

Conclusions

In short, IRBs confront a range of research integrity problems, broadly defined, and vary in how they learn of these lapses and respond. While many institutions have separate compliance offices, the boundaries and relationships between these entities and IRBs vary considerably. Many committees view integrity broadly, rather than narrowly, and themselves discover and monitor violations.

The lapses IRBs detect appear to be mostly minor, but they are not always. Boards discover studies that should have been submitted but weren't; they also discover undisclosed changes to protocols—to sample size, study arms, and timing of participant visits. Many of these problems are bureaucratic, involving only forms, and do not directly harm subjects. Other infractions, such as fabricating data, raise more concerns but are relatively rare. Though some critics have argued that most of the problems IRBs encounter concern "merely paperwork,"[18] other examples emerge here as well.

IRBs may learn of RI problems through continuing annual reviews, researcher self-reports, and random or for-cause audits. Complaints by staff or subjects appeared rare: at most no more than one to two times every year or two. The mechanisms of detection are limited. In the end, IRBs cannot catch all offenses.

In assessing these violations, IRBs seek to gauge *intent*, but often find it difficult. Although these lapses often appear unintentional, conscious or unconscious attitudes can underlie researchers' "sloppiness," and be difficult to decipher. Motivations for work-related behavior can stem from both social and psychological factors.[19]

Disregard for the rules may also result in part from perceived injustice.[9,20] Researchers may feel that increased regulation and paperwork have been unjustifiably imposed on them. Conformity may also be particularly hard for researchers, who, by definition, tend to be innovators, challenging accepted assumptions and ways of thinking.[21]

These interviewees raise questions of whether IRBs should be more fully and systematically involved in monitoring and responding to integrity issues, and if so, how. The IOM calls for institutions to enhance research monitoring, but to relieve IRBs of the burden of ensuring institutional compliance with rules and regulations (such as those concerning conflicts of interest) and to give those to a compliance or other office.[22] Such differentiation can, however, be hazy and challenging. IRBs review studies in detail and can potentially spot problems. To have other offices scrutinize studies as well could create a duplication of efforts, and thus a waste of limited resources. Yet separate compliance offices do not always disclose their decisions to IRBs, generating frustration, confusion, and inefficiency.

One could argue that according to the federal regulations, narrowly defined, monitoring RI does not lie within the scope of the IRB. But ethical violations can affect risks and benefits to subjects, and therefore arguably fall within the IRB's purview. IRBs also monitor researchers, and uncover and respond to lapses. Consequently, in practice, assessments of integrity can be closely linked to evaluations of how researchers report ongoing potential risks and benefits to subjects.

But if checking and assessing RI falls under IRBs' mandate, these functions pose dilemmas, such as whether boards should devote more resources to these activities. Frequently, discoveries of lapses now occur through limited mechanisms and serendipity. Especially as the amount and complexity of research increases, more support for such monitoring would appear important. Yet questions remain of *how much* monitoring is needed and *when* such resources should be used. More invasive research may warrant heightened scrutiny. Strikingly, though, these chairs often felt that industry-funded research requires less monitoring than did other studies, since industry funders were already overseeing it. Drug company scandals have, however, persisted. Such violations frequently relate to marketing, but can involve research as well. Hence, these assumptions and decisions about relative needs for assessment demand ongoing exploration and discussion.

Dilemmas emerge, too, about what thresholds and standards committees should use. The fact that an audit can almost invariably uncover problems suggests that more audits should perhaps be conducted, but it also raises questions of what kinds of violations justify additional expenditures. On the other hand, the standard in research ethics should not be "perfection." Clinical care involves the "art" of doctoring, with unpredictabilities and human judgments. "Perfection" is not always expected. Errors occur—one hopes, only minor ones. Whether a lowered expectation and standard should thus be employed in research, where findings and procedures are presumably objective and replicable, is debatable, and requires broad discussion.

Clarification of policies can also be beneficial—e.g., whether researchers need to notify IRBs of every minor change in a protocol, and if not, which minor alterations require review and approval (which can take weeks or months). Unfortunately, IRBs and investigators can define "mere paperwork" and "small changes" very differently. Researchers may consider certain changes "minor" that are actually more significant. Questions surface, too, of whether PIs can use data collected when protocols were noncompliant, and if so, when.

Larger strains underlie these issues: ultimately, how IRBs do and should decide whether to trust *vs.* closely monitor individual researchers. Trust is a complex and amorphous concept.[23] It can facilitate and streamline many interactions, but becomes more fragile as the size and complexity of enterprises burgeon. To assess whether trust is warranted, IRBs may need *evidence* (through monitoring), but confront quandaries of how much, and what kinds. In general, social systems establish formal rewards and punishments, as well as "unplanned and largely unconscious mechanisms which serve to counteract deviant tendencies."[12] These interviewees highlight the importance of understanding how institutions do or should try to identify cases of "deviance," and decide how many resources to use in doing so. The complex social systems within which IRBs operate, involving larger academic institutions, compliance offices, PIs, research staff, subjects, and outside federal agencies, therefore shape these issues. Understanding not only official formal regulations, but also day-to-day interactions and experiences, proves key—how policies and guidelines are in fact interpreted, applied, and shaped within these dynamic social systems.

The good news here is that, overall, the frequency of major RI violations appears relatively low. IRB critics might then assert that IRBs need not expand their monitoring activities, and/or can even decrease these. But these boards identify problems that otherwise would not be found. Researchers do not always self-regulate well. They may not know or correctly self-apply federal regulations, and are by definition conflicted. Unfortunately, the actual baseline frequency of lapses remains unknown. Such data are needed to gauge whether the rate and seriousness of these problems are high enough to warrant additional resources. Yet determining such rates of noncompliance is hard, as researchers may underreport and even hide errors. Indeed, how much IRBs in fact reduce concrete harms to subjects is unclear. Subjects may be hurt due to serious, unanticipated AEs in a study (e.g., previously unknown side effects of a drug), but these harms may not result from *ethical* lapses per se. Still, subjects' rights need to be protected.

Understandably, scientists may resent such monitoring; but research involves public trust, especially since taxpayers fund much of it. Such transparency and scrutiny are essential.

The fact that "whistleblowers" who report problems to IRBs may be penalized is also worrisome. Mechanisms to avoid such negative repercussions, though established by institutions, can prove insufficient. State protections can potentially help, but they have varied, and their effectiveness has been questioned.[24]

It is unknown whether the current relatively low frequency of complaints by *subjects* is appropriate. Staff and subject complaints may be low because of fears of backlash, but they could potentially improve research ethics within institutions. Arguably, committees should encourage subjects to provide more feedback (whether good or bad) concerning study participation. Complaints require investigation by the IRB, and hence resources, and may prove invalid. Nonetheless, such input could potentially yield valuable information. Subjects should perhaps be asked more routinely to complete "evaluation" forms about their participation, indicating how satisfied or dissatisfied they are, and whether their experiences could be improved. Such information could aid both researchers and committees.

Institutions can also promote research integrity in other ways. Within institutions, four patterns of motivation can promote organizational effectiveness: legal compliance (backed by use of penalties), use of rewards, self-expression, and internalization of organizational goals.[25] IRBs want researchers to internalize ethical values, but tend to encourage only legal compliance, integrity, and fear of repercussions, not rewards per se. Hence, investigators may not fully embrace this institutional goal. Perhaps IRBs can consider rewards (e.g., public announcements of successful IRB approvals, and papers). An individual's internalization of institutional values can depend on how much he or she is actively involved in organizational decisions, and sees the organization dispersing rewards fairly.[25] Unfortunately, PIs may see their primary goal (e.g., advancing research) as conflicting with that of IRBs. But ethical behavior can improve subject and community perceptions of researchers' work, facilitating investigators' goals.

To enhance integrity, IRBs and researchers need to work together more fully. To achieve this goal, members in each group need to improve their practices and attitudes in order to strengthen both science and subjects' rights.

CHAPTER 12

Researchers Abroad: Studies in the Developing World

In 1996, one of the world's largest drug companies, Pfizer, conducted a study in Nigeria in which 11 children died. The company gave 200 children with bacterial meningitis (a brain infection) either an effective treatment (ceftriaxone) or an experimental antibiotic (trovafloxacin or Trovan).[1,2] The families of the 11 deceased children sued. Pfizer produced a letter of approval from a Nigerian IRB at the hospital where the study was conducted. But the letter was in fact forged: the hospital had no IRB, and no Nigerian IRB had ever approved the study. And there was no proof that informed consent had been obtained. The subjects' parents said they did not know that their children were participating in a study. The researchers had also continued to administer the experimental drug to patients who developed negative side effects—side effects that eventually proved fatal. Nor did the investigators switch participants who weren't responding to the experimental drug over to the effective medication. Subsequent investigations revealed many flaws in the study's design, including a lack of adequate initial diagnoses. It also turned out that the company had used inadequate doses of the effective drug in order to increase the chances that the experimental drug would appear to perform better.

In 2010, 14 years later, WikiLeaks's founder, Julian Assange, released thousands of US State Department cables—one of which happened to reveal that Pfizer had in fact hired detectives to seek out evidence of corruption in order to smear the Nigerian Attorney General, Michael Aondoakaa, to pressure him to drop the lawsuit. Pfizer's investigators passed this information about alleged corruption to local media. Eventually, Pfizer settled out of court for $75 million.[3]

Poor study design, lack of informed consent, improper handling of adverse outcomes, distortion of findings, outright lying and forgery, blackmail: this notorious case illustrates a wide variety of ways that American researchers overseas may engage in unethical behavior to pursue profit. Unfortunately, scandals overseas, though typically less egregious, are not unusual. Between 2007 and 2011, for instance,

GlaxoSmithKline enlarged its Shanghai office from one to 460 employees to manage the increased number of studies they were conducting in China. But the company allegedly engaged in bribery and corruption, and failed to document key interactions with research subjects.[4,5] As pharmaceutical companies and the NIH fund ever more research in the developing world, IRB oversight has become increasingly challenging.

Three overlapping yet distinct problems exacerbate the difficulties of monitoring research in the developing world: the extreme poverty in many regions, the cultural differences in views of health and ethics between those countries and the United States, and the greater likelihood of corruption—whether among local officials or doctors, industry funders, researchers, or others. These concerns often exacerbate one another, as well as magnify the problems mentioned in previous chapters. The vast economic and cultural differences between certain industrialized and emerging economies can frequently result in fewer resources and less government oversight, facilitating corruption. In these and other countries, US IRBs therefore confront intensified challenges—sometimes along with researchers, and at other times alone. "We worry a lot about third world research when our faculty are the PIs," Judy said. "Just knowing what's right and reasonable for the country, or what could go wrong…is scary."

Why, then, embark upon research in the developing world? First, because poorer countries are beset by major public health problems that new drugs and protocols can potentially address. Pandemics of HIV/AIDS, malaria, and tuberculosis continue to rage overseas. Western countries are initiating studies on how to prevent HIV, for instance, through medications, microbicides, adult circumcision, and clean needles for drug users. Even the most altruistic of these efforts, however, can pose ethical dilemmas. For instance, many patients with HIV do not yet take medication, in part because of limited resources.[6] Quandaries surface of how much should be spent to prevent HIV-negative individuals from getting infected rather than treating patients who already harbor the virus.

Second, research is on the rise in the developing world because studies on diseases that affect *both* rich and poor nations are cheaper to conduct in the latter. Thus, drug companies increasingly conduct studies in emerging countries—not only to take advantage of lower costs, but often due to the less-scrupulous oversight.

Increasingly, developing countries have been establishing IRBs—generally called Research Ethics Committees (RECs)—but these committees frequently lack sufficient resources and training.[7,8,9,10,11] (For simplicity, I will use "IRB" to refer to both IRBs and RECs). A 2005 study of country representatives from the 46 member states in the WHO African Region found that approximately one-third of these nations did not have an IRB, though 80 percent of the respondents said an ad hoc review mechanism existed.[12] Frequently, however, these reviews were only by a few colleagues. The thoroughness and quality of these reviews is unknown. Moreover, separate studies have found that in Latin America,[10] Tanzania,[13] and South Africa,[14] most IRB members are male. Foreign researchers and IRB members see the US ethical review process as "unnecessarily burdensome" in time and difficulty.[15] Different cultures also hold varying conceptions and definitions of "selfhood," "autonomy," "justice," and "cures."[16]

Some critics have suggested that American investigators and IRBs are naïvely importing Western values, beliefs, and practices into other cultures, engaging in "ethical imperialism."[17] Wider debates rage concerning the degrees to which decision making in research ethics is or should be "universal" rather than shaped by local cultures. Some philosophers argue that ethics should not vary between contexts or societies, since "ethical relativism" may preclude criticism of another's position. But others counter that "ethics are local," not universal, and that a "common morality" does not exist.[14]

Certainly, participants in resource-poor countries are more likely to be vulnerable and/or have low education and literacy.[14] Many subjects do not understand US approaches to research ethics. One study, for instance, found that most participants in a malaria vaccine trial in West Africa do not comprehend key aspects of the informed consent.[18] Yet I found in a study that IRB members in the US are more likely than those in at least one developing country (South Africa) to think that subjects in the developing world *do* understand informed consent forms, risks and benefits, and placebos.[19] US IRBs may thus fail to appreciate the degrees to which study subjects in these other countries have trouble grasping these concepts.

Tensions and misunderstandings often arise between US and foreign researchers who are working together on the same protocol. In one study, 29 percent of US researchers thought that most research collaborators in foreign countries do not even speak or read English well.[20] In US-sponsored research, joint IRB reviews also can prove problematic.[21] A US IRB may approve a study that the developing country's IRB rejects, thus prompting critics to accuse the US IRB system of "ethical imperialism"—of exporting its values to other cultures.[22]

Overall, as indicated in Figure 12.1, US IRBs commonly face challenges in the developing world due to several broad sets of differences related to cultural and economic differences and often more prevalent corruption. Cultural difference frequently results in part from geographic distance, along with poor infrastructure and histories of colonialism, exploitation, and corruption.[23] As a result, American committees grapple with how best to interpret and apply the ethical principles in the Belmont Report (see Chapter 1). US IRBs vary from reviewing research in the developing world regularly to doing so rarely, if at all. In general, those boards that are more experienced in thinking through these problems have acquired a greater comfort doing so, but are also more aware of the potential pitfalls.

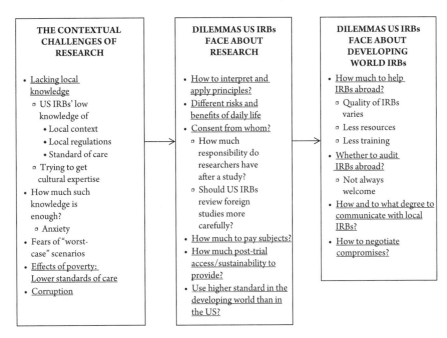

Figure 12.1 Issues Regarding US IRBs Reviews of Research in the Developing World.

Contextual Challenges

LACK OF LOCAL KNOWLEDGE

In trying to influence interactions between researchers and subjects in far-removed geographic, temporal, social, economic, and cultural milieus, US IRBs confront many uncertainties. These committees cannot readily anticipate what can "go wrong," nor do their own values necessarily reflect those of participants. In addition, both within and between developing countries, enormous variations exist in culture, resources, local researchers' experience, and infrastructure. US IRBs may be either overly or insufficiently concerned about such challenges. Some boards appear to adopt more of an "out of sight, out of mind" mentality, naïvely believing that participants will understand lengthy, complex consent forms. Other committees may worry about highly unlikely or unrealistic "worst-case scenarios," and take "extra precautions" that prove unnecessary and can in fact impede research. Unable to know fully or directly what is appropriate for a country, such committees may end up being overly paternalistic.

US boards often lack "local knowledge" about fundamental logistical details. An IRB in the local host country but not in the US may be aware, for instance, that the hospital where the proposed research is to take place is now closed. As Laura, the lawyer, said,

> There's local knowledge that we just wouldn't have known. Like, questioning a certain institution's ability to handle the research. Or the facility is under construction or renovation, and can't be used. Or the study involves prisoners or people who become imprisoned during the study.

Local knowledge can thus involve logistical and procedural concerns as well as ethical principles. PIs should possess these details but may not do so; or they may know them but fail to convey them adequately to the IRB.

US boards often try to obtain additional cultural expertise, but do not always sufficiently succeed. Scott, the IRB director, said,

> Sometimes our IRB has to go the extra mile and get someone familiar with the culture. For instance, elders of tribes may make the informed consent decisions for everyone in their group. We do our due diligence.

IRBs may remain unsure whether they themselves have gone far enough. "We always wonder," Nancy said.

Unfortunately, to know in advance the exact circumstances of a study in the developing world may be impossible. Even a highly responsible researcher who has done his or her best to be fully informed may arrive abroad and realize that the situation is far different than he or she anticipated. Committees vary in flexibility and in foreseeing, considering, and responding to these exigencies. Greg, the social scientist and chair, said,

> Researchers end up in a country, and realize that things aren't as thought, and they then have to make changes. We've worked closely with investigators at that point to . . . approve modifications, so they don't have to jump on a plane, come home, and cancel the research until then.

Given these unforeseeable obstacles, IRBs must trust investigators even more than in domestic research. As Robin said, "It's really left up to the PI to carry it out. We don't necessarily oversee things. We don't . . . do audits in our own country!"

In these settings, qualitative research, parts of which cannot be wholly specified in advance, can present invaluable data but also particular challenges. Robin continued,

> We struggle the most with qualitative or participatory-action research, where anthropologists go and blend themselves in the village, gathering

information. It's not a controlled clinical situation. They need to convey that they understand that when they collect qualitative information, *they* are the instrument, and their ability to understand the ethics and integrity issues are important. We're approving the *person* more than the process or study itself.

Here again, trust between the IRB and these researchers is essential but takes time to build, and thus may not always be robust at the outset. IRBs may struggle since they know that some faculty do not supervise students properly in such work—especially overseas. Robin added,

> They just kind of let their students go out there. So, we are more careful, scrutinizing what the student is doing. We make sure the protocol is much more precise.

US committees may also be unsure about relevant local laws and regulations. Laura, the lawyer, said, "You can have the best intentions to follow the local rules, but can't get a copy of them. The IRBs in a country may not even have a copy." International documents such as the Helsinki Declaration are available, but the host country's own relevant laws or regulations may not be. Such laws and regulations from all countries in the world are now being assembled, but these compilations are often incomplete or out of date. Even once such regulations are obtained, additional problems can arise because the same regulation or guideline may be interpreted differently within or between countries. Consensus between countries—at least in written regulations—is growing, but interpretations can still range widely. Communication between IRBs in the US and developing countries may also be poor or nonexistent.

And when is *dual* IRB approval needed? US investigators have often argued that since they are already getting IRB approval in the host country for a study abroad, they should not also need to obtain approval from their home institution's IRB. Some US IRBs require that they approve a study if one of their institution's researchers is a co-investigator, but not if he or she reports being "merely a consultant." Other committees might require approval only if the investigator plans to be an author on a published paper resulting from the research. This means that, during the actual trials, two researchers may be engaged in the same or similar tasks, yet only one of them requires IRB approval. Moreover, papers may have as many as 20 to 30 authors—some of whom may have relatively small roles. Simple one-size-fits-all approaches may not work well here; case-by-case consideration may be necessary.

For foreign research, even more than domestic studies, US IRBs need to trust PIs, but can face more challenges in doing so. Investigators,"may be following all the regulations," Cynthia, the Southern administrator, said, "but, we're not there, and don't know. We're hoping for the best...that our investigator has research integrity, and is only doing research appropriately."

Unfortunately, when IRBs discover problems, they may do so not through the PI but through a third party. Cynthia explained that China and India have become popular places for companies to conduct their research, but "it takes a long time to figure out if there were any human rights violations. Sometimes that information comes to us in a *Newsweek* article." The absence of information leaves many IRBs feeling uneasy. Enhanced communication between IRBs in the US and developing countries can help, but is often limited.

EFFECTS OF POVERTY: LOWER STANDARDS OF CARE

In the mid-1990s one of the fiercest recent research ethics controversies erupted concerning the standard of care in poorer countries. The AIDS Clinical Trial Group (ACTG) 076 study in the US and France (commonly known as 076) showed that providing zidovudine (also known as AZT) to pregnant women and for six weeks to the newborn dramatically decreased the odds of the infant being born with the infection from 25 percent to 8 percent.[24] Researchers then wanted to see if the medication would work as well in developing countries, where 95 percent of HIV-infected people reside, but where the medication was costly— US$800 per pregnancy—and hence, not widely available. But the investigators also wanted to determine if smaller doses could be just as effective, since more children could then be helped. The World Health Organization (WHO) launched such an initiative; and 15 of these studies, funded by the CDC, NIH, Joint United Nations Programme on HIV and AIDS, and others, also used placebos.[25]

If conducted in the West, this research could not have included a placebo, because AZT was already proven to be effective. But investigators argued that in the developing world, malnutrition, poverty, other infectious diseases, and higher rates of breast-feeding (which might also transmit the virus) might affect responses to both the virus and the treatment, and that these additional factors could not be properly evaluated without a control group. Thus, these scientists used a placebo. They contended that since the standard of care was no treatment at all—none of these patients would have received drugs outside the experi- ment—placebos were in effect equivalent, and therefore not unethical.

Critics, however, accused the researchers of having an ethical double stan- dard. If scientists could not use placebos in the West, they should not do so in poor countries just because they could.[26] Rather, if an effective treatment is not available in a developing country, researchers should seek to make it available. Moreover, is it ethical to provide interventions that are less than fully effective? This question also arose in the United States with the Kennedy Krieger study of lead removal: whether researchers could ethically place children in homes with only *partial* lead abatement. This question becomes even more pressing, however, with research in developing countries, which are more likely to lack basic treatments, and have lower standards. This debate continues over whether researchers should offer the best treatment in the local country, in the West, or something in between.

These assessments are difficult because the *standard* level of medical care in a developing country can be hard to ascertain. One researcher, for instance, wanted to study and improve the care that women received during pregnancy, and planned to provide ultrasounds to help detect fetal problems. Laura's IRB learned, however, that women in this country were already giving birth to more girls than boys—presumably due to the selective abortion of female fetuses. Thus, Laura feared that providing the ultrasound through the study might inadvertently further increase abortions. She asked the investigators,

> ... are ultrasounds really part of prenatal standard care in a country— or just part of the study—and if so, are they given once or twice, and when? The protocol wasn't clear. In a society where elective abortions often happen because of gender selection, we didn't want to be unintentionally contributing to girls getting aborted! We went back and forth with the PI to find out. We wanted to make sure that *elective* abortions were in the adverse event reports, so we could track them, and see if the ultrasound was contributing to gender elective abortions.

But frequently, even asking the right questions does not yield accurate or clear answers; and additional information and details take further effort and energy to acquire. As Laura elaborated,

> The PI answered that, "One early-stage ultrasound is standard." Now we were in an ethical dilemma: do we take his word for it? If not, how much of our resources do we put into independently finding more information? The PI's answer was fairly convenient, since in early ultrasound, you're not likely to know the gender. So we took his word, but insisted that he include elective abortions in his AE reporting. That's a kind of balanced, compromised solution, where we may not do *all* the due diligence that we should, but didn't totally close our eyes.

Given the many details beyond their control, US IRBs may simply have to "compromise," and seek the best plan they can.

CORRUPTION

Given cultural, economic, and political differences, and the lesser governmental oversight and transparency that often ensues, corruption can pose obstacles as well. As mentioned earlier, GlaxoSmithKline engaged in bribery and other corrupt practices in China, as have several other Western corporations. Corruption can operate at many levels, from national to local, and have many effects. It can severely undermine US IRBs' trust of certain research conducted abroad. IRBs that have detected corruption tend to do so at lower levels. "Money goes into the pockets of institutional officials," Laura said, sighing. In some developing countries, corruption is "a way of life," forcing IRBs to struggle how to proceed as a result—whether to accept it, and if so, to what degree. Financial deceit may include, for instance, kickbacks from drug manufacturers to pharmacists—even in studies funded by the US government. Laura continued,

> Corruption is usually off the record, on the QT. A study pharmacist dispensing HIV medication is...going to be offered kickbacks by the drug manufacturing companies to order from *them*. So, the price will be inflated because he's going to get some of it. But that is *grant* money! Or, a subcontracted institution has hardly any infrastructure for grants or contracts management, so the money goes right into somebody's personal bank account to buy a new car.

In some developing countries, kickbacks may simply be considered an inherent part of business transactions. A US IRB may aim not to eliminate, but merely minimize these practices. Laura added,

> Very respected people in development say it's just a part of doing business—that 5 or 10 percent is an acceptable rate of paying extra for corruption. If it's 15 or 20 percent, it's a problem. Bribes just sort of pave your way.

But, of course, US federal grants do not allow these costs. Many IRBs thus struggle with how much, if any, to accept, fearing the pernicious effects.

Dilemmas Faced by US IRBs and Researchers about Studies in the Developing World

HOW TO INTERPRET AND APPLY PRINCIPLES

Once they enter these challenging cultural and economic contexts, researchers face a series of quandaries, as do US IRBs. As Cynthia said,

The study may have gone through a local ethics review board, and may be appropriate according to their social customs. But by *whose* standards—theirs, or the US?

Clashes can ensue. Foreign IRBs may interpret regulations in ways that US boards or researchers disagree with—either too rigidly, or too loosely. IRBs abroad may not understand or follow key aspects of the regulations—for instance, that they can expedite reviews. Laura added,

> Some don't meet regularly, but just when they get protocols. It's pretty hard to run an operation with that level of uncertainty. They don't always understand that they have flexibility to do expedited reviews, so they're calling meetings when they don't have to.... They are often reviewing a study that doesn't need IRB review.

In part, they may not understand the regulations because, as in the US, they may have not had sufficient training.

DIFFERENT RISKS OF DAILY LIFE

The risks of daily life in the developing world and in the US can differ markedly. Committees struggle to decide *whose* daily risk to use as the standard in assessing risks. As Nancy said, "The life of an average healthy American is...very difficult as a standard to apply in international research." In addition, the risks of certain behaviors may be low in the US, but high elsewhere. In certain developing countries, Nancy pointed out,

> It would be extremely stigmatizing if anybody knew that you had undergone a psychological examination. It would mean that your doctor or somebody thought you were crazy.

That is a risk based on cultural differences, but there are also risks based on the quality of basic resources and physical resilience. If a study depends on clean water, for example, a lack of it could alter the potential risks and benefits, utterly compromising fairly straightforward research. Similarly, Nancy raised the example of nutritional supplements:

> Nutritional supplements aren't harmful to a healthy American, but could be harmful, because of malnutrition. We don't know whether to apply the standard of a healthy adult American, or a typical African villager.... In the end, we are just going to make a judgment call about

whether the people are going to be better or worse off, and how big we think the risk is.... That drives us crazy.

Other health behaviors, too, can have far different risks, benefits, and connotations in the developing world than in the US. For instance, studies have examined whether HIV-infected mothers should breast-feed or bottle-feed. Yet these behaviors have very different risks in resource-poor regions. In many foreign countries, women customarily breast-feed, rather than use formula. But breast milk can transmit the virus to the infants. Hence, villagers might assume a woman who uses bottles must be doing so because she is infected, which is highly stigmatized. Moreover, for bottle feeding, women may use powdered formula, mixing it with local water that may be unclean or contaminated with parasites. As Laura explained:

> On bottle-feeding, 80 percent of infants may have severe morbidity and mortality because of diarrhea. So, babies' chances of getting HIV through breast milk are less than dying of diarrhea from bad formula. How do you balance that, and honor the social norms around breastfeeding?

Laura added, "If she's been given all the information about both kinds of risk, and still decides to breastfeed, we have to honor that." IRBs must then decide how to respond, and may require that such studies bolster the educational support they provide.

Due to these different cultural, economic, and political contexts in the developing world, studies that might seem low risk and relatively harmless in the US can become problematic as well. Robin said,

> We're approving surveys and interviewing people on the street, but a study was going to ask about the political leader in the country. I don't know what's going on in that particular country. If they said that the political leader is terrible, or they are not so diplomatic in how they say it, could that put them at risk?

Surveys may target particular groups that face even greater dangers. As Nancy reported,

> I have seen research on Middle Eastern detainees in prisons, and relatives of terrorists and failed suicide bombers, and the information is extremely sensitive and the populations are incredibly vulnerable. Another IRB regards it as just an interview.

If such information were lost, stolen, or published without the proper safe-guards, these interviewees could be tortured or killed. These examples are of course extreme, but social scientists commonly study strife-ridden regions.

In certain parts of the developing world, even disclosing sponsorship of a study can raise concerns. Nancy added,

> You can't say this is being sponsored by the US government because nobody would participate, or you'd get really biased responses, because it would only be participants who like the US government. The assumption will be that it's sponsored by the CIA. We have tried hard to get the researchers to disclose sponsorship, but they feared they themselves would then be injured. So we decided researchers can say, "We can't tell you who's sponsoring this, and if that's a problem, please don't participate." It's vexing.

Defining and monitoring AEs is also frequently more challenging in poor countries than in the US. IRBs and researchers abroad may not monitor or report AEs properly. "Basically, it doesn't happen," Laura said. "Delays are very common." In part this is because AEs in the developing world can be hard to evaluate, and administrative support for tracking such information is limited. Poorly functioning bureaucracies may also foster more AEs. Pharmacies, for example, may incorrectly record and/or dispense drugs or doses. "No lasting harm to subjects," Laura said about one such instance, "but we were very worried." In addition, other ongoing dangers in daily life make AEs harder to pinpoint. Participants may also have more untreated health problems, and gauging whether the study itself caused or exacerbated these can be difficult.

CONSENT FROM WHOM?

Relationships between an individual and his or her group can vary widely, affecting decisions about who should consent for a participant, and how. IRBs thus face challenges in understanding cultural concepts of identity and of self. Laura saw this issue as "sticky":

> The *identity* of an individual is very different across societies. In the US, it's very "one person, one identity"—detachable from others. But in lots of societies, individual identity includes the kinship group, or having a husband, father, or chief condone a decision, or tell the individual what to do. The researcher has to go through these gatekeepers first—a tribal

chief, then maybe a head of household—to get permission to talk to the individual. These gatekeepers don't necessarily speak for the individual, but the researcher has to get to the individual…and let them know they can say no.

US IRB members may therefore worry that some research subjects in other countries are being coerced into participation. "Men, women, and children do not always have the same abilities to say yes or no," Cynthia said. "Women can't vote. Their ethics are based on their social structure." Other US IRB members may be concerned about the reverse: husbands or other men preventing women who want to participate in a study from doing so. These men may want women to be at home working rather than traveling to clinics for trials. Cynthia continued,

> Sometimes we worry that the women are coerced or pressured to say no, because their husbands don't want them to be away from home. We hear that from the field.

Yet although IRBs may fret about the possibility of undue pressure, their level of concern is likely to vary depending on a study's level of risk. Laura added,

> We tend to have low-risk studies, so I don't worry too much about women's freedom to say no; or, if the husband or the other men say, "Do this!", that the woman feels coerced. I don't worry about people being pressured into brain surgery.

The acceptability in other cultures of practices that are condemned in the US further complicates reviews. Laura, who has visited research sites in the developing world, continued,

> Women told me things that they wouldn't feel safe saying in the presence of men—even male investigators—about domestic abuse, which is common, and acceptable there.

If their HIV infection becomes known, for instance, women can be beaten or divorced or worse.

In other countries, the age of consent can also vary, both culturally and legally. Nancy reported,

> The question came up: what's the age of consent to participate in research? There wasn't even an answer to the question. Old enough to vote wasn't really the right test, since it was not a democracy.

Living independently of their parents was also not a useful test. None were living by themselves. The age of marriage was 16 for boys and 13 for girls, so we just decided to cave in and use the US standard of 18.

Yet, in a wholly different culture, that standard may not necessarily make sense. IRBs in some countries have blocked researchers from taking blood samples out of the country. Certain cultures consider blood to be an integral part of one's essence, and removing it to another country for unfamiliar laboratory analyses can violate this notion of sanctity. Anecdotally, researchers have at times been able to negotiate arrangements whereby they send back to the US part of each sample, but not all of it.

HOW MUCH TO PAY SUBJECTS: AVOIDING EXPLOITATION OR COERCION

One of the most difficult conundra IRBs face in reviewing research in the developing world is how much to pay participants. These committees seek to navigate between the Scylla and Charybdis of exploitation (paying too little) or coercion (paying too much). Many US boards simply try to defer these decisions to IRBs in the foreign country where the research is going to be conducted. "We need to know from researchers what the locals recommend," Olivia said, "what they think is appropriate. It may not be money at all, but something else." For instance, they may recommend small gifts.

Yet IRBs in the developing world are often themselves unsure how to proceed, partly because of uncertainties and assumptions about subjects' conscious and unconscious motives. US committees may incorrectly assume that their foreign counterparts know the answer, yet the local IRB members may come from dramatically higher socioeconomic and educational backgrounds than do most subjects, which can impede their full understanding of these participants' motives—just as it can in the US.

Additional Responsibilities of Researchers and IRBs

HOW MUCH RESPONSIBILITY DO RESEARCHERS HAVE AFTER A STUDY CONCLUDES?

Many investigators who travel to foreign communities solely to conduct studies have been accused of conducting "parachute research"—flying in, collecting their data, and departing, thus helping their careers but leaving their participants' lives and welfare unchanged. IRBs face quandaries of what to do to combat this possibility—*how much* ongoing assistance researchers should provide after the study or trial has finished—aid commonly referred to as "post-trial access or sustainability." For studies offering subjects effective therapy, for instance, IRBs must decide how much, if any, treatment researchers should offer after the study has concluded. As Laura said,

> Sustainability after a study leaves is a huge concern. We consider post-study access to a proven beneficial treatment. We are looking for an arrangement or contract for free or low-cost supply. You get into questions of who should get it…whether not just subjects, but the whole village.

These issues confront IRBs in the US as well, but can be even more charged when evaluating studies in poorer countries, given the severely limited health resources there.

In some instances, researchers may be able to pay for little, if any, ongoing care after the study ends. Laura continued,

> Is it OK if a researcher says, "I just can't give free treatment; we just don't have the money. It's just a three-year NIH grant"? We would then want to know, "What efforts have you made to push back on that, and work for the best possible deal?"

Still, there is little consensus among US IRBs as to how long to require researchers to provide free treatment after a study—whether for one, two, or three years.

SHOULD IRBS BE MORE RIGOROUS FOR STUDIES IN THE DEVELOPING WORLD THAN IN THE US?

Many US boards are suspicious of investigators conducting certain research in poorer countries, and therefore review these studies more cautiously than they do projects in the US. As Olivia said,

> There's a *higher* standard. What's the rationale for going to another country? Are we taking advantage of a population?…The answer "Because it's easier to do research there" is wrong.

But if committees consequently seek higher ethical norms and justifications, just how high is appropriate? They must gauge *how* reasonable, realistic, or aspirational a particular high standard is. IRBs may set a high bar with the hope that, realistically, at least *some* improvement will occur.

Committees may also encourage researchers to try to strengthen the capacity—the training, skills, and resources—of local researchers and health systems. Still, boards may remain unclear exactly how much enhancement to seek, and in what ways. Laura said,

> We've aimed high, insisting that our researchers help build capacity, to provide the best standards of care—like Western standards. As long as we keep aiming for the highest standard, and insisting that studies build capacity, that means a better chance of sustainability later, without us. If medication isn't available for herpes simplex, take it there! We understand we are shooting for the stars, and settle for the moon.

US committees may also encourage researchers to negotiate as optimal an arrangement as possible—especially when industry is involved. "We end up trying to find out what's the best possible outcome that we can structure," Laura said, "the best possible deal."

Through these efforts, the quality and integrity of research in several countries appears to be improving in recent years, but major gaps remain. As Laura described,

> For any FDA-regulated drug or device, you're going to have [a certain] level of scrutiny, because otherwise the FDA won't accept the data. So, it's catalyzed the training of in-country researchers in how to manage and clean data. But it still needs to grow.

HOW MUCH SHOULD IRBS HELP COMMITTEES ABROAD?

In response to the these challenges, several US IRBs have sought to assist not only researchers but IRBs in the developing world. In these countries the quality of IRBs/RECs and their reviews can vary enormously—as they do here—but be harder to ascertain from afar. These IRBs often have fewer resources and full-time staff and less infrastructure and training, and their performance may be monitored little, if at all.

IRBs in the developing world also may be wary of finding themselves simply approving US decisions automatically. Laura added,

> A lot of in-country IRBs are just not very confident. The classic concern is that they are rubber-stamping the Western IRB decision. They don't routinely stand up much to challenge our decisions, though there are a couple of exceptions.

A few US IRBs actively provide sample policies and forms. The NIH has funded Fogarty International Center programs to enhance training in research ethics in the developing world, assisting foreign IRBs.[27] IRB administrators from some countries have also traveled to the US to be mentored, but doing so takes money. Relationships and investments of time and resources by US IRBs can require years to bear fruit. The lack of skilled staff can itself become self-perpetuating. In poorer countries, IRB staff may be seen as lower-level clerical employees, not professionals. "Since professionalism of IRB administrators doesn't exist [in these countries]," Laura continued, "the job does not have a lot of appeal."

Whether to Audit IRBs Abroad

To increase their trust of IRBs in the developing world, some US IRBs attempt to monitor or audit these committees closely in some way. Yet such auditing can generate challenges and stress. Understandably, foreign committees do not always welcome outsiders' input or investigations. Audits often frighten foreign committees and researchers, who fear being scrutinized and judged. Developing world IRBs may also view US committees' scrutiny and audits as paternalistic. Some US IRBs therefore simply decide not to probe too closely what overseas IRBs are doing. On the other hand, the fear of upsetting or unsettling these foreign committees and uncovering problems is not necessarily a sufficient excuse to turn a blind eye. Still, extreme care and delicacy are vital. American committees can thus struggle with how much to pressure a committee abroad to conform to *their* procedures and standards. US IRBs may try to conduct friendly audits, but doing so can be hard, given sensitivities. "We always try to be as collegial as possible with PIs, and not be like an IRS audit," Laura said. "But it's always a continuous process. We're never really done."

US IRBs may also want to conduct site visits of developing-world IRBs but lack the necessary funding to do so. Given the challenges involved, American committees may simply be left feeling anxious about research abroad, especially initially, but decide to proceed nonetheless. Ongoing personal relationships—especially with researchers both here and in other countries—can promote mutual trust and education.

Conclusions

The recent increase in research conducted by US investigators in the developing world poses a host of ethical and logistical challenges, fueled by contrasting cultures, economics, and health standards. As in the US, developing world IRBs vary in resources, quality, and training. Frequently, health systems in these countries have lower resources and oversight, long-standing practices of inefficiency, and little transparency. US boards often have little knowledge of foreign local contexts, regulations, and standards of care. Risks and benefits in daily life can differ dramatically. US IRBs try to obtain relevant information about different cultures, but doing so can be difficult. Committees may be left fearing "worst-case scenarios."

A few studies have shown that IRBs in the developing world confront several obstacles, [7,8,9,10,11,12,13,14] but the men and women in my study highlight how IRBs in the US also face quandaries in reviewing developing-world studies. Cultural, legal, economic, and geographic distances exacerbate these dilemmas. Participants in research may speak different languages, and have little, if any, ability to read and write. In certain developing regions, over 80 percent of subjects may not understand basic concepts such as placebo, randomization, and the ability to withdraw from a study at any time. [28,29] Notions of "experiment," "treatment," "cure," "consent," "coercion," "under influence," "autonomy," "rights," and "identity" may not exist in certain cultures or differ markedly from views in the US. When two very different contexts collide, committees grapple with how to apply specific notions of justice. IRBs can face not only cultural and ethical differences but economic disparities as well. These gaps exist at all levels—from health systems (regarding corruption and long-term assistance) to individual subjects (concerning amounts of compensation). Countries differ, too, in broader business norms. In some countries, bribes and kickbacks are routine. Anecdotally, researchers may report such corruption to the FDA and other US agencies, but remain uncertain what then happens—whether other researchers are warned.

IRBs have difficulty, too, knowing when they sufficiently comprehend other cultural contexts—how much detail and due diligence are adequate, and how to decide. Committees, approving lengthy consent forms, may not all sufficiently acknowledge these deficits in their deliberations. In separate interviews I have recently been conducting, IRB members and researchers in the developing world have suggested that they feel very distant from US IRBs, which generally communicate only via formal memos—presenting decisions without the reasoning behind them. [30] Investigators in one developing country, for instance, as part of a radio advertisement to recruit participants for an HIV prevention study funded by the US government, wanted to use a popular song in the local language. The local IRB agreed, but the US IRB refused. The local researchers did not understand why the US committee objected. I asked the local researcher if perhaps because the US committee thought the song might unduly influence individuals to participate; but the researcher had no idea. The US board never gave an explanation. Moreover, though the US IRB may have feared undue influence from a song, no evidence exists that this view was justified. The US IRB personnel I interviewed frequently felt they had insufficient communication from IRBs abroad, but barriers to communication can clearly exist in both directions. [31]

How much US IRBs and researchers do or should assist foreign committees, and at what financial and logistical cost, is also unclear. Particularly given budget constraints, researchers and IRBs wonder how much NIH support they should be using to build and assist IRBs in emerging economies. One could argue that providing such assistance falls outside the purview of the IRB, but the Belmont Report dictates that committees and researchers follow the principle of justice. Still, how much IRBs should pursue it—especially how much they should use their limited resources to do so—remains fuzzy, and needs broad discussion.

These phenomena elucidate in microcosm the far wider challenges that arise as globalization continues to spread economic and social changes across every realm from business to universities. Yet given huge gaps between richer and poorer nations, with vast socioeconomic and cultural differences, these challenges need to be carefully and sensitively negotiated and addressed. US committees need to recognize that they may interpret and apply regulations in ways that do not make sense abroad. Given past histories of colonialization and exploitation, local populations in many of these countries may perceive IRBs' actions as paternalistic, making these committees' efforts counterproductive. But enhanced communication between IRBs in the US and in the developing world can potentially prove mutually beneficial and overcome fears and barriers. IRBs often communicate poorly, however, in part because they do so via the intermediary of researchers. Direct communication may help committees mutually inform each other about the challenges they confront.

US IRBs' attempts to affect downstream processes—interactions between PIs, staff, and subjects—are much harder to achieve in the developing world than at home. Committees may thus seek compromises and minimization of potential problems but remain anxious and possibly obsess over details.

Clearly, more research on these views is needed. Given the globalization of science, and the concomitant possibilities of abuse, more rigor, guidance, and standards in this area are also imperative.

PART

THE FUTURE

CHAPTER 13

Changing National Policies

As a researcher, I was initially wary of IRBs. In my years of conducting studies, they had delayed investigations—in my view, often unnecessarily—that many colleagues and I had sought to conduct. These committees had forced us to spend weeks and months of our time completing bureaucratic forms and awaiting replies. But as a doctor and as a son, I had witnessed firsthand the need to protect vulnerable patients. The interviews I conducted for this book helped me to see that, while the system certainly needs to be improved, neither side is entirely right or wrong. I now appreciate these committee members' perspectives and dedication far more than I did before; but I can also see more clearly the challenges they face and the unintended consequences of their actions, both good and bad. The problems and potential solutions are more complex than I had suspected.

Although researchers commonly refer to IRBs as "the Ethics Police," I came to see how this term does not accurately describe them. Nonetheless, the phrase clearly reflects many scientists' frustration, which these committees and others need to recognize and address much more fully.

In retrospect, the authors of the regulations 40 years ago embarked on a grand experiment. Now, almost a half century later, it is clear that they have succeeded in many ways, but that their work also needs to be revised and updated. Science advances ever faster, and can collide with moral principles. At times, investigators have violated ethical norms, but IRBs have also impeded science. In other instances, committees have approved studies that they should not have. Research ethics review is essential, but needs to change. Many IRB decisions are straightforward, but others are not, causing problems. IRBs are not all bad, and can do enormous good, but the *status quo* needs to be improved.

IRBs base too many of their decisions on idiosyncratic gut feelings. Due to scandals, OHRP shutdowns, and fear of lawsuits, many committees have become substantially more cautious. Scandals speak more loudly than do researcher complaints. Hence, IRBs have helped patients more than researchers, but at times still err, often because of COIs.

Unfortunately, debates about IRBs have become increasingly polarized. Certain criticisms of IRBs—for example, that they are "unconstitutional"—are too extreme, yet some IRB personnel also strongly oppose any significant changes to the status quo.

As shown in Table 13.1, the challenges presented here can be tackled at three levels: that of the federal government, the local institution, and the local IRB. At each of these layers, interviewees discussed possible new approaches and reforms.

I focus on possible federal improvements below, and possible local alterations in the following chapter. Unfortunately, major policy changes at the federal level face stiff obstacles. Twenty-three government agencies originally signed on to the Common Rule governing IRBs. Any modifications would presumably require coordination and agreement among all of these federal agencies—a huge, if not impossible, task. The Secretary's Advisory Committee on Human Resource Protections (SACHRP) has also proposed various changes. A few of these suggestions may have informed FAQs on the OHRP website,[1] but most of these recommendations have not been enacted. Ergo, this committee may often function

Table 13.1. **Suggested Changes Concerning IRBs: Federal Level**

- *Goals for change*
  - o Less idiosyncratic variation
  - o Less delay/less impediment to science
  - o More rigor of reviews
- *Mechanisms for change*
  - o Larger structural changes:
    - Centralization?
      - may offer several advantages and disadvantages
    - Different rules for social science research?
  - o Other changes:
    - More guidance and consensus (e.g., from OHRP, IOM, and/or others)
    - More case law/open, published precedents
      - Proprietary information can be redacted
    - External appeals process
    - More regionalization/centralization
      - Providing it is done well
      - Part of what is needed, not a "be all and end all"
    - More external (unaffiliated and non-scientific) members
    - Improved informed consent
      - Shorter summary documents to accompany longer forms
        - Yet many details need to be addressed

as a de facto "blue ribbon commission," allowing policymakers to "explore and address" a problem without actually enacting any significant alterations.

Still, improvements are possible. Policymakers' options fall across a spectrum, from clarifying existing regulations to centralizing IRBs and exempting much social science research.

No New Policies Needed

Most, though not all, of the interviewees here wanted little if any change in federal policy and were wary about proposed alterations—particularly any increased use of central IRBs (or CIRBs). A few believed that *no* policy changes at all were needed. Nathan, for instance, felt that the regulations represent the "minimum standard": "The government's done enough. The framework's there—all it requires are logical thinkers and effective implementers."

Others acknowledged problems with the current system but were unsure what to alter. They felt constrained by the status quo but were unclear what, practically, could be done. As Dwayne, a chair, said,

> I wish there could be less regulation and paperwork. It's become more and more burdensome for researchers. This is affecting all of medicine. It's very difficult to get things done. Layers of paperwork hinder the process. It definitely sends the wrong message. I tell colleagues, "Come to an IRB meeting. We're *not* out to get you, but are trying to obey the rules." But there is a frustrating dichotomy. I don't know the solution.

Many simply confessed that they did not have much sense of the larger policy issues and alternatives. "I am not sure," Jeremy, a chair, said, "if the alternatives would better address positives and negatives, and come up with a better balance."

CENTRALIZING IRBS

The most dramatic change proposed by the Obama Administration and others has been increased centralization of IRBs, about which these interviewees voiced strong opinions. Complaints of discrepancies in committee reviews of multisite studies has already fueled the centralization of some reviews in the US and elsewhere.[2] In Europe, central, regional, and local RECs often coexist, but conflict. The European Union has sought to harmonize reviews across countries, yet individual countries have disagreed about how and to what degree to unify processes and decisions.[3,4,5,6,7]

Centralization has been discussed in the US for more than a decade,[8,9] but thus far it has been instituted only to relatively limited extents[10] and has faced opposition. These CIRBs can be either governmental bodies or private, for-profit commercial entities: two varieties that differ both in purpose and in potential conflicts of interest. And yet both have been established as alternatives to local IRBs. For government-funded multisite studies, several models of CIRBs have been suggested, generally allowing local boards to accept, reject, or amend these central committee decisions.

Many universities have relied on certain for-profit IRBs when their own IRBs have become backlogged. The largest, Western IRB, located in Tacoma, Washington, has a solid reputation. The National Cancer Institute (NCI) has also created two CIRBs—one each for adult and pediatric cancer treatment research.[11]

One study found that CIRBs reduce time, staff effort, and costs,[12] but the quality of its reviews was, alas, not assessed. Among medical school IRBs, 24 percent have used a CIRB; 73 percent thought there was no reason to do so, however, since their local IRB worked efficiently.[13] Increased centralization will continue, but to what degree, how, and when is unpredictable. The impact, outcomes, and effectiveness of current CIRBs will help determine how much they are more widely adopted.

In 2009, the US Government Accountability Office (GAO) launched a "sting" operation of several for-profit CIRBs, sending them a fictitious protocol conducted by fictitious researchers for review. When one of these IRBs nonetheless approved the study, the GAO shut the company down. Yet some observers have argued that it is not the IRB's job to vet a researcher's credentials—that is, to see if he or she is fictitious (as was the case here) or legitimate.

Surprisingly though, no studies have examined how local IRBs view and experience their centralized counterparts.

The interviewees here were very aware of CIRBs; most had interacted with centralized, for-profit ones, and several had worked with governmental ones as well. Despite the limitations of local committees, however, *all* still favored local over centralized reviews. Their perceptions may not always have been wholly "accurate," but nevertheless reflected their views and experiences, and are thus vital to grasp.

Advantages of Centralization

A few interviewees explicitly acknowledged the advantages of CIRBs, but did so only rarely—not wholly as a substitute for their own committee. A handful felt that requiring one study to go through multiple IRBs squandered valuable resources. Charlotte, though an administrator and not a researcher herself, said,

> Busy scientists, trying to do really good science, should not be bogged down, having to go to four different IRBs. An awful lot of time is spent

jumping through bureaucratic hurdles. That's a waste of everybody's time. It would be nice if that could be streamlined somehow.

A few others supported CIRBs, but only in particular situations—for example, to avoid drug companies "gaming" the system. Industry may take advantage of smaller hospitals that are not closely tied to academic medical centers, have less experienced IRBs, and undertake research primarily for the money. Andrew therefore felt that CIRBs may be good for such other, smaller hospitals—but not for his own.

A few interviewees acknowledged possible advantages of using CIRBs if local boards were then allowed to accept, reject, or modify the reviews. Kevin, the health care provider and chair, said,

> I don't want to lose individual input at the level where the study takes place. The CIRB established by NCI with adults represents one of the more logical approaches to review, taking relatively little time, and still allowing local input. We still have an option of altering, overriding, or rejecting the central CIRB action.

Jack, the rural physician and chair, also saw benefits to the NCI CIRB. The reviews,

> mostly from the NCI's cooperative group studies, have helped streamline our work. The discussion notes are high quality, and we can choose to accept their reviews. That would be a good way of reviewing studies regularly.

Perceived Advantages of Local IRBs

Yet as we saw earlier, most IRBs felt that only local reviews reflect local community values. A few interviewees took a more balanced, nuanced view that the current system has both strong advantages *and* disadvantages that need to be carefully weighed. "We have a very decentralized system," Laura said. "That gives a lot of responsibility and flexibility to local IRBs, which is a blessing and a curse." Yet in the end, these interviewees, too, favored the continuation of local reviews.

LOCAL KNOWLEDGE OF SUBJECTS

In supporting decentralized over centralized boards, almost all these men and women cited the advantages of "local knowledge." Indeed, only a local IRB may know certain unstated details about a protocol, such as the fact that a particular institution primarily serves a particular population. As Cynthia, the administrator, said,

> In one study of parenting skills for moms, the rationale was to show how young moms, living alone without the benefit of several generations to

help them, didn't know anything about comfort care—lullaby singing, story-telling, rocking chairs with fussy babies. But the hospital they picked was a *private* hospital that only accepts *private pay patients*. The patients who could benefit most from the study were indigent patients in clinics. We asked: are *those* individuals really going to be at this private hospital? One co-investigator saw patients only at that hospital, and had quite a bit of influence. We urged them—we cannot insist that a study be conducted at a specific hospital. But if the objectives are for a particular population who can't take advantage of the study, I think it's within the IRB purview to say, "Would you be willing to offer this study to people who are not patients there—advertise it through clinics or hospitals where these other patients would be able to access it?" ... Their objective was well stated, but that's where the *local oversight* comes in—if you didn't know that that hospital only accepted private pay patients.

Only a local IRB might also know that a particular hospital serves a vulnerable population, necessitating that the protocol contain *extra* protections. As Martin, a researcher and chair, explained,

If I am going to recruit all my patients from a certain psychiatric center, a colleague here in town would know *exactly* what I'm talking about, and who those patients are—and their demographics. That kind of *local knowledge*. If you are accused of a crime, you want to be judged by a jury of your peers, not by somebody who has the same demographic from halfway across the country.

Martin draws analogies to a jury and suggests that the "peers" who presumably constitute it represent not demographics alone, but other characteristics—shared membership in, as well as knowledge of a community. He sees importance in knowing details about a particular population—having a sense of familiarity that is concrete, not abstract:

The farther away you get from the actual group of subjects, the harder it is for a committee to judge the risks and benefits. So in our IRB, we are thinking about whether it's ethical and reasonable to do a study of new asthma treatments for young black children in our city. This is not abstract. We all know exactly who's involved, what the lives of those individuals are like, what the protocol could offer them. An IRB in another state could not make as informed a decision.

Ideally, centralized or regional IRBs should be able to request and assess such details, but Martin's comment highlights challenges that CIRBs face.

PROTECTING "OUR OWN" SUBJECTS

Many interviewees feel they have not only local knowledge but local responsibilities—particular bonds with, and duties to protect, subjects at their own institution. As clinicians, they may feel obligations toward the specific communities of patients they serve, as well. Jeremy, the physician and chair, said,

> With the local approach, we absolutely feel committed to the subjects in *this* area. A lot of them are *our patients*. They are from the community that we are committed to serving. That commitment couldn't be higher. I would worry that if the IRB became more regionalized, de-personalized and, particularly, for-profit, that would go away at little bit.

Thus, for IRBs, professional, social, and geographic closeness can heighten senses of moral obligation.

As suggested earlier, IRBs often feared centralized bodies as "anonymous bureaucrats in Washington." This attitude reflects a sense that linkages with a local community are important; and a general wariness of federal government involvement. As Dwayne, the rural researcher and chair, said,

> Centralized IRBs may be a solution, but we really want to know what's going on on *our* campus—what's being said, conveyed, to *our* community and participants. It would be hard for people to say, "Oh, this was approved by some anonymous body, so it should be OK."

Some see centralization as a perilous step toward unresponsive, uncaring authority. Phil said,

> If people have face-to-face relationships, they can sit and say, "Look, here's what we're talking about." If it becomes regionalized or centralized, it's going to become like a Soviet-style bureaucracy. It's bad enough now!

LOCAL KNOWLEDGE OF RESEARCHERS

Local knowledge can also include an awareness of local scientists' personalities and past lapses, or other relevant behavior. Scott, the IRB director, said,

> The most effective IRBs are those in an institution where the reviewers are familiar with the work and integrity of the researcher. That is the

most important element, other than the actual research proposal itself.
What's this researcher's *track record*? Has he been shot down once or
twice? Regional IRBs might get reports of that info, but don't have the
personal understanding, feel, and flavor that's needed for a heightened
level of review.

He suggests an elevated standard here—a "heightened level of review"—that
only a local IRB can provide. Yet questions arise of what this level consists of:
how "heightened" it is; when it is needed and/or feasible, and to what degree; and
in what ways knowledge of the researcher does or should influence assessments.
Scott and others also evoke notions of "feel" and "flavor," suggesting subjective,
almost aesthetic qualities involved.

Such local knowledge about researchers can include not only subjective
impressions concerning these scientists' integrity, but also suspicions concerning
their views of, and respect for, the IRB. For instance, local researchers may try to
pressure committees, which can then make the board wary of them in the future.
An IRB may feel that such researchers' efforts indicate disrespect. Scott added,

> When a PI tried to exercise his power as a vice-dean, and convince the
> IRB to review a study favorably, his future submissions were questioned.
> It's an integrity issue: he's exercising a position of influence, which con-
> tributes to the appearance of coercion.... That happens rarely.... It's
> usually low-risk research. The PI may use the "no harm, no foul" prin-
> ciple: "I did all this research without IRB review. I now know I need IRB
> approval. But no one got hurt. What's the big deal? Give me retroac-
> tive approval." Obviously, we can't. But it doesn't stop there. One person
> came back and said, "You're going to screw me up, ruin my publication,
> and tarnish my reputation."

The IRB may then examine such an investigator's subsequent studies more
closely. As Scott continued, "That PI is willing to try and convince his peers to
make an exception for him because of who he or she is." Personal knowledge
about a local scientist can thus potentially sway how a committee assesses his or
her protocols. Yet prejudice may exist either positively or negatively. Questions
also surface of how important such past experiences should be—whether this
sort of added caution might ever go too far, and whether each protocol should
instead be reviewed afresh, solely on its own merits.

"CURBSIDE CONSULTS" WITH RESEARCHERS

Though federal regulations originally made IRBs local bodies so that these committees would reflect local standards and laws, additional, unintended benefits

emerged—under the present arrangement, PIs can interact with their IRB both formally and informally, thereby potentially facilitating the process. Knowing the local "gatekeeper" (i.e., the IRB) has advantages. Jack argued, "I don't think it was the intent, but the *practical* outcome of local IRBs is that PIs bounce stuff off me all the time." IRB members can interact with PIs informally and in person, rather than through the constraints of formal memos back and forth. Such informal 10-minute verbal communication can allow researchers to present possible approaches (e.g., "What if I did X?"), get immediate feedback, and then make better decisions as a result. Such conversations can significantly shape studies early on, clarifying what research the IRB may find ethically problematic. Informal local feedback has the advantage, too, of being readily available, whereas an exchange of memos might take weeks, or even months. Jack added:

> Researchers say, "What do you think of this?" I say, "I can tell you: 'We're going to make you do *this*,' 'Say X.' 'No, you can't give the pharmacist a finder's fee to identify how many patients are getting this drug.'" Or, we'll get an informed consent, and say, "Our IRB likes to see the wording a certain way. E-mail me, and we'll send it back to you." It is good to have the local cooperative mechanism.

A sense of *mutual* commitment and trust can thereby be increased.

Curbside consults can allow researchers, too, to explore the possibility of making small changes to protocols already approved—for example, making exceptions to include patients who do not exactly fit the preestablished criteria or timeline. These alterations might alter not the direct risks or benefits to the subject, but rather the indirect social benefits of the research. Local IRBs can thus readily communicate their concerns to PIs. Jack added,

> The most frequent curbside thing I have to deflect, and say "OK, we need paperwork for this," is: "This patient fits the study really well, except for this one really little glitch. Can I put him in the study anyway? The protocol says within four weeks. It's been four weeks and three days." That's when I push back.... Researchers then say, "It doesn't really make any difference, but I had to write something in the protocol." I answer: "If that rule was important enough to write down, why is it OK to break it? If it's OK to break it, maybe you should rewrite the rule to reflect *reality*." I do that a lot—not so much trying to protect the subject from risk, but *protecting the science from damage*. If you make all these exemptions, you are going to dilute the science.... It puts the science at risk. Usually, it's not serious, but a couple times I've said, "This is the fifth time you've asked me about this. Rewrite the protocol, rather than making all these

exemptions. If this is an important rule, you can't break it." They then have to convince me that it's OK. Because otherwise, thinking ahead, the paper's method section says "patients will have had a CT scan no more than four weeks ago." And I'll say, "That's not true." This is small stuff, but it's of a piece of real falsification of data.

The content of the disagreement here does not concern differences in local community values, but illustrates how local IRBs can potentially facilitate the *process* of informal interactions, allowing far more immediate and effective "give and take." These closer, more frequent interactions can also enhance investigators' research ethics, and potentially diminish the odds of scientists making potentially problematic changes without notifying the IRB.

Local chairs' interactions with colleagues may enable the IRB, too, to hear about a researcher's difficulties and struggles, potentially enhancing committees' understandings of the strains these researchers confront. Jack added, "I hobnob with colleagues. I hear the woes of our local cancer investigator over audits in big cooperative studies." Such strengthened mutual understanding can help mollify tensions.

At institutions that focus on just one medical specialty, disease, or organ— whether pediatrics, cancer, diabetes, or the brain—IRBs will also understand that specific area of medicine extremely well, which can be helpful. As Katherine, an IRB administrator from such a specialty institution, said:

> We are a small institution, and can be very flexible with PIs, especially with administrative approval for a lot of the research. A lot of researchers here would be upset if we did away with our IRB. Here, people understand this specific area of research—the terms and concepts.

Still, regulations mandate that all IRBs have appropriate specialization for reviewing all protocols.

DESIRES FOR LOCAL AUTONOMY AND COMFORT

Committees may also oppose centralization because they want to review protocols on their own, to become as familiar and comfortable as possible with the issues involved. They don't trust that another IRB's review would be the same or as good as their own. As Charlotte, the administrator, said,

> Each IRB has *its own learning curve*, and comes to its own sense about an issue. I could call up the IRB administrator [elsewhere] and say, "We've been through this.... This is how it is." They would say, "Thank you very much. We're going to go figure it out for ourselves." Like anybody, we

don't like other people telling us how to run our own shop—although it should count for something that another IRB has approved it. I don't know how you can streamline that. It is inevitable.

IRBs may therefore want to undergo their own complex cognitive and emotional decision-making processes.

Giving up control can generate anxiety and wariness. As Judy said, "We are now *ceding* some of our reviews to the central IRB for NCI studies. There is a big resistance to doing it for all studies—to give *up that control*." Hence, local control, comfort, and potential liability, rather than community values, may underlie IRB preferences for local review.

Perceived Problems with Centralization: Differences between CIRBs

Several interviewees perceived problematic variations between CIRBs. Difficulties could arise with these entities due not to the underlying concept of such centralization, but instead to the specific realities of who exactly was on each committee, what training members had, and how "reasonable" they were. Chairs and members of CIRBs, like those of local IRBs, could have their own personalities and idiosyncrasies. A centralized committee could easily prove to be *stricter* than a particular local one. Troy, a researcher and chair, had had this experience:

> In our city, research involving people covered by Medicaid and Medicare has to go through a city IRB, which puts more control on you. It requires more and more time and paperwork, and can get crazy, particularly for behavioral research. They often set an even *tighter* set of rules, and just keep coming back with more questions in whatever you do. The city IRB is primarily laypeople, and they are very, very thorough. Some of these members have four pages of handwritten notes on a very small study. It's too much.

Individual CIRBs may themselves differ significantly. For example, a few interviewees felt that the centralized pediatric cancer board is not as good as the adult one. Kevin, the health care provider and chair, said,

> A model is only as good as the quality of the reviewer. I have absolutely rejected, refuse to become a part of, a similar program with Children's Oncology Group because the quality just isn't there.

He felt that the pediatric CIRB has produced overly complicated consent forms and is less open to input from local institutions. "It has a sort of *dictator* syndrome. No one gives them feedback; while the *adult* CIRB listens to feedback, and is not like that."

Kevin continued, complaining about the consent forms used by the pediatric CIRBs:

> The quality of the consent forms, the way they present information, pales in comparison to the adult CIRBs. The Children's Group forms are not user-friendly enough, and do not convey information as it could be. Perhaps the pediatric group has bent over too far backwards, offering complex charts with medical jargon of potential drug side effects. Some of the consent forms just leave my head spinning. They present *facts*, not *information*.

This distinction between facts and information highlights the different functions of each of these categories: Information is meant to "inform," to create a sense of understanding in the recipient's mind, whereas "facts" implies nothing about the recipient whatsoever. Yet, as we saw, to decide how to "inform" subjects and determine what is sufficiently "user friendly," rather than merely "present facts," can be hard.

Several other interviewees also preferred the adult to the pediatric CIRB—particularly since local committees can choose to accept or alter the adult board's reviews—prompting local support of at least some centralization. Kevin thought that the adult CIRB took time and sought input, while the pediatric group failed to do so:

> Four years before the adult CIRB launched, they asked for input. They had draft after draft of how to go about doing what they wanted to do. They did it very cautiously . . . to test the waters, and it turned out very well. I think the Children's Oncology Group was simply pressured to follow suit, but did so without having the requisite background and preparation.

Perceptions of the pros and cons of centralization depend in large part, too, on the specifics of how much each IRB permits local committees to modify or reject reviews. Troy, the chair, said,

> We've worked very well with the adult CIRB because it leaves the local IRBs a lot of room to make changes. We're very happy with that. Other large-scale regional IRBs have not seemed all that great. Limited numbers of people have oversight, and are not involved with the institution. They don't know the *institutional*, let alone the local culture. The adult CIRB differs from the others. It's national, looking at huge cancer

studies all over the country; so they develop a standard of what they expect, and what's in the consent. Local IRBs can then modify it.... It's probably very effective.

Hence, the *details* of how more centralized models work are important. *The national debate thus needs to evolve beyond simply central vs. local review, to examine to what degree, and how exactly different models might operate.* Troy also feels that knowledge of local institutional culture is important as well (though it is not the intent of the regulations).

Multisite studies may also vary in structure. In some cases, a primary-site IRB takes the lead, and the other sites' committees agree to cede to it. Institutions could also potentially decide in advance to rely on another institution's IRB, but then reject particular reviews. Katherine, an IRB administrator, said that her IRB agreed to make an exception to its usual practice and accept an outside review because her IRB was an "add-on," and did not want to be inappropriately determining the overall multisite study.

> We accepted their consent form and protocol.... But that was an *exception* to the rule.... Really the *only* one, because we were at the point, otherwise, of being the tail wagging the dog. The other medical center was taking the lead, and doing most of the research. Our researchers just sort of tagged along.

Yet other local boards may not want to cede any control to a more central institution. Yielding responsibility may be hard legally, ethically, and emotionally, raising fears.

Not only governmental, but also private, for-profit CIRBs provoked a broad array of opinions. While some interviewees relied on and respected such entities, others questioned how these bodies could sufficiently glean local communities and values. Concerns arose, too, that for-profit entities might have conflicts of interest, since they are paid to review and approve studies. Stephen felt that these for-profit IRBs "primarily do their business with drug company sponsors. So, the very people that are paying them are the ones that they are regulating."

As members of local IRBs, almost all interviewees were strongly wary or critical of for-profit boards—fearing lower standards among these for-profit competitors, and often an implicit threat. Martin, a chair, said,

> I'm not really sure what standards these so-called private IRBs uphold, where a doctor doing a study out of their private practice would just pay money and get some IRB to approve it. My impression is that the standards are not as high. I've been involved in many multi-site trials, and

someone said, "That design isn't going to fly with the university's IRB, but *the private IRBs will accept it.*"

The potential profit motive of private IRBs concerns many. Kevin, a health care provider and chair, said,

> I am against them. They're in it for the money, for rapid turn-around time. PIs say to me, "Every time I change a word in the consent form, it costs me $1,000," and these PIs are therefore reluctant to make changes.

For-profit IRBs are generally also not local, and make no pretense of being so.

Are Local IRB Members Biased in Their Views of CIRBs?

In part due to the psychological and legal issues mentioned earlier, IRBs often appeared *biased* in favor of local control. In citing the benefits of local review, many interviewees seemed to have little, if any, sense of the status quo's potential costs to investigators—that for multisite studies, reviews by multiple local IRBs can vary considerably for idiosyncratic reasons, consuming enormous additional resources and time. Martin, the chair who stated earlier that it was easier to judge risks and benefits that are closer (*vs.* "farther away"), added, "I like the current model. I'm not sure why. I've never been on regional IRBs."

As an investigator, he participated in a multisite research group in which he felt that IRBs varied little, except over phrasing.

> I'm involved in a consortium, and don't see a lot of difference between what's acceptable at one institution *vs.* another. There are usually arguments over wording here and there, but not the basic risk *vs.* benefit analyses of a protocol.

Although one might expect all researchers in multisite studies to favor CIRBs, he does not—perhaps because he has long been an IRB member. Yet his statement undermines his earlier notion—that local community values play important roles here—and conflicts with the data that show discrepancies frequently involve more than wording alone. He and others also appear to downplay or not consider or weigh the possible logistical and other burdens to PIs involved.

MORE REGIONAL IRBS?

In debates over whether to establish more CIRBs, several interviewees suggested that an alternative would be simply to have more *regional* rather than national boards, gathering more local information. For instance, Troy, who saw a current "city-wide" IRB that reviews certain protocols as "too strict," nonetheless perceived potential advantages in wider use of such municipal-wide entities—though not this *particular* one. Statewide IRBs are also possible. Unfortunately, some states have only one major medical center, or one major one and a few smaller ones, and hence smaller institutions worry about the largest hospital or university dominating or in effect ruling the CIRB.

CONCLUSIONS ABOUT CIRBS

The men and women here thus suggest advantages and disadvantages of both local and centralized committees. Overall, however, these local IRB chairs, administrators, and members overwhelmingly supported local over centralized boards. These men and women felt that local committees can better provide local knowledge of subjects and of PIs, and "curbside consults" with scientists that can facilitate mutual trust, potentially decreasing researcher noncompliance. Local committees may also appreciate local institutional culture much more. While a few respondents acknowledged that the current system can impede multisite studies, and that centralization could potentially streamline work and reduce duplication of efforts, ultimately all interviewees supported continuing local IRBs in some form.

Significantly, these men and women highlight how the quality of CIRBs can range markedly. Many of these individuals have had experience with the centralized reviews of for-profit IRBs, the NCI for adult oncology trials, and the Pediatric Oncology Group, and felt that whoever happens to be on the committee profoundly influences the nature and outcome of CIRB deliberations. Both local and CIRBs therefore appear to have unintended consequences, good and bad, that need to be recognized far more fully.

These interviewees felt that local knowledge of subjects and researchers, longstanding informal interactions with these PIs, and consequent trust and "comfort" are vital. Investigators may interact more fully and informally, and hence effectively, with local rather than central IRBs. In general, relationships can depend on both the quantity and quality of information exchanged. Communication early in a process can avoid difficulties later (e.g., researchers investing efforts on approaches the IRB will eventually reject). Local IRBs can potentially provide informal "curbside consults" that establish and maintain mutual confidence, enhancing the protection of study participants. Hence, informal interactions in an institution, established over time, can be critical.

Such social bonds affect not only colleagues and researchers but patient populations as well. IRB chairs and members, many of whom are themselves physicians, feel a sense of commitment to "their patients" (i.e., those of their institution), and thought that entrusting these patients to a distant, "anonymous" CIRB represents an abdication of this responsibility. Belonging to a community can thus generate deeply personal, social, and moral bonds that can enhance protection of subjects. Yet desire for such local linkages can fuel opposition to CIRBs. Presumably, however, an ethical obligation to safeguard subjects as much as possible should exist on central committees as well, and extend to participants elsewhere, too. Hence, IRB members should not protect subjects at their home institutions more than CIRB members should safeguard the rights and well-being of study participants at another medical center. Nevertheless, individuals may feel special loyalty to their own community.

Local IRBs' close knowledge of researchers and patients does not appear to have been the intent of the regulations. Rather, committees were established to reflect local community values and laws. Nonetheless, enhanced communication and trust between IRBs and researchers, committee awareness of details about subject populations, and commitment to these individuals are valuable.

Still, tradeoffs ensue. Local IRBs may enhance reviews (by providing local knowledge of subjects and PIs) and/or generate costly and unnecessary discrepancies. But it is not clear how to balance the advantages of local IRB reviews (unintended by the regulations) against the disadvantages (inter-IRB discrepancies). Whether the advantages of local review offset the consequent problems, and whether a reformed system could yield these benefits while avoiding these disadvantages, is not yet evident. The answers to many dilemmas here are not simply empirical but also normative—involving values, varying levels of faith in scientists, and fears of abuse.

Within the US, whether community values in fact ever significantly differ in ways that do or should shape specific IRB decisions—and if so, when and how often—are also unknown. No empirical evidence has ever been presented to support this assertion. The fact that institutional and personality issues can play roles is not surprising, given the complex dynamic social processes involved. But while proponents of local review frequently claim that relevant community values vary significantly, the examples that the men and women provide appear here instead to reflect differences in local knowledge, and presumptions about others' discomfort with sex, which may be inaccurate and merely reflect prejudices and homophobia, and were presumably not the intentions of the regulations' authors.

Reasons for favoring local IRBs appear to stem not from objective evidence of improved human subject protection, but largely from opinions and emotional discomfort. Still, despite this absence of evidence of significant differences in local community values, IRBs support this rationale, because it is suggested in 45 CFR 46, and appears to justify their efforts, existence, and expense. Nonetheless, enhanced local knowledge of subject populations and researchers can heighten caution in reviewing certain protocols. Increased cognizance of their lives can arguably help protect subjects indirectly—even if not measurably and directly.

These interviews also underscore several other potential disadvantages of centralization. While IRB critics may see centralization as a panacea, certain problems appear likely to persist. CIRBs may not be any more objective than local IRBs—both can be shaped by the particular views or predilections of chairs and members.

These interviewees express, too, suspicion of "anonymous government bureaucracies." This same apprehension underlies broader fears of "big" government generally, and beliefs in "state rights." Yet, local IRBs may consequently resist centralization, impeding the potential spread and efficiencies of such broader review. Given concerns—whether valid or not—that CIRBs will insufficiently incorporate local knowledge, other models may be advantageous—perhaps having local reviewers contribute to CIRB discussions. But how exactly such mechanisms would operate—for instance, in multisite studies being reviewed by a CIRB—and whether such "dual reviews" would decrease expenses and discrepancies, and if so, how much need to be studied by establishing and evaluating such programs. These interviewees may also be biased. They receive support—even if it is only part of their salary—for their work in the *status quo*, which they may therefore be invested in continuing.

Current arguments about local *vs.* central reviews do not appear to reflect these complexities, but should. National debates need to shift from focusing simply on a binary decision of local *vs.* centralized IRBs, to explore specifically how different models (including regional ones) do and could function, what the relative advantages and disadvantages of each are, how to balance these, what obstacles might arise in implementing any change, and whether and how these barriers ought to be overcome. We need to consider carefully the difficult tradeoffs here—for instance, when, if ever, the benefits of local IRB knowledge offset the delays and obstacles of multiple local IRB reviews. Debates have not generally addressed these dilemmas, but need to.

Centralized boards may work particularly well in areas with relatively small pools of expertise, but still need to interact with PIs closely, frequently, and effectively. At local IRBs, interactions may be informal, based on long-standing relationships and mutual trust. In establishing such relationships, CIRBs face obstacles. To build these bonds at a federal level may be hard. Federal bureaucrat responses would presumably be "official" in ways that local "curbside consults" are not. Still, CIRB reviews can potentially incorporate additional local knowledge in certain ways. Hence, options need not simply be dichotomous—local *vs.* central, all or none. Rather, CIRBs could seek enhanced local input. Further studies can explore more fully, as well, the roles and effects of informal communication; and ways and frequencies of local IRB alterations of CIRB reviews.

Questions emerge, too, as to which studies should be reviewed through central, regional, or local boards. While many proponents push CIRBs for large multisite studies, smaller and single-site studies might then be left wholly to local review, and be prey to local biases and impediments. Subjects in multisite *vs.* other studies might then receive different kinds and degrees of protection. Questions then arise of exactly what sized studies justify a CIRB.

While some critics herald centralization as a virtual cure-all, these interviews emphasize the importance of more nuanced understandings of how precisely these and other models may best be used, and the intricate tradeoffs and uncertainties entailed. Given local IRBs' resistance to CIRBs as structural solutions, altering local committee attitudes may be more achievable—helping board members become more cognizant of their own potential assumptions and biases.

DIFFERENT RULES FOR SOCIAL SCIENCE RESEARCH?

The federal government could change policies regarding not only CIRBs, but also social science research as well. Interviewees here highlight needs to consider separate rules for much social science research, but what these new regulations should say remains unclear.

Given social scientists' complaints of being unduly burdened administratively by IRBs, the Obama Administration has proposed changing the regulations so that researchers would not have to submit low-risk studies to IRBs for continuing re-review every year (which requires time and effort), but instead could do so less frequently. This change seems straightforward and would reduce administrative burdens on both investigators and IRBs, and hence aid research.

The Obama Administration and others have also suggested excusing all minimal-risk, particularly behavioral and social science research from IRB review and letting researchers make these determinations for themselves. Yet questions arise about this possibility. Not all such research is uniform; and PIs' beliefs that their own research is of minimal risk are not all correct.

Several men and women here feel that the current regulations are flexible enough to accommodate social science research. Many IRBs defend their committee as acting flexibly, and see no problems in how they interpret regulations, though they at times cite problems in how *other* boards apply these statutes. Still, these interviewees tend to argue, the system as a whole is adequate. Indeed, one chair dubs the notion that "the regulations are flexible for social science research" the "*OHRP party line.*" Yet a few others also point out examples of IRBs hampering science. In the end, the regulations cannot be readily divorced from problematic interpretations of them. Discussions of whether and how these policies should be altered need to consider any current suboptimal implementations of regulations by IRBs.

Moreover, proposals to allow certain researchers to self-assess minimal risk are problematic. If it were up to PIs to decide whether they require IRB review, with its additional bureaucratic burdens and potential alterations to their protocols, their decisions would be inherently biased. Just as physicians poorly estimate their own COIs,[14] so, too, many researchers may not be entirely objective in evaluating the potential harms of their own experiments.

Certain minimal-risk studies should surely be exempt from full IRB review, but which protocols should fit this category needs careful consideration. Experiments involving deception, for instance, need more prudent review, yet receive little attention in the Obama Administration's Advance Notice of Proposed Rulemaking (ANPRM) and other proposals for change. Self-regulation may also be problematic for minimal-risk studies in which investigators interact with subjects more than simply administering surveys (e.g., involving support groups or role-playing). The ANPRM asks whether all surveys should be excused from any IRB review unless they "involve topics that are emotionally charged, such as sexual or physical abuse."[15] But, especially among vulnerable persons, appropriate researcher training and sensitivity can be important for a far broader array of surveys—for example, concerning stigmatized behaviors (such as homosexuality, unprotected sex, or drug use), mental illness, sexually transmitted diseases, life-threatening diseases such as cancer, and deaths of family members. Without anyone else reviewing their self-assessments, researchers may be biased in stating whether their questionnaires and procedures are sufficiently sensitive. Moreover, the topics that some participants may find sensitive cannot always be fully predicted. Stanley Milgram and Philip Zimbardo (in the Stanford prison experiment) were surprised that their studies upset study subjects. Qualitative semistructured interviews and other surveys may probe sensitive areas *indirectly*, further complicating these self-assessments.

On the other hand, egregious cases of unanticipated dangers from minimal-risk research like Milgram's and Zimbardo's are relatively uncommon, though they are often cited in support of the status quo (which requires that many minimal risk studies be submitted and reviewed by IRBs—even if only on an "expedited" basis). We need to understand to what degree these egregious examples are the exceptions rather than the rule.

Under the changes proposed by the Obama Administration and others, IRBs would retrospectively audit a small sample of "excused" social science studies, but the likelihood of catching egregious violations by this method is relatively small. Defenders of this proposal argue that subjects in social science experiments who feel injured could potentially sue the researchers and the university, but such legal actions can be extremely costly. Vulnerable research subjects, in particular, may lack the resources, courage, or savvy to pursue such litigation.

Another option would be for all institutions to establish separate IRBs that specialize in reviewing social science. A social scientist and IRB chair, Phil, thought this specialization would be ideal because otherwise, "we spend time just making sure that other people understand our language in social science. Sometimes our students run amuck—just using words that other IRB members don't understand."

SMALLER-SCALE FEDERAL CHANGES

More Guidance

Several interviewees were wary of large regulatory changes such as CIRBs and categorically excusing social science research, but felt that clarifications in policy and changes at other smaller levels are doable and can often help. In particular, additional government *guidance* can reduce ambiguities and tensions. As Joe, the chair, said,

> The federal government or OHRP needs to step in, and give some *guidance*. They don't have to say, "It's gotta be *this* way," but they have to provide *more guidance* than there is now. The regulations basically say: it's up to you to interpret things. But what is "slight increase over minimal risk" in pediatric studies? On a whole host of issues, we have absolutely no guidance, which contributes to very heterogeneous reactions of IRBs handling exactly the same studies.

Nonetheless, Joe opposed CIRBs: "Investigators think a central IRB will make things go faster. But it doesn't really solve problems." Instead, he and a few others wanted more concrete governmental input on how to interpret and apply current regulations. He continued, "I'd rewrite the policies: make them more specific. They are vague on purpose, but that leaves universities trying to figure out for themselves how to apply them."

Even if the regulations per se are not changed, OHRP could nevertheless help resolve many of these vagaries, further clarifying terms. As suggested earlier, federal or other external input could provide examples of how the guidelines should be applied in specific situations—e.g., concerning placebos and educational studies. "The more guidance that we can get," Stephen said, "the more helpful it is—particularly with real-life applications."

Many IRBs, however, feared that any new guidelines would be seen as fixed mandates by regulators and take on lives of their own. As Pam explained,

> Whenever they put something out and say, "Oh it's only guidance—not required"; AAHRPP [The Association for the Accreditation of Human Research Protection Programs] will still hold you to it.

New rules, and even clarifications, can also have unintended side effects. Diverse IRBs implement and apply new rules differently. "The more rules you make," Phil explained, "the more unanticipated consequences." More guidance could potentially mean less flexibility for IRBs, but that need not be the case. The government can clarify terms, provide examples of appropriate interpretations, and help standardize responses, while still letting local IRBs make decisions.

NOT HAVE IRBS REVIEW MINOR CHANGES?

Currently, PIs need to obtain IRB approval for any change—no matter how small—that they make in a study. Such amendments should be done in an expedited way. Nonetheless, some IRBs can take weeks or months to review such small alterations. OHRP could, however, also dictate that PIs can make minor changes in protocols without advance IRB approval, especially in minimal-risk studies. Such a change would ease administrative burdens for both IRBs and PIs. Questions arise, however, as to whether or not researchers would accurately self-assess whether the changes they seek are indeed all minor such that the alterations do not affect the ethics involved. PIs might, for instance, say that adding blood tests to a survey study is minor, when that is not the case, given questions of what the tests would examine, and who would see the results. Research can be conducted to assess how well PIs would make these judgments appropriately.

MANDATING MAXIMUM TURNAROUND TIMES

OHRP could also specify that IRBs must respond to PIs within a set period of time—for example, three or four weeks. Granted, many committee approvals will require additional clarifications from PIs and further communications back and forth. Hence, final approval would at times take longer. But establishing a time limit could help facilitate the process, relieve tensions with researchers (who feel unduly delayed), and perhaps incentivize committees to respond as swiftly as they can.

External Members

Other, smaller alterations in regulations and standards appear relatively easy to enact. For instance, IRBs could also potentially include more than one unaffiliated, non-scientific member. IRBs commonly say they have difficulty retaining and recruiting effective such members. But pooled resources and assistance to these individuals, including some from better-resourced institutions, can address these problems. Unfortunately, one or both of these potential roles have been diluted since the OHRP has determined that one person can occupy the role of both "nonaffiliated" and "non-scientific" member (e.g., a nurse at the hospital, or an employee's sister, or a clergyperson). This policy should be reexamined. In addition, IRBs and researchers should, on their own, engage more robustly in recruiting members from communities of patients and study participants. Understandably, given past abuses (e.g., Tuskegee), some groups are wary of research. But IRBs were established to help, and these committees need and welcome input. Patient

groups and diverse communities should consider the benefits of having representatives join IRBs, and encourage individuals who are potentially interested to do so.

Informed Consent

In several ways, processes of consent can be improved. Shorter summary documents can preface and introduce more detailed forms. Still, the content as well as
the form of these condensed statements needs attention and consensus, to determine what exactly they should include and exclude. Importantly, the central tension of whether these documents are legal or informative needs to be resolved.
At present, they in fact often serve both purposes—as legal and informative. But
if that is the case, it should be acknowledged and confronted head-on—not dismissed or denied. Other modalities, such as videos and interactive online media
can be used as well to communicate relevant information. Independent, trained
third parties could also obtain consent, but those require resources. Such efforts
are, however, needed if we are to take informed consent seriously and not treat
it merely as a formality. Templates, too, can help, if they are flexible and not too
legalistic. Many of these documents are still at too advanced a level to be understood by lay people. OHRP or others need to monitor these levels vigorously and
establish what changes are essential and when "enough is enough."

Accreditation

AAHRPP has begun accrediting IRBs and assessing programs' formal structures, although not the content of these committees' decisions themselves (e.g.,
how these committees define, interpret, and weigh risks and benefits). Increased
accreditation of IRBs constitutes another possible change at the national level.
The federal government or other groups could potentially encourage or require
such certification, which could help address certain issues. But the accreditation
procedure could also be made much more efficient and helpful, and examine the
content of decisions, not only logistical operations.

Several IRB members cited the advantages of having this certification.
"Accreditation is definitely worthwhile: you fill in all these gaps that you weren't aware
of," Scott, a director, said. "It forces us to self-evaluate our procedures and policies."

But others felt that the accreditation movement began too early and has not
functioned as well as hoped, generating problems. The process consumes time
and resources, leaving less for other purposes. Even Scott, who likes accreditation, nonetheless admits, "It can be a pain because they ask for checklists and
additional aspects to an application—way over the top."

Moreover, the credentialing process examines a committee's standard operating
procedures (SOPs); this assessment can potentially help improve certain aspects of
the logistics, but it also heightens the focus on paperwork. The process has led some

PUBLISHING DECISIONS AND DEVELOPING
A BODY OF CASE LAW

Since institutional memory is generally poor—hard both to establish and to maintain—IRBs, together with OHRP, PRIM&R, AAHRP or other organizations could also build and help disseminate a solid body of "case law". These organizations could facilitate its use, communicating more effectively and fully with IRBs across the country, and posting online more vetted interpretations and applications of principles to specific cases. OHRP could also establish a hotline to assist boards by responding to questions rapidly. As Robin explained:

> OHRP can post more FAQs or guidance of specific examples. That's how it's done in the law. You apply the law in a particular situation. Then, the decision in that case is published in a law reporter. The next person that comes along will look at the different cases, and try to see where his or hers fits in, and then publish it in another law report. This is how case laws and guidance could be built up. It's almost like paradigm cases: looking at cases where it's clearer, then working your way into the current situations.

As with the law, in building and publishing a body of established precedents, other IRBs, organizations and scholars could comment, and committees could then refer to this corpus in making decisions. Organizations such as PRIM&R could help determine and define the appropriate categories or aspects of decisions to be included—for example, amounts of compensation awarded across studies, or cases in which the risks of a particular procedure (such as a spinal tap) are thought to be justified by a study's benefits. Over time, collecting and referring to this information could significantly help reduce unnecessary idiosyncrasies in decisions both within and between committees. Basic questions around which disagreements persist—for example, whether a blood draw constitutes minimal risk or not—could potentially be resolved.

The legal system similarly confronts ambiguities and differences in interpretation, but avoids many pitfalls by being more transparent, and by seeking and drawing on documented precedents and appeals. In the absence of these mechanisms, many IRBs can become rigid, believing that their own interpretations are incontrovertible and the only ones possible.

Making IRB minutes publicly available (with redaction of proprietary or confidential information) can also significantly increase consistency. Minutes would include outcomes and rationales, not identifying who said what. IRBs may argue that confidentiality precludes such openness, and that PIs and funders won't like it; but sensitive information can be redacted, and researchers and grantees may in fact prefer such enhanced transparency and openness.

The fact that many IRBs appear to be duplicating each other's efforts in developing policies and procedures highlights potential needs for more widely available and accessible "templates" and guidelines that can assist institutions.

Dissemination of explicit "best practices" can also be beneficial. Committees could more fully and systematically share effective strategies they have individually developed. As Liza said,

> When I have an issue, I don't first see if there's guidance on it but instead call other IRBs I respect, before reinventing the wheel: "How do *you* handle this?" Formalizing [such communication between IRBs about specific issues]—as "best practices"—would probably help more than a guidance document.

A listserv, IRB Forum, exists[17] for discussions, but not all IRBs use it, and some do not want to reveal publically their uncertainty or lack of knowledge or confidence. OHRP could also create websites for posting or disseminating such materials. However, achieving consensus on what optimal practices indeed constitute "the best" can be hard. Liza explained,

> PRIM&R [Public Responsibility in Medicine and Research] has not wanted to do that, nor I think should. Who's to determine whether something is the best practice? Five people will look at it, and say, "That person doesn't understand the regulations."

But, if each IRB is to maintain the independent authority that it does, this problem needs to be solved. An open forum of experts can address these differences and establish consensus—or at least the areas in which agreement can be reached and determine clear points on which divergence exists and why (i.e., on what such continued difference depends). If IRBs cannot reach consensus because of personal and idiosyncratic reasons, such discrepancies have arguably gone too far, and need to be reduced.

EXTERNAL APPEALS

Local IRBs generally have enormous power, interpreting regulations as they see fit, despite the scientific, social and economic costs involved. Another crucial organizational change is therefore the establishment of a mechanism of external appeals, as allowed with judicial courts. The physician and bioethicist John Lantos[18] has also suggested the establishment of an auditable and transparent "appellate" IRB to allow investigators to then appeal local IRB decisions at a higher administrative level. Such a mechanism could be established through, for instance, OHRP. The fact that researchers dissatisfied with their reviews have no means to contest their IRB's decision, except by returning to this same committee breeds bitterness and resentment. Interpretations shape the law, too; but courts permit formal outside reassessments. "In the law, you can appeal," Robin said, "and ultimately, get it to the Supreme Court. Then, *that's* final." The Supreme Court's nine judges are rarely unanimous, but serve as the final arbiters. This appellate board could publish its decisions (with appropriate redactions) that could then be publicly examined and critiqued. The ANPRM asked in Question 28 whether such appeals mechanisms should be established.[15] The answer is yes. However, over the past several years, proposals for such an appellate system have received little support. Local IRBs may resist, rather than readily accept these alternative models. Yet, the present lack of an appeals process may bolster IRBs in underplaying the impediments posed by variations between committees, fueling idiosyncrasies in decisions, and hence hampering research.

Appeals courts might not only resolve many questions, but also foster accountability. Such a final arbiter would still confront uncertainties, but would set clear, published standards and precedents that IRBs and researchers could thus find, cite, and follow. These external review mechanisms would take researchers' time, but offer important correctives, and incentivize IRBs to review decisions carefully. Such external review bodies can be regional or centralized.

As with the Supreme Court, the Appellate IRB would not necessarily have to make a decision about every case. Researchers who wish to obtain an external review would have to complete forms describing their reasons. The external reviewers could then assess these requests to decide which applications appeared justified. This process of applying for appeals could be open and transparent. The publications of external review board decisions would assist in furthering consensus concerning contested parts of protocol reviews. Investigators requesting appeals would also need to consider their desires carefully, knowing that the request might become public.

A skeptic may argue that "each case is unique" and that publishing such precedents will thus not be helpful. But in law, too, cases are each unique, with details that are not all generally applicable to other situations. Transparent documentation of how principles have been weighed against each other and applied in particular situations can thus provide enormous benefits. Researchers would probably request an outside review only rarely, because they would have to devote time and effort to it. The case may get published, and afterward, the PI would still have to continue to interact with his or her own IRB, which could then be awkward. Moreover, unsuccessful efforts to externally overturn an IRB's decision may carry a bit of a stigma within one's institution. Nevertheless, the availability of this option may make researchers feel less powerless and stuck, and IRBs more careful.

Another mechanism for external appeals, which could be adopted even if a national system of appeals is not established, would be for IRBs to act as such as external review bodies for each other. Institutions could set up reciprocal arrangements with each other (with confidentiality protections to safeguard researchers' ideas). Simply the *possibility* that another IRB might later review a particular decision could encourage boards to ensure that their decisions appear reasonable not only to themselves but to a wider audience as well—thereby encouraging the notion of greater standardization.

OHRP could also dictate or guide more fully other aspects of IRB functioning—for instance, that IRBs review material within a set period (e.g., four weeks) of submission by researchers. Establishing such parameters could help assuage researchers' frustrations and tensions.

As with the SUPPORT study (comparing oxygen levels among premature infants), OHRP's decisions have at times generated controversy; but open, transparent discussion of these issues—of when and why disagreements occur and how best to resolve these—can advance the field most fully.

The ANPRM asks, too, whether IRBs should report to OHRP when they are more restrictive than the regulations in certain ways—specifically, when they decide that review of a study can be expedited.[15] But the system's efficiency could be improved as well if IRBs report to OHRP other ways in which they may deviate. Committees could report publically, for instance, the median lengths of time between submission and approval of protocols (including the lengths of time that both PIs and IRBs take to respond to each other), and numbers of appeals (if a system that allows them is established). As IRB submissions are increasingly electronic and online, such data may even be relatively easy to provide.

In sum, broad changes in national policy have been proposed—from centralizing of IRBs to exempting much social science research from review and requiring accreditation of boards and personnel. Proposals by Obama and others may have certain benefits, but will also have unintended consequences that we need to anticipate and consider. Federal policy in these realms can be an important instrument of change, but it remains a relatively crude one—all regulations on such a grand scale depend on implementation, often leaving loopholes, and creating unintended consequences. Moreover, even new regulations would simply establish a foundation; local IRBs could choose to be more stringent. In the end, federal-level policy reforms are important, but insufficient alone. Other, local-level improvements are also essential.

CHAPTER 14

Conclusions

OTHER CHANGES

I was initially drawn to studying IRBs because my conflicting experiences as a son, a physician, and a researcher had left me perplexed. Now that I have finished this study, I still have questions, but these have changed and sharpened. The dilemmas involved in research are far more intricate than I had anticipated; nevertheless, many clear improvements are clearly possible.

Fixes at the national level can help, but, as we saw, we need far more nuanced understandings and approaches at other levels as well. First, we must all recognize that the challenge of defining, interpreting, and weighing abstract principles, ambiguous policies, and competing future risks and benefits by a committee is in its own right *a complicated and often idiosyncratic human process.* These boards grapple with decisions that involve profound philosophical, moral, and political dilemmas. IRB personnel are highly committed, but many of the questions they consider are largely unknowable: if we could predict the results of a study, we wouldn't need to conduct it in the first place.

Even after policymakers contemplate potential federal changes, ambiguities and difficulties will no doubt continue, and these need to be better recognized and considered. From the Ten Commandments to the New Testament, from Confucius, Socrates, Plato, Aristotle, and Augustine to Kant, JS Mill, Karl Marx, and John Rawls, thinkers have offered varying ethical frameworks with which to consider how we should behave toward one another. All these writers have pondered moral tensions that take on new dimensions in these contemporary bioethical conundrums.

Second, IRBs need to be seen more holistically—as part of far larger and constantly evolving systems. This view must take into account at times erratic and dissonant directives from federal agencies, implicit and explicit pressures from drug companies and local institutions, and varied cooperation from researchers. *These dynamics—combined with the experiences, personalities, and beliefs of whoever happens to be at a particular committee meeting—all shape IRB deliberations.*

Unfortunately, the stakeholders involved with IRBs have competing goals. Employees at federal agencies, responsible to the Congress and the president, face certain constraints. Corporations seek profit. Academic institutions seek to advance knowledge while garnering grants. Researchers aim to propel science forward while earning a living, and to further their own careers. IRB personnel try to protect subjects while reviewing colleagues' work and interpreting and weighing vague terms. A medical center's size and history, as well as particular IRB chairs' personalities and clout, can influence how committees and researchers negotiate these strains. Committees must monitor colleagues while simultaneously winning their cooperation. Not surprisingly, committees' decisions around the same protocols and issues vary.

In many ways, IRBs are unique, working at complex intersections of science, politics, sociology, psychology, money, and ethics. These boards resemble juries but, operating as they do without a judge or the possibility for appeal, they have more power. They also resemble NIH grant-review committees and journal reviewers in certain regards, but with dramatic exceptions. Governmental staff members guide federal grant committees. NIH councils make final funding decisions, and are overseen by Congress. For journal articles, editors make the ultimate adjudications. For both journal articles and grants, the criteria are usually strictly scientific, hinging not on ethical judgments but on fixed numerical criteria (e.g., statistical significance and power). Subjectivities exist, but are more muted. Determinations of how much possible harm is worth how much potential benefit involve moral intuitions; statistical calculations do not.

As Henry Beecher[1] suggested in his 1966 presentation of unethical published studies, PIs cannot wholly be left to police themselves. Rather, some kind of external group that includes scientific peers must do so. Unfortunately, the consequent establishment of ethics committees also introduced the seeds of potential discord. In the 40 years since then, the research enterprise has grown exponentially in size and complexity, and yet over these past four decades, the regulations have not significantly changed: enhanced cooperation and integration must now be developed.

IRBs frequently confront the inherent tensions between researchers' need for scientific freedom and study participants' need for protection. Many committees maintain supple, open stances. Others see the regulations fairly rigidly, failing to question their own views and ignoring the costs of their decisions to PIs—or, conversely, they do not go far enough in monitoring their colleagues' research, due to various conflicts of interest. Yet, while IRBs tend to see their decisions as rooted in local community values—and thus as legitimate, unassailable, and implicitly objective—this claim almost always turns out to be incorrect.

When I began this study, a social scientist asked me whether IRBs differ by whether they are located at private *vs.* state universities, or small *vs.* big institutions. I found that these factors can affect decisions, but not systematically in any one clear direction. IRBs do not differ according to fixed, black-and-white, objective dichotomous categories—such as whether the institution is public or private, or has more or less than a certain fixed amount of grant support. Rather, more subtle and dynamic local micro-ecologies flourish here. IRBs interpret and apply abstract ethical terms and ambiguous regulations with relatively little guidance or case law—that is, precedents of difficult cases on which a consensus has been reached, publically analyzed, and deemed appropriate. And yet many IRBs deny the impact of these all-too-human factors and claim unwavering authority, based on local community values.

How then should we proceed? Proposals by President Obama and others address a few but not all of these concerns and, as of this writing, the fate of these possible reforms remains unclear. Eventually, some of these proposals may be enacted, but which, to what extent, and with what outcomes is wholly unpredictable.

Centralization occupies much of the debate about the future of IRBs, and will probably increase for certain studies; yet many challenges will persist. Of course, CIRBs, too, may be subjective, potentially reflecting the preferences of individual chairs or vocal members who happen to be present at a meeting. Local review also has several advantages—reflecting not local community values, as is often posited, but local knowledge. Controversies will surely continue.

Yet regardless of whether, how, and to what degree federal agencies revise certain regulations, the perspectives limned here will remain crucial. The existence of discrepancies does not mean that local IRBs should be eliminated. Rather, current debates should be reframed to probe how we can and should improve ethical oversight, given the potential costs to science; how much discrepancy should be tolerated in return for how much "extra precaution"; how the pros and cons of these and other proposals should be weighed, and by whom (i.e., by IRBs, researchers, university administrators, federal policymakers, and/or others).

Some critics have argued that IRBs need to be more "efficient," but what that means—whether they should be quicker, use fewer resources, review more studies, or do so less rigorously—is unclear.

Whatever transpires at the federal level, ethical problems cannot be solved by rigid federal rules alone; the Obama Administration's proposed policy alterations will not fully resolve these tensions any more than the Nuremberg Code or the Belmont Report did. Indeed, the Declaration of Helsinki gets revised every two to four years. Fortunately, as seen in Table 14.1, many local institutional, committee,

Table 14.1. **Suggested changes concerning IRBs—Local level**

- *Institutional level*
  - o Having more well-trained staff who could make independent decisions about key issues
  - o Providing appropriate compensation to IRB members
- *IRB level*
  - o More transparency
    - ▪ Open doors: being as responsive and accessible to researchers as possible
      - ▪ Inviting and encouraging researchers to attend IRB meetings
    - ▪ Establishing institutional memory and a body of case law
    - ▪ Changing attitudes
      - ▪ Recognizing inherent subjectivity in interpretations and applications of principles and terms
      - ▪ Acknowledging the costs of IRB idiosyncracies to research
  - o More and different training
    - ▪ Reaching consensus and standardization on definitions, interpretations, and applications of key terms and principles
    - ▪ Requiring testing of IRB personnel to demonstrate adherence to these standards
  - o Increasing IRB willingness to be studied
- *Researcher level*
  - o Changing attitudes
  - o Enhancing understandings of purposes of ethical principles and regulatory oversight
  - o Not "blaming the messenger" (i.e., the IRB)
  - o Avoiding inattentive and sloppy submissions to IRBs
- *Public level*
  - o Enhancing public education

and researcher improvements are possible, involving both formal structures and informal interactions.

Multiple-pronged efforts are vital. As we saw in the last chapter, some alterations can start on national levels, but individual IRBs must all strongly adopt and value such efforts—in part because in the end, the interpretation and implementation of any modifications will be local. Changes must be not only top-down, but bottom-up. *Perhaps most important, institutions and IRBs need to instill and foster a culture to uphold not just the letter, but the spirit of the law—to promote the principles of bioethics beyond the narrowest possible definitions of the regulations alone. Universities need to develop and nurture a culture of not merely compliance, but of shared ethical policies and mission.*

The most effective reforms will be those in which this larger mission will be visible, and in which both IRB members and scientists can see gains themselves. Such improvements are not only possible, but essential.

IRBs Must Change

IRBs must recognize that they are part of the problem. Many boards have begun to see the need to improve, but they still have a long way to go. They must not only make procedural reforms; they must also shift their own and others' perspectives.

Many committee personnel have become part of a larger IRB community—a pro- fession and in some ways an industry, "the IRB world"—and these committees, both individually and as part of this larger group, must change.

ESTABLISHING INSTITUTIONAL MEMORY AND A BODY OF CASE LAW

In addition to establishing a national body of case law, committees should also seek to establish more of an institutional memory internally—a systematic way of keeping track of what they did or did not approve in the past. Establishing such a tracking system may require some additional resources, but since IRBs are now commonly switching to electronic record keeping, such cross-referencing becomes increasingly feasible and achievable.

Presumably, many precedents will become national in scope. If additional, locally specific issues arise that are not included, IRBs can at least keep track of their own responses, expanding their institutional memory in order to guide future or fellow committees within the same organization, reducing discrepan- cies. It would of course be difficult to track every detail of a protocol, but critical areas where substantial variations and idiosyncrasies emerge could be noted and followed.

THE IMPORTANCE OF BEING RESPONSIVE AND ACCESSIBLE

Committees must become more transparent. As we saw earlier, relationships between IRBs and PIs could be improved if additional committees adopted more of an "open door" policy. Many IRBs prohibit researchers from communi- cating with individual members, requiring instead that all communication to be sent to anonymous "IRB mail" addresses, without mentioning any individual staff member's names. Others insist that PIs deal only with IRB staff, not chairs or members. Similarly, committees often communicate with researchers only by memo, which unfortunately stiffens and formalizes exchanges. Curbside consults and other verbal interactions can help PIs to be more prepared for the review ahead of time.

INVITING RESEARCHERS TO ATTEND IRB MEETINGS

As many committees do not now invite to their meetings the PIs whose protocols are being reviewed, another beneficial reform would be for all IRBs regularly to include rather than exclude investigators from these discussions. While some committees do routinely invite researchers to these meetings, many other boards refuse to do so, since individual members fear they may then feel uncomfortable expressing opinions. But this exclusion, aimed at protecting committee members from feeling pressured by PIs, incurs serious costs. As an unintended consequence, PIs then feel unfairly judged by an anonymous and arbitrary authority—a faceless power—which can fuel their resentment. In contrast, transparency would heighten mutual trust, responsibility, cooperation, and respect. Researchers who attend these meetings would leave the room during voting, but they would see that reviewers' concerns are not arbitrary or personally motivated. They could also potentially provide their perspectives and responses to committees' concerns, facilitating communication. Reviewers themselves could then also learn from the PI about whether and how they may inadvertently be impeding the science. For this reform to work, however, all parties will obviously have to act responsibly and respectfully. *Such openness would serve to foster trust, and potentially highlight a benefit of local, as opposed to centralized, IRBs.*

CHANGING IRBS' ATTITUDES

IRBs must do far more to acknowledge and incorporate the complex realities involved in their work—to see more clearly how much they are engaged in *highly variable exegesis*. If PIs are slow to acknowledge that IRBs are following federal regulations, committee members are slow to acknowledge that they are often not *merely* following those regulations; IRBs have significant discretionary power, even if most of them are loath to admit it. Researchers certainly recognize the power of these boards, and for IRB members to deny it is philosophically and sociologically naïve. Committees need to admit that they vary for reasons that are not based on their Federal mandate, and that such significant variations are thus frequently unjustified, given the social and scientific costs.

Many IRB personnel acknowledge that "personalities" may be involved in their decisions, and yet they still appear to believe that they arrive at *the one and only* acceptable answer—that, in other words, their decisions are not just inherently valid but also, once made, essentially incontrovertible—rather than being partly the result of an "art." If there were only one acceptable answer, of course, differences between IRBs who evaluate the same studies would not be as frequent as they are. These differences do not necessarily indicate that any one of the IRBs is in error, but these variations do highlight how the review process can be a highly interpretive endeavor.

ACKNOWLEDGING THE COSTS OF IRB WORK TO RESEARCH

Boards also need to acknowledge more frequently the *costs* of some of their decisions to researchers in both scientific time and resources, and hence the potential decreased *social benefits* of local IRBs' interpretations of regulations. Some costs are inevitable, but others are not, and may be unnecessarily burdensome. IRBs analyze the risks and benefits of the work of researchers, but not of their own processes and decisions. This omission fosters tension and grief.

IRBs have critical functions and power; they must therefore grasp more fully the degrees to which they possess and can therefore misuse their authority. They must institute more effective checks and balances. Trust, on which research ethics depends, is hard to build and easy to impair. More mutual respect is vital. At times, IRBs do themselves a disservice by alienating PIs—which can have the undesired result of eroding researchers' commitment to protecting subjects.

At the same time, IRB power *is* limited. Perhaps for this reason, many committees place an enormous emphasis on the bureaucratic procedures involved in research, and obsess over what they think they can control—the consent form. As an alternative to ballooning paperwork and administrative oversight, PIs and IRBs can work together to build additional mutual trust, yet doing so requires effort on both sides.

And so how much power *should* IRBs have? If some subjectivity is inevitable, how much is acceptable? Clearer guidelines and the other mechanisms for improvement are critical. Ethics is, however, often messy, and will still always require deliberations. Hence, greater humility on both sides is essential as well. To protect subjects as best as possible, recognition of both these phenomena and the benefits of such consistency is crucial. The lack of such acknowledgment harms researchers' relationships with IRBs and their commitment to closely following IRB regulations.

Needs for More thorough and Standardized IRB Training

IRB attitudes will not be easy to change, and hence, committees need to be incentivized to pursue uniformity, rewarded for pursuing standardization, and admonished for straying too far. Currently, the burdens of committee variations fall on scientists, not IRBs. Boards have little desire to yield autonomy, and may fear that recognizing this subjectivity may undermine the legitimacy of their decisions—that acknowledgement that more personal, rather than community factors mold committee decisions may prompt researchers to question these reviews.

Standardized education and tests for IRB personnel can also increase consistency within and between committees. OHRP, PRIM&R, AAHRP, scholars and other relevant stakeholders can seek to arrive at consensus concerning how particular protocols or research scenarios should be reviewed—how to define, interpret, apply and balance the regulations in reviewing these studies, and/or articulate the limits of desired or acceptable differences in approaches. *IRB chairs, members and administrators could then take tests to assess their rates of concurrence with these agreed-upon standards.*

Similarly, for many years, psychiatrists would disagree on whether they thought particular patients had major depression—or other diagnoses—or not. Some psychiatrists felt that certain patients surely had a disorder, while other providers were unsure, or thought not. This variability impeded treatment and research. Consequently, over several decades, investigators rigorously developed and tested clear criteria and rating scales to determine whether a patient in fact demonstrates certain symptoms and conditions. The Diagnostic and Statistic Manual (or DSM) and various rating scales resulted—a set of carefully defined criteria to determine whether an individual warranted a certain diagnosis or not. Since then, countless psychiatrists have been trained to use these criteria, reaching consensus about diagnoses, and if not, clarifying the evidence required to resolve disagreements.

Likewise, criteria could be developed for IRBs to determine whether, for instance, a particular procedure or study is more than minimal risk, whether a protocol's benefits outweigh its risks, and whether a consent form adequently explains the key elements of a study, is written at too high a level, or is good enough (i.e., how "obsessive" to be). Such standards regarding the content of IRB decisions will not necessarily be easy to develop. The DSM has taken several decades, expanding, and guiding, and being shaped by, empirical studies, and revised periodically to reflect new research and clinical findings. But, especially as research continues to grow over upcoming decades, trying to develop agreed-upon standards in IRB decisions is vital.

Remarkably, though PIs, to conducts studies, must regularly undergo testing about research ethics, no such requirements exist for IRB chairs, members or staff. Though recently, some IRB staff take an exam to become a "certified IRB professional", this testing, while important, is not mandated, has not been taken by thousands of IRB personnel, and does not go far enough to seek consensus concerning the content of IRB reviews (i.e., focusing not merely on knowledge of the language of the regulations—though that is obviously important—but on how to *interpret and apply these* in particular instances). Exams on such content could crucially help reduce IRB variations.

Analogously, as professionals, physicians, for instance, seek to agree as much as possible, not disagree, on how to treat particular diseases. One doesn't want doctors all to act idiosyncratically. So, too, IRB personnel, in seeking to be considered professionals, should strive to achieve far more standardization regarding not only memorization of the verbiage of the regulations and relevant administrative procedures, but the content of IRB decisions. As we saw, while some observers may argue that IRB accreditation adequately addresses these issues, it focuses on harmonizing IRB forms and processes—not on outcomes.

Hence, all IRB members, staff, and chairs could be required to undergo rigorous training and testing using such standardized protocols, to make sure that they arrive at the accepted consensus. Granted, there may be a few small areas in which different "taboo" cultural practices may make some IRB members uncomfortable. Yet as mentioned earlier, the only topic where such possible differences appeared possibly to emerge here regarded studies of sexual behavior among gay men—specifically concerns that *other* IRB members may be homophobic. That is, one interviewee in a large city with many gay men thought that studies of sexual HIV-risk behavior might make IRBs *elsewhere*—in conservative rural areas—uncomfortable. However, his perception may not be wholly accurate. Another interviewee in a conservative state thought that some IRB members were uncomfortable reviewing a study about attitudes toward homosexuality, though insisting that the subject matter did not cause the problem. National attitudes towards lesbian and gay issues are, however, rapidly changing. Moreover, even if some individuals in more conservative vs. more liberal areas of the country may differ in comfort about homosexuality, no evidence exists that attitudes might vary among these more liberal areas—e.g., among New York, California, Massachusetts or Washington. In addition, principles of justice should, arguably, prevail over any unfair discriminatory attitudes in IRB decisions. Importantly, in this study of IRBs across the country, no other examples arose reflecting local community differences. Standardized tests could potentially exclude this or other such topics, if necessary, and if found. But all the other differences between IRBs that appeared here did not reflect differences in local community values or law. Importantly, such standardized tests can thus help minimize unnecessary variations.

More standardization will help, but won't guarantee uniformity of outcomes by 100% of boards. Still, these efforts can foster more consistency and transparency, and awareness of the costs of idiosyncratic variations, and thus be beneficial. Some critics may argue that the amount of consensus will be limited, but such efforts at agreement should at least be undertaken to guage whether in fact such limits exist, and if so, where and why, and whether and how these can be addressed.

Many IRB personnel will surely oppose this suggestion of such required tests. No one likes to take tests. But such examinations could motivate IRBs to try to reach consensus on many issues, furthering the notion that efforts at consistency in interpretations are valuable. Details would have to be established, but such an approach should at least be considered, as this mechanism could help decrease inefficiencies in the system, and thereby improve researchers' perceptions, trust and relationships toward IRBs, and decrease tensions. Through these mechanisms, interpretations may still vary, but as much as possible should be more systematized and accountable.

Such training could be stipulated on a national level, supported by national organizations such as PRIM&R and AAHRP, and/or adopted by institutions and IRBs themselves.

These reforms would reassure PIs and relieve IRB committees of considerable pressure. Interviewees repeatedly voiced their frustration at the lack of guidance provided for their decision making; often they felt that they were struggling for clarity in a void. Any new systems that help to streamline or accelerate the reviewing process will aid committees and researchers alike.

IRBs Must Allow More Research on Themselves

This project has revealed that more studies of IRBs are urgently needed—and yet conducting such research, as I learned, is very difficult. To advance science while protecting subjects' rights, more research on IRBs themselves is crucial to understand how and why they in fact vary, As individuals, some IRB chairs and members are willing to discuss their experiences, yet research on IRBs as a whole has been seriously stymied. Board chairs and administrators have completed short quantitative surveys about logistical issues, but have often resisted or blocked being studied through observations or tape recordings of their own meetings, claiming that such research would require consent from all members and staff, PIs, and funders whose studies are being reviewed at a meeting. Yet to get 100 percent of all of these groups to agree and provide informed consent is essentially impossible. If even one committee member declines, the research cannot proceed. Some IRB chairs and administrators have said that for *even one* of them to complete a questionnaire about the IRB, the researcher should first have to obtain IRB approval from all board members and staff.

Douglas Diekema, chair of an IRB, criticized the suggestion, based on these interview data, that IRBs varied for reasons other than differences in local community values; and he defended deviations between IRBs. He dismissed the value of these interviews with individual chairs, members, and staff and asserted that "disparities among IRBs cannot be assessed meaningfully without looking at the actual decisions of different IRBs considering the same protocol."[2] Yet Kathleen Dziak and others have performed such assessments, and found wide variations between committees. She found, for instance, that IRBs varied in whether they allowed an opt-out process for potential participants, or required an opt-in mechanism—impeding the comparison of data between sites.[3] Such comparison studies are also difficult to conduct, however, since IRBs may review a study differently if they know their assessment of a study is being investigated for its uniformity with other committee's decisions.

Diekema added that to assess reasons for deficiencies between IRBs, studies that directly observe IRBs are needed:

> To truly understand why different IRBs make disparate decisions will likely require an anthropologic methodology where trained observers embed themselves within IRBs in multiple institutions and evaluate the deliberations and decisions of those IRBs....We will need to go beyond surveys and interviews to a systematic evaluation of the actual work that IRBs do.[2]

Yet, unfortunately, many IRBs have consistently thwarted such efforts (i.e., by requiring that IRB members, researchers, and funders sign informed consent). They have seemed to feel that there is nothing in it for them. But that view is extremely short-sighted, hampering the need to improve relationships with researchers *and* the protection of subjects as a whole.

Indeed, I have conducted research for two decades, interviewing patients and physicians about highly sensitive, stigmatized issues that could easily cause discrimination, including their own HIV infection and genetic diseases, illicit sexual activities, drug use, incarceration, depression, and suicidality. Yet the only one of my protocols that my IRB deemed more than minimal risk—and therefore the only one for which I was required to appear before the entire board to explain, justify, and defend—was this study of IRBs. "What are you going to do with all this sensitive data?" they asked. I answered that of course I would treat it the same way I treated sensitive data on all these other, equally sensitive issues, but the IRB still seemed nervous, and asked me many further questions.

Committees urgently need to change, and not only to permit but to encourage researchers to study and observe them, in order to improve the status quo. Such efforts are vital to enhance knowledge, transparency, and trust.

Researchers Must Change

At the same time, some researcher complaints about the status quo appear to reflect both resistance to the regulations and rationalization. After all, IRBs are not "the enemy," but instead mandated committees generally struggling to do their best to protect subjects. Though some boards may show too little flexibility, and even consciously or unconsciously abuse their power, most do not and instead are well intentioned.

Why, then, do so many PIs complain about and even hate IRBs? In part, these researchers are blaming the messengers for the message—chastising IRBs for the federal requirements—even though these committees are only carrying out their duty. Many investigators have only hazy ideas of the complexities involved, or assume that the sorts of transgressions that triggered the development of the current regulations are all now in the distant past. Unfortunately, this assumption is incorrect. PIs owe it to not only IRBs but also to themselves and their research subjects to better understand why and how these committees function.

Only a small fraction of researchers deliberately flout the IRB and the federal rules. When this does happen, however—whether for professional or monetary gain—the consequences can be either negligible or very grave (e.g., resulting in injuries or death). When serious violations occur, both subjects and the general public expect scientists to face repercussions. Researchers must recognize that their rogue, sloppy, or careless colleagues—as much as the federal government or their own IRBs—are in part responsible for the tightened implementation of regulations that can ensue.

Even so, because most researchers *do* strive to follow the rules, they do not perceive themselves as needing policing; many of them therefore feel unfairly treated and judged even *before* submitting a protocol, and so can be resistant and defensive from the outset. Unfortunately, IRBs cannot exempt researchers from scrutiny simply because these investigators state that they are doing everything they should be; "bad apples" cannot be easily identified in advance. Committees can't know for sure which investigators will behave ethically and which will not.

Many PIs also fail to appreciate that, even when well intentioned, they often have significant blind spots. As suggested by the asthma study at Johns Hopkins in which Ellen Roche died, the gene therapy experiment that killed Jesse Gelsinger, and research on the Havasupai, some investigators feel that their studies are ethically fine when that is not the case. Like all humans, PIs may be unaware of their own biases, or be able to rationalize them, subtle though these may be. Hence, examining a study from the outside is key.

Unfortunately, some PIs submit sloppy or incomplete protocols. Sometimes these deficiencies are signs of the researcher's frustration or excessive carelessness; at other times, it is merely an oversight. In either instance, it can seem disrespectful to their IRBs, exacerbating strains. Researchers must learn to recognize that such deficiencies are discourteous not only to the IRB but to colleagues, too: poor protocol submissions can reduce the trust and productivity of a committee, and therefore hurt the research community as a whole.

At the same time, many researchers believe that they must follow whatever suggestions an IRB makes on a study—that investigators cannot push back, for fear of offending the IRB or not getting their study approved. In fact, these interviews taught me that committees frequently make suggestions or express concerns that are *negotiable,* not incontestable. Researchers sometimes fail to realize this fact, and instead feel obliged to change their study to incorporate all the input they receive from their committee—even if it mars the study—simply to get the protocol approved. But many of the IRB personnel I spoke with were amenable to communicating better with researchers. Hence, investigators should inform their IRB when they think the committee has gone too far; PIs should defend aspects of their studies that boards unwittingly threaten. Researchers often fear their IRB, but should not; open dialogue is key.

Last, scientists may want to police *one another* more—encouraging their staff and colleagues to abide by the highest possible ethical standards for both moral and practical reasons. In any respected institution, academic excellence and humane treatment of participants should not be seen as opposing goals. Likewise, failures to uphold proper standards, even by a small number of investigators, heighten scrutiny of *all* researchers—whether within a particular institution or nationally—imposing costs on everyone. A less antagonistic relationship with IRBs is in researchers' best interests.

Public Education

If these committees don't fully recognize how they are seen by PIs, and researchers have crude understandings of these boards, it is not surprising that *the general public knows next to nothing about IRBs.* We all expect that medical knowledge will continue to advance, and that we will all be protected from any missteps. All of us have been or will be patients at some point in our lives, and have benefited from scientific advances that preceded us. *It therefore behooves all of us—whether as patients, family members of patients, doctors, nurses, researchers, policymakers, journalists, or members of the wider community—to try to better understand the complexities of these issues and the possible solutions.* Those of us who agree to participate in research should not only read the forms we have been given, but also ask questions when aspects of the study are unclear.

Future Scholarship

These interviews suggest several directions for future studies. Exploration of the lived experiences of IRB members, as undertaken here, has yielded critical perspectives and insights; future investigations should use both narrative and quantitative approaches to probe IRBs further, both in the US and abroad. Such studies might examine, for instance, how frequently committees construe and apply regulations differently due to particular psychological and institutional factors, and whether and how educational or other interventions can reduce problematic IRB variations. Interviewees did not appear to differ systematically in their views based on their roles (e.g., chairs *vs.* administrators), gender, or other straightforward sociodemographic factors; but future research can probe such possible differences among larger samples. Elucidation of how various forces affect IRBs can enrich our understandings of ethical decision making among IRBs—and, more broadly, in medicine, public health, and other realms.

These men and women readily discussed their difficulties but rarely spoke of studies that they ill-advisedly approved. They may be less aware of such errors, or feel uncomfortable discussing such cases. They also may see these problematic results as stemming from researchers' failures to describe or conduct the study properly rather than from the committee's failure to anticipate problems during its own deliberations. Future investigations can also assess IRBs' retrospective views of such problematic studies.

The interviews in my own study have several potential limitations. Interviewees spoke to me at one point in time, rather than over a longer period. I did not directly observe their IRBs, or inspect their written records; or interview medical school deans, hospital presidents, or other leaders at each institution—all of which would have been very difficult, if not impossible, to do. I was, however, able to draw on my own three decades of experience observing, interacting, and corresponding with these committees. Subsequent research can try these other methods. These approaches may be difficult, given in part IRBs' resistance to being observed, but they should still be attempted. In the meantime, the 46 IRB personnel here provide insights on many critical issues.

These interviews dramatically highlight the need to adopt more humanistic, and balanced approaches, incorporating in appropriate ways the humanities and social sciences far more into efforts to understand and improve IRBs and to advance science while protecting human participants. These individuals illuminate not only how interpretations of ethical principles can vary widely, but also how complex the psychology and sociology of power are—how and why people embedded in different social systems often interpret the same moral principles differently (and justify their positions), but may not see themselves as doing so.

Academic medical centers aspire toward objective science—not subjective human values and experience. A positivistic model of ethics currently seems to prevail concerning IRBs, too—the "check the box" mentality that one and only one definitive set of changes to a protocol makes it ethical, and that an IRB's decision, once made, is the sole determination possible, and thus incontestable. Yet this rigidity poses problems. Rather, we need to consider carefully the roles and vagaries of individual and institutional desires, beliefs, and norms. The fact that IRBs can vary in how they interpret and apply the regulations in reviewing a particular study should not be seen as inherently bad. Instead, IRBs and policymakers should strive hard to reduce unjustified idiosyncrasies, and to achieve consensus on how IRBs *should* apply the regulations in particular protocols or scenarios. Subjectivity exists in clinical medicine, too; but the medical profession works hard to establish and follow standards of care. So, too, should IRBs.

The process *is* subjective and perhaps must be, but the answer isn't to deny that fact, but to acknowledge its dangers and build on its strengths. Some variations in interpretations will surely persist in certain areas, but we should ensure that when that is the case, the discrepancies are appropriate. We should not automatically accept these differences as inescapable and unproblematic. Future scholarship and efforts at consensus can assess, too, when and how much variation is acceptable or inevitable. We need to recognize that many IRB decisions are not objective, but rather get negotiated and shaped in varying contexts; and we need to seek to reduce any idiosyncrasies that may result. It will be important, but not necessarily easy, to decide whether any particular discrepancies are necessary, and if so which—how much objectivity or subjectivity is appropriate, especially when discrepancies arise. A strong case will have to be made that idiosyncrasy is needed in a review, rather than representing an easy, comfortable default position. Ignoring these tensions and the need for close intercommunication, explanation, and negotiation has contributed to many of the problems PIs now face.

BROADER IMPLICATIONS

These men and women shed light on not only IRBs but also broader aspects of society, ethics, science, power, and decision making today. In other areas, too, many policymakers and observers seek technocratic fixes without understanding the underlying problems and moral tensions involved and the need to initiate other, subtler attitudinal changes as well.

Interpreting Ethical Principles

Just as Freud's *Interpretations of Dreams* and Clifford Geertz's *Interpretation of Cultures* each opened up new ways of thinking about these respective phenomena, so, too, I think, we need to explore far more the *interpretations of ethics*. Many philosophers and others have tended to see ethical principles as simply involving universals that are either present or absent in particular arguments. The interviewees here, however, illustrate how these principles *get interpreted and applied* in variable ways, molded by broader social, institutional, and psychological influences. This is not by any means to say that all interpretations are equally strong, valid, or well-reasoned: some interpretations are better than others. At the same time—given the vast uncertainties inherent in assessing the possible future risks, benefits, and outcomes of a scientific investigation—more than one interpretation and application of principles by an IRB may be valid. Individuals respond differently to uncertain dangers, fears, and conflicts, such as that between control *vs.* trust. No one person's or committee's conclusions involving interpretations and applications of competing abstract principles are necessarily always *solely* correct, with all others wrong. Processes of group consensus can restrain extreme views but also take on lives of their own, swayed by chairs or particularly vocal members (especially, on many IRBs, white male physicians. See Bell et al in Chapter 2.). Judges, too, regularly disagree, and the field of bioethics is rife with opposing views on many issues. Likewise, IRBs disagree. Over time, as science continues to expand, further understanding of how and why they vary will be increasingly important.

I am by no means advocating so-called ethical relativism. Rather, I am suggesting that, given the substantial unknowns in gauging the potential risks and benefits of studies that have not yet been conducted, social and psychological factors may yield different decisions on similar cases. For a given study, IRBs in a single location might each arrive at a different decision that may each appear well reasoned and supported by the limited available evidence. The idea that only one objective, correct IRB decision exists in every situation is *incorrect*.

Some of these views may meet resistance. Some IRB personnel will surely argue that their decision about a particular contested protocol is the only valid approach. And yet, as a field, bioethics has been criticized for tending to focus on universal principles and ignoring how these get interpreted and applied in specific local contexts.[4] "Universal principles" are vital, but problems arise when we refuse to acknowledge that these ideas are still subject to differing interpretations and applications. Increasingly, therefore, many patients, clinicians, and scholars are trying to bridge these gaps, stressing the importance of narratives and language in optimizing patient care.[5] They face resistance but are beginning to narrow the rift. Similar efforts are crucial in research ethics, too.

Notions of Power

The interviewees here also highlight issues that have received relatively little attention concerning power: how individuals or organizations may feel they possess little or no power, even as they are viewed by others as having it. Many observers may assume that such denials of possession of power are disingenuous, but that was not my sense here. Rather, many of these interviewees genuinely seemed not to see themselves as having power, and their surprise that they were perceived otherwise was itself surprising to me, illustrating the intricacies of these dynamics. Those with perceived power may feel it is absent, or only small, or justified. The fact that people seen by others as having force and authority do not feel they possess it underscores needs to grasp more fully the manifold meanings of "power." Many people commonly employ this term as if it indicates an absolute object, not in many cases a relative phenomenon, based on individual perceptions.

IRBs also appear at times to misunderstand and abuse their perceived power without realizing it. The lack of an appeals process bolsters them, insulating them from feelings that they might be wrong. Their views can, in turn, foster self-righteousness, antagonizing researchers. Well-meaning people can thus wield tremendous clout, and yet remain oblivious of the unintended consequences. These phenomena, too, deserve far wider analysis and discussion.

OUR FUTURE

As a researcher, I am still at times maddened by IRBs. In the end, even after speaking to all of the men and women here and listening to their views, I still sometimes feel imposed on and frustrated by these committees. That frustration is greatly mitigated, however, by the fact that I now understand far better their *raison d'etre*, perspectives and constraints. More and earlier scientific breakthroughs might have helped cure my father's leukemia; and yet in retrospect, a more holistic and humanistic approach to his illness might have helped us make a better choice about his final months. Certain distinctions are much sharper for me now: science will continue to improve and extend our lives, but it will also continue to require assistance from countless research subjects and frequently involve risks with little, if any, reward for the individuals involved. I have more questions now than when I started, but I hope that this work will spark further discussion and exploration of these mounting quandaries.

Some IRB personnel may feel threatened by these findings and suggested improvements. Just as many researchers rebuff criticisms of their work by IRBs, some committee members will no doubt dismiss the critique here, arguing that it does not apply to them. Indeed, Diekema expressed exactly this view—that the IRB chairs, members, and staff I spoke with can be discounted because only studies that directly observe IRBs are relevant (though, as we discussed, IRBs have largely blocked such studies). Of course, the paucity of data on IRBs generally is—as I have argued throughout—a compelling reason for far more in-depth studies. It is not, however, an excuse for doing nothing until those studies are completed. That stance simply reinforces researchers' belief that IRBs are more interested in their own power than in the greater good, and inhibits efforts at informed, meaningful reforms.

One of the most valuable findings here has been that the two seemingly divergent critiques of IRBs—that they are either overly protective of subjects, or not protective enough—are *both* valid in different instances. It is critical for all of us to recognize that they can be reconciled; and these interviews suggest tangible ways of addressing each of these opposing problems. We need clearer and more rigorous and reflective thinking about IRBs; better, more sophisticated training of IRB personnel, to ensure that they can address these social and philosophical intricacies; and more transparency, open doors, external appeals, institutional memory, case law, standardization, and efforts to avoid COIs. As much as possible, these boards should seek to enhance themselves and the system as a whole—to gain the trust and cooperation of researchers and subjects. To do less is, arguably, to fail at their very mission. At the same time, as explained above, researchers, institutions, and federal agencies need to change, as well. *Resistance on both sides needs to soften for true improvements to occur.*

At the same time, given the ambiguities of ethics, law, science, language, nature, and human interactions, vagaries and negotiations are inescapable. I have become cautious of easy answers or quick fixes. These are human processes—fuzzy and complex. Just as laws continually evolve and courts grapple to apply them, IRBs will be needed to adjudicate studies in the coming decades. Although standardization will help, it is not a cure-all. To proceed, then, we need models that are based not solely on science, law, or ethics, but are instead multidisciplinary, integrating the humanities with natural and social science. Much of research ethics is, and will always need to be, done by consensus, and negotiated over time by a complex array of researchers, ethicists, and others. We should strive to reach the best consensus we can. Much depends on this balance.

As Sir Winston Churchill said about democracy, the current system is flawed—"the worst system...except for all the others."[6] Still, these limitations should then be addressed fully and frankly—not dismissed with claims that the system is running better than it in fact is, or than it could be. Ultimately, all of us—as present and future patients, or scientists or subjects—need to deepen our appreciation of these issues. How we balance these tensions is up to us. The more we understand how to do so, the better off we will all be.

APPENDICES

Appendix A

ADDITIONAL METHODOLOGICAL INFORMATION

Chapter 1 presents a brief overview of the study methods I used. More fully, I randomly selected 60 academic and nonprofit research institutions by choosing every fourth one on a list of US institutions ranked by the amount of NIH funding they received. I interviewed IRB leaders from 34 of these 60 institutions (a response rate, as social scientists term it, of 55 percent). In some cases, I interviewed both a chair/director and an administrator from an institution (for instance, when the chair thought that the administrator might better be able to answer certain questions). I also asked half of these leaders (every other one on the list) to distribute information about the study to members of their IRBs in an attempt to recruit one member of each committee to be interviewed as well. Many, perhaps most, committees do not release membership lists, instead keeping them secret, so I could not contact these individuals directly. I don't know if these leaders distributed the information and I only asked them twice—some researchers e-mail and phone potential study subjects additional times to try to increase participatory rates. In the end, I interviewed 7 other members (6 regular members and 1 community member). Each interview took approximately one to two hours.

The interviews focused on participants' views of research integrity (e.g., PIs' noncompliance with regulations), IRB responses (e.g., auditing), and factors involved in decisions, but shed important light as well on many other, broader issues that arose concerning IRBs' decisions, and interactions and relationships with PIs. Relevant sections of the interview guide are in Appendix B, through which I sought to obtain detailed descriptions of the above issues. From a theoretical standpoint, Clifford Geertz has advocated studying aspects of individuals' lives, decisions, and social situations not by imposing theoretical structures, but by trying to understand these individuals' own experiences, drawing on their own words and perspectives to obtain a "thick description".[1] In the methods, I have adapted elements from grounded theory.[2] My approach was thus informed by techniques of "constant comparison" in which data from different contexts are compared for similarities and differences, to see if they suggest hypotheses. This technique of "constant comparison" generates new analytic categories and questions, and checks them for reasonableness. During the ongoing process of in-depth interviewing, I considered how participants resembled or differed from each other, and the social, cultural, and other contexts and factors that contributed to differentiation. Grounded theory also involves both deductive and inductive thinking, building inductively from the data to an understanding of themes and patterns within the data, and deductively, drawing on frameworks from prior research and theories.

I drafted the questionnaire, drawing on prior research I conducted and published literature. Transcriptions and initial analyses of interviews occurred during the period in which the interviews were being conducted, enhancing validity, and these analyses helped shape subsequent interviews. The Columbia University Department of Psychiatry Institutional Review Board approved the study, and all participants gave informed consent.

Once the full set of interviews was completed, subsequent analyses were conducted in two phases, primarily by myself and a trained research assistant (RA).

In phase I, we independently examined a subset of interviews to assess factors that shaped participants' experiences, identifying categories of recurrent themes and issues that were subsequently given codes. We read each interview, systematically coding blocks of text to assign "core" codes or categories (e.g., instances of IRB tensions with PIs; and interactions with OHRP and FDA). While reading the interviews, a topic name (or code) was inserted beside each excerpt of the interview to indicate the themes being discussed. We then worked together to reconcile these independently developed coding schemes into a single scheme. Next we prepared a coding manual, defining each code and examining areas of disagreement until reaching consensus between them. New themes that did not fit into the original coding framework were discussed, and modifications were made in the manual when deemed appropriate.

In phase II of the analysis, we then independently performed content analyses of the data to identify the principal subcategories, and ranges of variation within each of the core codes. The subthemes identified by each coder were reconciled into a single set of "secondary" codes and an elaborated set of core codes. These codes assess subcategories and other situational and social factors. Such subcategories include specific types of tensions with PIs (e.g., PIs complaining about the IRB to institutional leadership), or specific types of problems concerning industry funding, such as studies of "me-too drugs" or "postmarketing studies"), or specific types of differences in interpretations (e.g., different definitions of "minimal risk" or "social benefit").

Codes and subcodes were then used in analysis of all of the interviews. To ensure coding reliability, two coders analyzed all interviews. Where necessary, multiple codes were used. The coders assessed similarities and differences between participants, examining categories that emerged, ranges of variation within categories, and variables that may be involved.

We examined areas of disagreement through closer analysis until consensus was reached through discussion. We checked regularly for consistency and accuracy in ratings by comparing earlier and later coded excerpts.

To ensure that the coding schemes established for the core codes and secondary codes are both valid (i.e., well grounded in the data and supportable) and reliable (i.e., consistent in meaning), they were systematically developed and well documented.

Through this process, we were able to explore "cases" of problems that arose (e.g., difficult decisions IRB chairs faced), to examine the range and patterns of issues that emerged.

Appendix B

SAMPLE SEMISTRUCTURED INTERVIEW QUESTIONS

I. Background Information:

- Are you an IRB Chair? Administrator? Member?
- Gender: *(1) Male (2) female*
- Highest educational level attained:
  (1) *High school/equivalent*
  (2) *Bachelor's*
  (3) *Some graduate*
  (4) *Masters*
  (5) *Ph.D.*
  (6) *M.D.*
  (7) *Other*

- Would you describe yourself as:
  (1) *African American*
  (2) *Caucasian*
  (3) *Latino*
  (4) *Asian American/Pacific Islander*
  (5) *Other:*

- How many years have you been on the IRB?
- How many hours/week do you spend working on IRB matters?
- How did you come to be in your current IRB position?
- Are you actively involved in research yourself? If so, what role(s) do you play (e.g., PI, co-I)? What kinds of projects are you involved with (e.g., clinical trials, epidemiologic studies)? What percentage of your time do you spend doing research?
- Are you compensated in any way for your work on the IRB? If so, how?

II. Research Integrity Problems

A. GENERAL

- How do you define RI?
- Do RI issues arise on your IRB? If so, how?
- What sorts of RI issues have you faced on the IRB?
- What do you think is the responsibility of the IRB concerning RI?
- How have decisions about RI been made in your IRB?
- Can you think of a recent case in which RI issues were discussed? What were the issues?
- What has been the most difficult case concerning RI that you have faced? What kind of issues arose?
- Have your concerns about RI issues changed over time? If so, how?
- Do you think IRBs should have more of a role in monitoring or responding to RI? If so, how?
- Do you think IRBs and PIs view RI differently or apply RI standards differently, and if so, how?

B. NONCOMPLIANCE

- Have you seen problems in researcher noncompliance with IRB regulations or mandates? If so, what kinds of problems?
- How comfortable are you with PI self-reporting?

C. CONFLICTS OF INTEREST (COI)

Financial COI

- How do you define a COI?
- Does the nature of the funder of the research (e.g., commercial vs. government or foundation) affect your review of protocols? If so, how?
- Has your IRB discussed protocols involving financial COI in the past year? If so, what kinds of conflicts were discussed? In what ways were they resolved?
- How adequately do you feel PIs self-report COI? Has your IRB ever challenged a PI's arrangement with industry sponsors? If so, why?
- Have you ever requested that financial arrangements between sponsors and PIs be disclosed to potential participants? Why?

Nonfinancial COI

- Has your IRB ever discussed nonfinancial COI? If so, how? What kinds of issues were discussed? How were they resolved?
- Have you seen nonfinancial COIs interfere with RI? If so, how?
- What do you think are the best ways of "managing" COIs?

- What have been the most difficult kinds of issues involving COI that your IRB has faced in the past year?
- How do you think nonfinancial COIs should be managed?
- Some people have argued that universities should not allow "even the appearance of COI"—Do you agree?

D. ADVERSE EVENTS

- How do you and your IRB handle adverse events?
- How often are adverse events discussed at your IRB? How are these addressed?
- Do you think PIs report adverse events in a complete manner? Within an appropriate time frame?

E. OTHER RESEARCH INTEGRITY ISSUES

- What kinds of problems with PIs' plans for data collection have you seen in the past year?
- What kinds of problems with PIs' plans for data storage have you seen in the past year?
- How often have you found problems with PIs' reviews of the literature in documents that the PIs have submitted to the IRB in the past year?
- What kinds of problems in RI related to PIs' collaborations with other PIs or institutions have you observed in the past year?
- What kinds of issues concerning RI have been the most difficult that you have faced, and how were these resolved? What other RI problems do you encounter?

F. FACTORS INVOLVED

IRB Characteristics

- What are the barriers and facilitators in IRBs monitoring and addressing RI problems?
- Have your views or approaches toward RI been affected by your experiences or education? If so, how?
- What administrative support is available to your IRB?
- Do you and other members of your board feel able to keep up with the workload satisfactorily?
- What training have you had relevant to your work on the IRB? Was it helpful? Why or why not?
- Have you had formal ethics training? What was the nature and duration of the training? Has it been helpful to your work on the IRB? Why or why not?
- Do you perceive any grey areas or problems weighing issues about RI? If so, how?

- Have you or other IRB members ever recused themselves from deliberations?
- What kinds of "serious or continuing" violations of regulations have you seen or heard about?
- Have you ever felt conflicts in addressing RI issues?

PI Characteristics
- Is your IRB more cautious about some researchers than others? Why?
- Would you like additional data about PIs or studies concerning RI? If so, what?
- In general, do PIs:
  - Treat your IRB with respect?
  - Take advantage of opportunities to be educated about relevant policies?
  - Maintain accurate records?
  - Respond in a timely and appropriate way to IRB requests?
- Does your knowledge of the PI affect how you look at his or her protocols? And if so, how?

Institutional Characteristics
- Have you served on IRBs in more than one institution?
- Do you think institutional contexts or settings affect IRBs' roles and decisions regarding RI? If so, how?
- How do you think your IRB is seen within your institution?
- What kinds of conflicts, if any, has your IRB faced with your institution? Have these conflicts been resolved?
- Have you or your IRB ever had input from your institution concerning RI? If so, how?
- Does your institution have a compliance office? If so, how does it interact with your IRB? How well does that work? What problems have come up?
- Does your institution have a COI committee? How does the IRB interact with it? How well does that work? What problems have come up?

G. IRB RESPONSES TO RI PROBLEMS
- What kinds of actions have you or your IRB taken concerning RI?
- Approximately how much time is spent discussing RI issues at meetings? Do you think the amount is too much, too little, or adequate?

Audits
- Do you think your IRB should do: more audits, fewer audits, or about the same as at present?
- Have you ever decided to audit a study because of your concerns about it? On what information were the audits focused? Has your IRB discussed the audits? If so, in what context? What kinds of issues arose?

Sanctions
- Has your IRB discussed sanctions against PIs? If so, what kinds of issues arose? Were any sanctions actually implemented? Why?

Reporting of Problems
- Has your IRB ever discussed reporting RI problems to an outside agency? If so, what kinds of issues arose?
- Has your IRB ever been involved in an investigation of a protocol at your institution by an outside agency? If so, for what *kind* of problem? What was the outcome?
- Do challenges arise in reporting problems to outside agencies? If so, how?

III. Implications

- Would any structural or institutional changes help your IRB's ability to monitor RI? If so, what?
- Would your IRB benefit from more training in monitoring or responding to RI? If so, how? In what form (e.g., conference, printed materials, website)?
- Do you think a centralized IRB rather than local IRBs would have advantages concerning RI and other areas? If so, what?

IV. Other Issues

- What do you think makes an IRB work well or not in monitoring and responding to RI?
- In ensuring RI, what do you think constitutes a "good" IRB chair and what should be their roles?
- Has your IRB been accredited or considered getting accredited?
- Do you have any other thoughts about these issues?

Thank you very much for your participation.

Appendix C

ACRONYMS

45 CFR 46	Also known as "The Common Rule"—Basic federal policy concerning the protection of human subjects in government-funded research
AAHRPP	Association for the Accreditation of Human Research Protection Programs
ACTG	AIDS Clinical Trial Group
AE	Adverse event
ANPRM	Advanced Notice of Proposed Rule-Making
CIOMS	Council for International Organizations of Medical Sciences
CIRB	Central IRB
CIP	Certified IRB professional
CME	Continuing Medical Education
COI	Conflict of interest
CRO	Contract research organization
DSMB	Data Safety Monitoring Board
DSMP	Data Safety Monitoring Plan
EU	European Union
FDA	Food and Drug Administration
HIPAA	Health Insurance Portability and Accountability Act of 1996
HR	Human resources
HHS	Department of Health and Human Services
ICU	Intensive Care Unit
IND	Investigational new drug
IOM	Institute of Medicine
IRB	Institutional Review Board
JCAHO	The Joint Commission on Accreditation of Healthcare Organizations

MRI	Magnetic resonance imaging
NA/NS	Nonaffiliated/nonscientific member
NGO	Non-governmental organization
NICU	Neonatal Intensive Care Unit
NIH	National Institutes of Health
NSF	National Science Foundation
OHRP	Office for Human Research Protections
OIG	Office of the Inspector General
OMB	Office of Management and Budget
OPRR	Office for Protection from Research Risks
ORI	Office of Research Integrity
PHS	United Stated Public Health Service
PI	Principal investigator
PRIM&R	Public Responsibility in Medicine and Research
QA	Quality assurance
QI	Quality improvement
RA	Research assistant
RCR	Responsible conduct of research
REC	Research Ethics Committee
RI	Research integrity
R01	Research Project Grant
SACHRP	Secretary's Advisory Committee on Human Research Protections
SOPs	Standard operating procedures
SUPPORT	Surfactant, Positive Pressure, and Oxygenation Randomized Trial
STD	Sexually transmitted disease
TB	Tuberculosis
WHO	World Health Organization
WMA	World Medical Association

SOURCES

Figures

Figure 5.1: Klitzman R. How IRBs view and make decisions about consent forms. *Journal of Empirical Research on Human Research Ethics* 8.1 (2013): 8–19.

Figure 7.1: Klitzman R. Local IRBs vs. federal agencies: Shifting dynamics, systems, and relationships. *Journal of Empirical Research on Human Research Ethics* 7.3 (2012): 50–62.

Figure 10.1: Klitzman R. The ethics police? IRBs' views concerning their power. *PLoS One* 6.12 (Epub 2011, Dec 13): e28773.

Figure 10.2: Klitzman R. From anonymity to "open doors": IRB responses to tensions with researchers. *BMC Research Notes* 5.1 (2012): 347.

Figure 11.1: Klitzman R. Views and experiences of IRBs concerning research integrity. *Journal of Law, Medicine and Ethics* 39.3 (2011): 513–528.

Tables

Table 1.1: Klitzman R. Views and experiences of IRBs concerning research integrity. *Journal of Law, Medicine and Ethics* 39.3 (2011): 513–528.

Table 3.3: Klitzman R. How IRBs view and make decisions about coercion and undue influence. *Journal of Medical Ethics* 39.4 (2012): 224–229.

ACKNOWLEDGMENTS

I am very grateful to many people who made this book possible. Most of all, I am deeply indebted to the men and women whom I interviewed and who shared their experiences and insights with me. I am grateful, too, to the National Institute of Nursing Research; the Ethical, Legal and Social Implications Program of the National Human Genome Research Institute (R01-NG04214); the National Library of Medicine (5-G13-LM009996-02); and Jean McEwen, Joy Boyer, and Elizabeth Thompson for supporting this project. I especially want to thank Peter Ohlin, who had faith in this book from the outset and has been wonderfully supportive throughout. His colleagues at Oxford, including Lucy Randall, Christian Purdy, Jeremy Wang-Iverson, John Hercel, Michelle Kelly, and Susan Lee have also been a pleasure to work with.

I would also like to thank Alice Truax, as well as Warren Stone, Rénee Fox, Mark Olfson, Ric Hamlin, Melanie Thernstrom, Stewart Adelson, Robert Kertzner, Elaine Larson, Ilene Wilets, Marcia Moyer, and Patty Volk for their valuable input; and Patricia Contino, Kristopher Abbate, Jennifer Teitcher, Brigitte Buquez, Cydney Halpin, Felisha Miles and Meghan Sweeney for all their assistance with this manuscript.

Portions of this material appeared in a different form in *Science, Academic Medicine, The Journal of Law, Medicine and Ethics, Journal of Medical Ethics, Clinical Trials, PLOS One, BMC Medical Ethics, American Journal of Bioethics—Primary Care, IRB*, and *Journal of Empirical Research in Human Research Ethics*.

NOTES

Chapter 1

1. Moses H, Martin JB. Biomedical Research and Health Advances. *NEJM* 364.6 (2011): 567–571.

2. Dorsey ER, de Roulet J, Thompson JP, Reminick JI, Thai A, White-Stellato Z, Beck CA, George BP, Moses H. Funding of US biomedical research, 2003-2008. *JAMA* 303.2 (2010): 137–143

3. National Institutes of Health. The NIH Almanac: Appropriations (April 4th 2014). Available at http://www.nih.gov/about/almanac/appropriations/part2.htm

4. Massey DS, Tourangeau R. Where do we go from here? Nonresponse and Social Measurement; *The Annals of the American Academy of Political and Social Science* 645 (2013): 222–236.

5. General Accounting Office. *Scientific Research: Continued Vigilance Critical to Protecting Human Subjects* (Publication No. GAO/HEHS-96-102). Washington, DC: General Accounting Office, 1996.

6. Goldman J, Katz M. Inconsistency and institutional review boards. *The Journal of the American Medical Association* 2.248 (1982):197–202.

7. Eaton WO. Reliability in ethics reviews: some initial empirical findings. *Canadian Psychology* 24.1 (1983):14–18.

8. Doob AN. The reliability of ethical reviews: Is it desirable? *Canadian Psychology* 24.4 (1983):269–270.

9. Olfson M, Marcus SC. Decline in placebo-controlled results suggests new directions for comparative effectiveness research. *Health Affairs* 32.6 (2013): 1116–1125

10. Dziak K, Anderson R, Sevick MA, Weisman CS, Levine DW, & Scholle SH. Variations among Institutional Review Boards in a multisite health services research study. *Health Services Research* 40.1 (2005): 279–290.

11. Silverstein M, Banks M, Fish S, Bauchner H. Variability in institutional approaches to ethics review of community-based research conducted in collaboration with unaffiliated organizations. *Journal of Empirical Research on Human Research Ethics* 3.2 (2008): 69–76.

12. Greene SM, Geiger AM. A review finds that multicenter studies face substantial challenges, but strategies exist to achieve Institutional Review Board approval. *Journal of Clinical Epidemiology* 59 (2006): 784–790.

13. Newgard CD, Hui S-H, Stamps-White P, Lewis RJ. Institutional variability in a minimal risk, population-based study: Recognizing policy barriers to health services research. *Health Services Research* 40.4 (2005):1247–1257.

14. Finch SA, Barkin SL, Wasserman RC, Dhepyasuwan N, Slora EJ, Sege RD. Effects of local institutional review board review on participation in national practice-based research network studies. *Archives of Pediatric Adolescent Medicine* 163.12 (2009): 1130–1134.

15. Mansbach J, Acholonu U, Clark S, Camargo CA. Variation in institutional review board responses to a standard, observational, pediatric research protocol. *Academic Emergency Medicine* 14 (2007): 377–380

16. Ravina B, Deuel L, Siderowf A, Dorsey ER. Local ORB review of multicenter trial: Local costs without local context. *Annals of Neurology* 67.2 (2010): 258–260.

17. Veatch R. Problems with Institutional Review Board inconsistency. *The Journal of the American Medical Association* 248.2 (1982):179–180.

18. Office of Inspector General. *Institutional Review Boards: Their role in reviewing approved research* (DHHS Publication No. OEI-chapter-01-97-00190). Washington, DC: US Government Printing Office, 1998a.

19. Office of Inspector General. *Institutional Review Boards: Promising approaches* (DHHS Publication No. OEI-chapter-01-91-00191). Washington, DC: US Government Printing Office, 1998b.

20. Office of Inspector General. *Institutional Review Boards: The emergence of independent boards* (DHHS Publication No. OEI-chapter-01-97-00192). Washington, DC: US Government Printing Office, 1998c.

21. Office of Inspector General, Department of Health and Human Services. *Institutional Review Boards: A time for reform* (DHHS Publication No. OEI-chapter-01-97-00193). Washington, DC: US Government Printing Office, 1998d.

22. Office of Inspector General. *Protecting human research subjects: Status of recommendations* (DHHS Publication No. OEI-chapter-01-97-00197). Washington, DC: US Government Printing Office, 2000a.

23. Office of Inspector General. Recruiting human subjects: Pressure in industry-sponsored clinical research (DHHS Publication No.

OEI-chapter-01-97-00195). Washington, DC: US Government Printing Office, 2000b.

24. Levine RJ. Institutional Review Boards: A Crisis in Confidence. *Ann Intern Med.* 134 (2001): 161–163.

25. Burris S. Regulatory innovation in the governance of human subjects research: A cautionary tale and some modest proposals. *Regulation & Governance* 2.1(2008): 65–84.

26. Sansone R, McDonald S, Hanley P, Sellbom M, Gaither GA. The stipulations of one institutional review board: A five year review. *Journal of Medical Ethics* 30 (2004): 308–310.

27. James JT. A new, evidence-based estimate of patient harms associated with hospital care. *Journal of Patient Safety* 9.3 (2013): 122–128.

28. Emanuel EJ, Menikoff J. Reforming the regulations governing research with human subjects. *New England Journal of Medicine* 365 (2011):1145–1150.

29. Burman W, Daum R. Grinding to a halt: The effects of the increasing regulatory burden on research and quality improvement efforts. *Clinical Infectious Diseases* 49 (2009): 328–335

30. Burris S, Moss K. US health researchers review their ethics review boards: a qualitative study. *Journal of Empirical Research on Human Research Ethics* 1.2 (2006):39–58.

31. Moreno J, Caplan A, Wolpe P, the Members of the Project on Informed Consent, Human Research Ethics Group. Updating protections for human subjects involved in research. *The Journal of the American Medical Association.* 280.22 (1998): 1951–1958.

32. Fitzgerald DW, Wasunna A, Pape JW. Ten questions for institutional review boards when reviewing international clinical research protocols. *IRB: Ethics & Human Research* 25.2 (2003):14–18.

33. Prentice E, Antonsen D. A protocol review guide to reduce IRB inconsistency. *IRB: A Review of Human Subjects Research* 9.1 (1987): 9–11.

34. Pollack A. Rule changes proposed for research on humans. *The New York Times*, July 24 2011, http://www.nytimes.com/2011/07/25/health/research/25research.html. Accessed April 16 2013.

35. Koerner AF. Communication scholars' communication and relationship with their IRBs. *Journal of Applied Communication Research* 33.3(2005): 231–241.

36. Fleischman AR. Regulating research with human subjects—is the system broken? *Transactions of the American Clinical and Climatological Association* 116 (2005): 91–102.

37. Bledsoe CH, Sherin B, Galinsky AG, Headley NM, Heimer CA, Kjeldgaard E, Lindgren J, Miller JD, Roloff ME, Uttal DH. Regulating creativity: Research and survival in the IRB iron cage. *Northwestern University Law Review* 101.2 (2007): 593–642

38. Edwards KL, Lemke AA, Trinidad SB, Lewis SM, Starks H, Snapinn KW, Griffin MQ, Wiesner GL, Burke W, GRRIP Consortium. Genetics researcher's and IRB professionals' attitudes toward genetic research review: a comparative analysis. *Genetics in Medicine* 14.2 (2012): 236–242.

39. Campbell EG, Weissman JS, Clarridge B, Yucel R, Causino N, Blumenthal D. Characteristics of medical school faculty members serving on institutional review boards: Results of a national survey. *Academic Medicine* 78.8 (2003): 831–836

40. Lind J. A treatise of the scurvy. *A Treatise of the Scurvy in Three Parts. Containing an inquiry into the Nature, Causes and Cure of that Disease, together with a Critical and Chronological View of what has been published on the subject.* London: A. Millar, 1753.

41. Baron JH. Sailors' scurvy before and after James Lind—a reassessment. *Nutrition Reviews* 67.6 (2009):315–332

42. Weindling P. *Nazi Medicine and the Nuremberg Trials: From Medical War Crimes to Informed Consent.* United Kingdom: Palgrave Macmillan, 2005.

43. Seluykh A. US researchers broke rules in Guatemala syphilis study. *Reuters,* August 29, 2011. http://www.reuters.com/article/2011/08/29/us-usa-guatemala-syphilis-idUSTRE77S3L120110829. Accessed April 16 2013.

44. Rothman D. Were Tuskegee & Willowbrook "studies in nature" *The Hastings Center Report* 12(1982): 5–7.

45. World Medical Association. Declaration of Helsinki as amended by the 64th WMA General Assembly, Fortaleza, Brazil, October, 2013.

46. McCoy AW. Science in Dachau's Shadow: Hebb, Beecher, and the development of CIA psychological torture and modern medical ethics. *Journal of the History of Behavioral Sciences* 43.4 (2007): 401–417.

47. Mashour GA. Altered states: LSD and the anesthesia laboratory of Henry Knowles Beecher. *Bulletin of Anesthesia History* 23.3 (2005): 11–14.

48. Beecher HE. Ethics and clinical research. *NEJM* 274 (1966): 1354–1360.

49. Surgeon General's directives on human experimentation. *The American Psychologist* 22.5 (1967): 350–355.

50. Milgram S. Behavioral study of obedience. *Journal of Abnormal and Social Psychology.* 67.4 (1963): 371–378.

51. Zimbardo PG. On the ethics of intervention in human psychological research: With special reference to the Stanford prison experiment. *Cognition* 2.2 (1973): 243–256.

52. Coughlin SS, Etheredge GD, Metayer C, et al. Remember Tuskegee: Public Health Student Knowledge of the Ethical Significance of the Tuskegee Syphilis Study. In: Coughling, SS. *Ethics in Epidemiology and Public Health Practice: Collected Works.* Georgia: Quill Publications, 1997.

53. National Research Act, Pub. L. No. 93-348, 88 Stat. 342 (July 12, 1974) (codified as amended in scattered sections of 42 U.S.C.).

54. Department of Health, Education, and Welfare, *The Belmont Report: Ethical principles and guidelines for the protection of human subjects of research*, Washington, DC: OPRR Reports, 1979. Available at: http://ohsr.od.nih.gov/guidelines/belmont.html.

55. US Department of Health and Human Services, 45 C.F.R. § 46 (2009) Available at: http://www.hhs.gov/ohrp/humansubjects/guidance/45cfr46.html. Accessed December 27, 2012.

56. Bartlett EE. International analysis of institutional review boards registered with the US Office for Human Research Protections. *Journal of Empirical Research Human Research Ethics* 3 (2008): 49–56.

57. Abbott L, Grady C. A systematic review of the empirical literature evaluating IRBs: What we know and what we still need to learn; *Journal of Empirical Research on Human Research Ethics* 6.1 (2011): 3–20.

58. Bell J, Whiton J, Connelly S. *Final report: Evaluation of NIH Implementation of Section 491 of the Public Health Service, Mandating a Program of Protection for Research Subjects*. Arlington, VA: James Bell Associates, 1998.

59. Monmaney T. VA Hospital's Ethical Nightmare. *Los Angeles Times*. March 25, 1999. http://articles.latimes.com/1999/mar/25/news/mn-20845. Accessed September 12, 2013.

60. Weiss R. US Halts Human Research at Duke. *Washington Post*. May 12, 1999: Page A1. http://www.washingtonpost.com/wp-srv/national/daily/may99/duke12.htm. Accessed December 27, 2012.

61. Amber D. Case at VCU brings ethics to forefront. *The Scientist*, May 1, 2000. http://www.the-scientist.com/?articles.view/articleNo/12810/title/Case-at-VCU-Brings-Ethics-To-Forefront/. Accessed May 1, 2013.

62. Steinbrook R. The Gelsinger case. In: Emanuel EJ, Grady C, Crouch RA, et al., eds. *The Oxford Textbook of Clinical Research Ethics*. New York: Oxford University Press, 2008.

63. Office of Information and Public Affairs. CPSC Announces Final Ban On Lead-Containing Paint (September 2, 1977). U.S. Consumer Product Safety Commission.

64. Mastroianni AM, Kahn JP. Risk and responsibility: Ethics, Grimes v. Kennedy Krieger, and public health research involving children. *American Journal of Public Health* 92.7 (2002): 1073–1076

65. Chisolm JJ. Removal of lead paint from old housing: The need for a new approach. *American Journal of Public Health* 76.3 (1986): 236–237.

66. Tiller J. Easing lead paint laws: A step in the wrong direction. *Harvard Environmental Law Review* 18 (1994): 265–276.

67. Ross, L. F. In defense of the Hopkins lead abatement studies. *The Journal of Law, Medicine & Ethics* 30.1 (2002): 50–57.

68. *Grimes v. Kennedy Krieger Institute, Inc.,* 782 A.2d 807, 366 Md. 29 (2001).

69. Pollak J. The lead-based paint abatement repair and maintenance study in Baltimore: Historic framework and study design. *Journal of Health Care Law and Policy* 6 (2002): 90–110.

70. Rosner D, Markowitz G. With the best intentions: Lead research and the challenge to public health. *American Journal of Public Health* 102.11 (2012): e19–e33

71. Stipulation of Dismissal, Hughes v. Kennedy Krieger Institute, Inc., Case No. 24C99000925 (Circuit Ct. Baltimore City, May 13, 2003) (No. 125).

72. Markowitz G, Rosner D. *Lead war: The politics of science and the fate of America's children.* Berkeley and Los Angeles: University of California Press, 2013.

73. Harmon A. Havasupai case highlights risks in DNA research. *The New York Times,* April 24, 2010. http://www.nytimes.com/2010/04/22/us/22dnaside.html. Accessed April 16, 2013.

74. Krumholz HM, Ross JS, Presler AH, Egilman DS. What have we learnt from Vioxx? *BMJ* 334 (2007): 120–123.

75. Meier B. In guilty plea, OxyContin maker to pay $600 million. *New York Times.* May 10, 2007. http://www.nytimes.com/2007/05/10/business/11drug-web.html?pagewanted=all&_r=0. Accessed February 7, 2014.

76. Van Zee A. The promotion and marketing of OxyContin: Commercial triumph, public health tragedy. *American Journal of Public Health* 99.2 (2009): 221–227.

77. Godlee F, Malone R, Timmis A, Otto C, Bush A, Pavord I, Groves T. Journal policy on research funded by the tobacco industry. *BMJ* 347 (2013): f5193.

78. Musk AW, De Klerk NH. History of tobacco and health. *Respirology* 8 (2003): 286–290.

79. The Bayh-Dole Act. Pub. L. No. 96-517 (December 12, 1980). Available at http://www.gpo.gov/fdsys/pkg/CFR-2002-title37-vol1/content-detail.html. Accessed July 22, 2013.

80. Moses H, Dorsey ER, Matheson DH, Thier SO. Financial anatomy of biomedical research. *JAMA* 294.11 (2005): 1333–1342.

81. Shiffman J. Donor funding priorities for communicable disease control in the developing world. *Health Planning and Policy* 21.6 (2006): 411–420.

82. Institute of Medicine (US) Committee on Assessing the System for Protecting Human Research Participants; DD Federman, KE Hanna, LL Rodriguez, eds., *Responsible Research: A Systems Approach to Protecting Research Participants.* Washington DC: National Academies Press, 2003.

83. NBAC, the DHHS Office of Inspector General, the General Accounting Office, the Advisory Committee on Human Radiation Experiments, the President's Commission for the Study of Ethical Problems in Medicine and Biomedical and Behavioral Research, and the National Commission for the Protection of Human Subjects of Biomedical and Behavioral Research, as cited in *Responsible Research: A Systems Approach to Protecting Research Participants.* Washington DC: National Academies Press, 2003.

84. Prentice E, Antonsen DA. Protocol review guide to reduce IRB inconsistency. *IRB: A Review of Human Subjects Research* 9.1 (1987): 9–11.

85. Department of Health and Human Services. Human subjects research protections: Enhancing protections for research subjects and reducing burden, delay, and ambiguity for investigators. *Federal Register* 76 (2011): 44512–44531.

86. Gray, BH. *Human Subjects in Medical Experimentation: A Sociological Study of the Conduct and Regulation of Clinical Research* (1975). Huntington, NY: R.E. Krieger.

87. McNeill P, Berglund C, Webster I. Reviewing the reviewers: A survey of institutional ethics committees in Australia. *Medical Journal of Australia* 152.6 (1990): 289–296.

88. Hayes GJ, Hayes SC, Dystra T. A survey of university institutional review boards: characteristics, policies, and procedures. *IRB: A Review of Human Subjects Research* 17.3 (1995): 1–6.

89. Klitzman R. How IRB leaders view and approach challenges raised by industry-funded research. *IRB* 35.3 (2013): 9–17.

90. Meslin EM, Lavery JV, Sutherland HJ, Till JE. Judging the ethical merit of clinical trials: what criteria do research ethics board members use? *IRB: A Review of Human Subjects Research* 16.4 (1994): 6–10.

91. Lidz CW, Simon LJ, Seligowski AV, et al. The participation of community members on institutional review boards. *Journal of Empirical Research on Human Research Ethics: An International Journal* 7.1 (2012):1–6.

92. Klitzman R. Views of the process and content of ethical reviews of HIV vaccine trials among members of US Institutional Review Boards and South African Research Ethics Committees. *Developing World Bioethics* 8.3 (2008): 207–218.

93. Stark LJM. *Behind Closed Doors: IRBs and the Making of Ethical Research.* Chicago: University of Chicago Press, 2011.

94. De Vries RG, Forsberg, CP. What do IRBs look like? What kind of support do they receive? *Accountability in Research* 9.3-4 (2002):199–216.

95. Geertz C. *Interpretation of Cultures.* New York: Basic Books, 1973.

96. Klitzman, R., The importance of social, cultural and economic contexts, and empirical research in examining "undue inducement." *American Journal of Bioethics* 5.5 (2005): 19–21.

97. Acton B, Emerich J, Dalberg E. *Lectures on Modern History*. Charleston, SC: Nabu Press, 2012.

98. Orwell G. Politics and the English Language (1945). In: Carey J, ed. *George Orwell Essays*. New York: Everyman's Library, 2002:954–967.

99. Kafka F. *The Trial: A New Translation Based on the Restored Text* (1914). Trans. by Breon Mitchell. New York: Schocken Books, 1999.

100. Kafka F. *The Castle* (Posthumous 1926). Trans. by Mark Harman. New York: Schocken Books, 1998.

101. Kahneman D, Slovic P, Tversky A, Eds. *Judgment Under Certainty: Heuristics and Biases*. Cambridge: Cambridge University Press, 1982.

Chapter 2

1. US Department of Health and Human Services, 45 C.F.R. § 46 (2009) Available at: http://www.hhs.gov/ohrp/humansubjects/guidance/45cfr46.html. Accessed December 27, 2012.

2. Campbell EG, Weissman JS, Clarridge B, Yucel R, Causino N, Blumenthal D. Characteristics of medical school faculty members serving on institutional review boards: Results of a national survey. *Academic Medicine* 78.8 (2003): 831–836.

3. De Vries RG, Forsberg CP. Who decides? A look at ethics committee membership. *Healthcare Ethics Committee Forum*. 14.3 (2002): 252–258.

4. Bell J, Whiton J, Connelly S. *Final Report: Evaluation of NIH Implementation of Section 491 of the Public Health Service Act, Mandating a Program of Protection for Research Subjects*. Arlington, VA: James Bell Associates, 1998.

5. Klitzman R. Views of the process and content of ethical reviews of HIV vaccine trials among members of US Institutional Review Boards and South African Research Ethics Committees. *Developing World Bioethics* 8.3 2008: 207–218.

6. Lantos J. "It is time to professionalize Institutional Review Boards." *Archives of Pediatrics & Adolescent Medicine* 163.12 (2009): 1163–1164.

7. Office of Human Subjects Research. Chapter 3. IRB Membership: Conformance with Regulatory Requirements (45 C.F.R. 46.107 and 21 C.F.R. 56.107). (Revised March 3, 2013) Available at http://ohsr.od.nih.gov/irb/Attachments/Chapter3.htm.

8. Anderson EE. A qualitative study of non-affiliated, non-scientist institutional review board members. *Accountability in Research* 13.2 (2006):135–155.

9. Porter JP. How unaffiliated/nonscientist members of institutional review boards see their roles. *IRB: Ethics and Human Research* 9.6 (1987): 1–6.

10. Allison RD, Abbott LJ, Wichman A. Roles and experiences of nonscientist Institutional Review Board members at the National Institutes of Health. *IRB: Ethics and Human Research* 30.5 (2008): 8–13.

11. Sengupta S, Lo B. The roles and experiences of nonaffiliated and non-scientist members of institutional review boards. *Academic Medicine* 78.2 (2003):212–218.

12. Rothstein WG, Phuong LH. Ethical attitudes of nurse, physician, and unaffiliated members of institutional review boards. *Journal of Nursing Scholarship* 39.1 (2007): 75–81.

13. Schrag ZM. *Ethical imperialism: Institutional review boards and the social sciences, 1965-2009*. Baltimore: The Johns Hopkins University Press, 2010.

14. Fox R. Training for uncertainty. In: Merton RK, Reader G, Kendall PL., Eds. *The Student Physician*. Cambridge: Harvard University Press, 1957.

15. Freidson E. The changing nature of professional control. *Annual Review of Sociology* 10 (1984):1–20.

16. Klitzman R. *In a House of Dreams and Glass: Becoming a Psychiatrist*. New York: Simon and Schuster, 1995.

17. Schuppli CA, Fraser D. Factors influencing the effectiveness of research ethics committees. *Journal of Medical Ethics* 33.5 (2007): 294–301.

18. Cooper-Thomas HD, Anderson A. Organizational socialization. A new theoretical model for future research and HRM practices in organizations. *Journal of Managerial Psychology* 21.5 (2006): 492–516.

19. Kammeyer-Mueller JD, Wanberg CR. Unwrapping the organizational entry process: Disentangling multiple antecedents and their pathways to adjustment. *Journal of Applied Psychology* 88.5 (2003):779–794.

20. Greene SM, Geiger AM. A review finds that multicenter studies face substantial challenges but strategies exist to achieve institutional review board approval. *Journal of Clinical Epidemiology* 59.8 (2006): 784–790.

21. Stair TO, Reed CR, Radeos MS, Koski G, Camargo CA; MARC investigators. Variation in institutional review board responses to a standard protocol for a multicenter clinical trial. *Academic Emergency Medicine* 8.6 (2001): 636–641.

22. Dyrbye LN, Thomas MR, Mechaber AJ, et al. Medical education research and IRB review: an analysis and comparison of the IRB review process at six institutions. *Academic Medicine* 82.7 (2007): 654–660.

23. National Institutes of Health. NIH Budget: Research for the People. (Revised September 18, 2012) Available at http://www.nih.gov/about/budget.htm/. Accessed September 25, 2013.

24. Lidz CW, Simon LJ, Seligowski AV, et al. The participation of community members on institutional review boards. *Journal of Empirical Research on Human Research Ethics: An International Journal* 7.1 (2012):1–6.

25. Savulescu J, Crisp R, Fulford KW, Hope T. Evaluating ethics competence in medical education." *Journal of Medical Ethics* 25.5 (1999): 367–374.

26. Rogers AS, Israel E. Smith CR, et al. Physician knowledge, attitudes, and behavior related to reporting adverse drug events. *Archives of Internal Medicine* 148.7 (1988):1596–1600.

27. Campbell EG, Weissman JS, Vogeli C, et al. Financial relationships between institutional review board members and industry. *NEJM* 355.22 (2006): 2321–2329.

28. Levinsky NG. Nonfinancial conflicts of interest in research. *NEJM* 347.10 (2002): 759–761.

29. Mello MM, Wolf LE. The Havasupai Indian tribe case—lessons for research involving stored biologic samples. *NEJM* 363.3 (2010): 204.

30. Beecher H. Ethics and clinical research. *NEJM* 274.24 (1966): 1354–1360.

Chapter 3

1. Hoyert DL, Xu J, Division of Vital Statistics, Centers for Disease Control and Prevention. Deaths: Preliminary data for 2011. *National Vital Statistics Reports* 61.6 (2012).

2. Martin JA, Hamilton BE, Ventura SJ, Osterman MJK, Mathews TJ, Division of Vital Statistics, Centers for Disease Control and Prevention. Births: Final data for 2011. *National Vital Statistics Reports* 62.1 (2013).

3. Vermont Oxford Network. *Vermont-Oxford Network Expanded Database Summaries.* Burlington, Vermont (2012).

4. SUPPORT Study Group of the Eunice Kennedy Shriver NICHD Neonatal Research Network. Target Ranges of Oxygen Saturation in Extremely Preterm Infants *NEJM* 362 (2010): 1959–1969.

5. Office for Human Research Protections. Letter to the University of Alabama at Birmingham. March 7, 2013. http://www.hhs.gov/ohrp/detrm_letrs/YR13/mar13a.pdf. Accessed March 27, 2013.

6. Public Citizen. Letter to the Honorable Kathleen Sebelius. April 10, 2013. http://www.citizen.org/documents/2111.pdf. Accessed February 27, 2014.

7. Editorial Board. An Ethical Breakdown. *The New York Times.* April 15, 2013. http://www.nytimes.com/2013/04/16/opinion/an-ethical-breakdown-in-medical-research.html?_r=0. Accessed December 27, 2013.

8. *The American Journal of Bioethics* 13.12 (2013): Full issue.

9. Macklin R, Shepherd L. Informed consent and standard of care: What must be disclosed. *The American Journal of Bioethics* 13.12 (2013): 9–13.

10. Wilfond BS, Magnus D, Antommaria AH, Appelbaum P, Aschner J, Barrington KJ, Younger S. The OHRP and SUPPORT. *NEJM* 368 (2013): e36.

11. Wendler D. What should be disclosed to research participants? *The American Journal of Bioethics* 12 (2013): 3–8.

12. Whitney SN. The python's embrace: Clinical research regulation by Institutional Review Boards. *Pediatrics* 129 (2012): 576.

13. Tin W, Milligan DW, Pennfather P, Hey E. Pulse oximetry, severe retinopathy and outcome at one year in babies of less than 28 weeks gestation. *Archives of Disease in Childhood. Fetal and Neonatal Edition* 84 (2001): F106–F110.

14. Lantos JD. Learning the right lessons from the SUPPORT study controversy. *Archives of Disease in Childhood. Fetal and Neonatal Edition* 0 (2013): F1–F12.

15. Rich W, Finer NN, Gantz MG, Newman NS, Hensman AM, Hale EC, Auten KJ, Schibler K, Faix RG, Laptook AR, Yoder BA, Das A, Shankaran S; SUPPORT and Generic Database Subcommittees of the Eunice Kennedy Shriver National Institute of Child Health and Human Development Neonatal Research Network. Enrollment of extremely low birth weight infants in a clinical research study may not be representative. *Pediatrics* 129.3 (2012): 480–484.

16. Epstein L, Landes WM, Posner RA. Are even unanimous decisions in the United States Supreme Court ideological? *Northwestern University Law Review* 106.2 (2012): 699–714.

17. Liptak A. Justices agree to agree, at least for the moment. *The New York Times.* May 27, 2013. http://www.nytimes.com/2013/05/28/us/supreme-court-issuing-more-unanimous-rulings.html?_r=1& Accessed February 7, 2014.

18. Freedman B. Equipoise and the ethics of clinical research. *NEJM* 317.3 (1987): 141–145.

19. Joffe S, Miller FG. Equipoise: Asking the right questions for clinical trial design. *Nature Reviews Clinical Oncology* 9 (2012): 230–235.

20. Miller FG, Brody H. Clinical equipoise and the incoherence of research ethics. *Journal of Medicine and Philosophy* 32 (2007): 151–165.

21. Kahneman D, Tversky A. Judgment under uncertainty: Heuristics and biases. *Science* 184 (1974): 1124–1131.

22. Fox R. Training for uncertainty. In: Merton RK, Reader GG, Kendall PL. *The Student Physician.* Cambridge, MA: Harvard University Press, 1957: 207–241.

23. Redelmeier D, Rozin P, Kanheman D, Understanding patients' decisions: Cognitive and emotional perspectives, *JAMA* 270: (1993): 72–76.

24. Elstein AS. On the origins and development of evidence-based medicine and medical decision making. *Inflammation Research* 53, Suppl 2 (2004): S184–S189.

25. Klitzman R. Views and approaches toward risks and benefits among doctors who become patients. *Patient Education and Counseling* 64 (2006): 61–68.

26. Kong A et al. How medical professionals evaluate expressions of probability. *New England Journal of Medicine* 325 (1986): 740–744.

27. Bergus GR, Levin IP, Elstein AS. Presenting risks and benefits to patients: The effect of information order on decision making. *Journal of General Internal Medicine* 17 (2002): 612–617.

28. Skloot R. *The Immortal Life of Henrietta Lacks*. New York: Broadway Paperbacks, 2010.

29. Shamoo AE. Ethically questionable research with children: The Kennedy Krieger Institute lead abatement study. *Accountability in Research* 9 (2002): 165–175.

30. Appelbaum P, Lidz C, Klitzman R. Voluntariness of consent to research: A preliminary empirical investigation. *IRB* 30 (2009): 10–14.

31. U.S. Department of Health and Human Services. Human subjects research protections: Enhancing protections for research subjects and reducing burden, delay, and ambiguity for investigators. *Federal Register* 76.143 (2011): 44512–44531.

32. Fleischman A, Levine C, Eckenwiler L, et al. Dealing with the long-term social implications of research. *The American Journal of Bioethics* 11.5 (2011): 5–9.

33. Melo-Martin D. IRBs and the long-term social implications of research. *The American Journal of Bioethics* 11.5 (2011): 22–23.

34. Mello MM, Wolf LE. The Havasupai Indian tribe case—lessons for research involving stored biologic samples. *NEJM* 363.3 (2010): 204–207.

35. Olson J, Tosto P. Dan Markingson had delusions. His mother feared the worst would happen. Then it did. *St. Paul Pioneer Press*, May 18, 2008,http://www.twincities.com/ci_9292549?IADID=Search-www. twincities.com-www.twincities.com&nclick_check=1. Accessed October 10, 2013.

36. Davies E. Investigating the fallout of a suicide. *BMJ* 347 (2013): f6039.

37. US Department of Health and Human Services, 45 C.F.R. § 46 (2009). Available at: http://www.hhs.gov/ohrp/humansubjects/ guidance/45cfr46.html. Accessed December 27, 2012.

38. Department of Health, Education, and Welfare. *The Belmont report: Ethical principles and guidelines for the protection of human subjects of research.* Washington, DC: OPRR Reports, 1979. Available at: http://ohsr.od.nih. gov/guidelines/belmont.html.

39. Coleman CH. Vulnerability as a regulatory category in human subject research. *Journal of Law, Medicine & Ethics* 37.1 (2009): 12–18.

40. Council for International Organizations of Medical Sciences (CIOMS). *International ethical guidelines for biomedical research involving human subjects* (2002). Available at: http://www.cioms.ch/publications/ guidelines/guidelines_nov_2002_blurb.htm.

41. World Medical Association (WMA). Declaration of Helsinki. (2008) Available at: http://www.wma.net/en/20activities/10ethics/10helsinki/.

42. Stevenson A, Siefring J, Brown L, et al, eds. *Oxford English Dictionary.* Oxford: Oxford University Press, 2002.

43. Fox RC, Swazey J. *Observing Bioethics.* New York: Oxford, 2008.

44. Shah S, Whittle A, Wilfond B, Gensler G, Wendler D. How do institutional review boards apply the federal risk and benefit standards for pediatric research? *Journal of the American Medical Association* 291 (2004): 476–482.

45. Berger RL. Nazi science: the Dachau hypothermia experiments. *NEJM* 322 (1990): 1435–1440.

46. Rothman SM, Rothman DJ. *The Willowbrook wars.* Piscataway, NJ: Aldine Transaction, 2005.

47. Emanuel EJ. Ending concerns about undue inducement. *Journal of Law Medicine and Ethics* 32 (2004): 100–105.

48. US Department of Health and Human Services. Office for Human Research Protections (OHRP). Available at: http://www.hhs.gov/ohrp/ index.html.

49. Sullivan MA, Birkmayer F, Boyarsky BK, et al. Uses of coercion in addiction treatment: clinical aspects. *American Journal of Addiction* 17 (2008): 36–47.

50. Newton-Howes G, Mullen R. Coercion in psychiatric care: Systematic review of correlates and themes. *Psychiatric Services* 62 (2011): 465–470.

51. Wertheimer A, Miller FG. Payment for research participation: A coercive offer? *Journal of Medical Ethics* 34 (2008): 389–392.

52. Largent E, Grady G, Miller FG et al. Money, coercion and undue inducement: attitudes about payments to research participants. *IRB* 34.1 (2012a): 1–8.

53. Largent E, Grady G, Miller FG et al. Misconceptions about coercion and undue influence: reflections on the views of IRB members. *Bioethics* (2012b): ePub.

54. Dickert N, Grady C. What's the price of a research subject? Approaches to payment for research participation. *NEJM* 341 (1999): 198–203.

55. Klitzman R, Albala I, Siragusa J, et al. Disclosure of information to potential subject research recruitment web sites. *IRB* 30 (2008): 15–20.

56. Klitzman R, Albala I, Siragusa J, et al. The reporting of monetary compensation in research articles. *Journal of Empirical Research on Human Research Ethics* 2 (2007): 61–67.

57. Barber B. *Science and the social order*. Glencoe, IL: Free Press, 1952.

58. Merton RK. *Social research and the practicing professions*. Lanham, MD: University Press of America, 1982.

59. Douglas M. *Purity and danger*. London: Routledge & Kegan Paul, 1966.

60. McMillan J. Coercive offers and research participation: A comment on Wertheimer and Miller. *Journal of Medical Ethics* 36 (2010): 383–384.

Chapter 4

1. Pronovost P, Neeham D, Berenholtz S, Sinopoli D, Chu H, Cosgrove S, Sexton B, Hyzy R, Welsh R, Roth G, Bander J, Kepros J, Goeschel C. An Intervention to decrease catheter-related bloodstream infections in the ICU. *NEJM* 355 (2006): 2725–2732.

2. Kass N, Pronovost P, Sugarman J, et al. Controversy and quality improvement: Lingering questions about ethics, oversight, and patient safety research. *Joint Commission Journal on Quality and Patient Safety* 34.6 (2008): 350–353.

3. Gawande A. A lifesaving checklist. *New York Times*, December 30, 2007. http://www.nytimes.com/2007/12/30/opinion/30gawande.html?_r=1&oref=slogin. Accessed October 17, 2013.

4. US Department of Health and Human Services, 45 C.F.R. § 46 (2009). Available at: http://www.hhs.gov/ohrp/humansubjects/guidance/45cfr46.html. Accessed December 27, 2012.

5. Fargen KM, Frei D, Fiorella D, et al. The FDA approval process for medical devices: an inherently flawed system or a valuable pathway for innovation? *Journal of NeuroInterventional Surgery* 5.4 (2013): 269–275.

6. Fins JJ, Mayberg HS, Nuttin B, et al. Misuse of the FDA's humanitarian device exemption in deep brain stimulation for obsessive-compulsive disorder. *Health Affairs* 30.2 (2011): 302–311.

7. Gunsalus CK, Bruner EM, Burbules NC, et al. The Illinois White Paper—improving the system for protecting human subjects: counteracting IRB "mission creep." *Qualitative Inquiry*. 13.5 (2007): 617–649.

8. Hamburger P. The new censorship: institutional review boards. *Supreme Court Review* 271 (2004): 271–354.

9. Schrag, Z. *Ethical Imperialism: Institutional Review Boards and the Social Sciences*. Baltimore: Johns Hopkins University Press, 2010.

10. Edwards KL, Lemke AA, Trinidad SB, et al. Attitudes toward genetic research review: Results from a survey of human genetics researchers. *Public Health Genomics* 14.6 (2011): 337–345.

11. Balk EM, Bonis PA, Moskoqitz H, et al. Correlation of quality measures with estimates of treatment effect in meta-analyses of randomized controlled trials. *JAMA* 287.22 (2002): 2973–2982.

12. Olivo Sa, Macedo LG, Gadotti IC, et al. Scales to assess the quality of randomized controlled trials: A systematic review. *Physical Therapy* 88.2 (2008): 156–175.

13. Juni P, Witschi A, Bloch R, Egger M. The hazards of scoring the quality of clinical trials for meta-analysis. *JAMA* 282.11 1999: 1054–1060.

14. Lindsey D. Using citation counts as a measure of quality in science: Measuring what's measurable instead of what's valid. *Scientometrics* 15.3–4 (1989): 189–203.

15. Morse JM, Barrett M, Mayan M, et al. Verification strategies for establishing reliability and validity in qualitative research. *International Journal of Qualitative Methods* 1.2 (2002): 1–19.

16. Groneberg-Kloft B, Fischer TC, Quarcoo D, et al. New quality and quantity indices in science (NewQIS): The study protocol of an international project. *Journal of Occupational Medicine and Toxicology* 4 (2009): 16.

17. RAND Corporation. RAND's standards for high-quality research and analysis. (2011) Available at http://www.rand.org/standards/standards_ high.html Accessed September 24, 2012.

18. Groneberg-Kloft B, Quarcoo D, Scutaru C. Quality and quantity indices in science: Use of visualization tools. *Science and Society* 10.8 (2009): 800–803.

19. Emanuel EJ, Miller FG. The ethics of placebo-controlled trials—a middle ground. *New England Journal of Medicine*. 345.12 (2001): 915–919.

20. Howick J. Questioning the methodological superiority of "placebo" over "active" controlled trials. *The American Journal of Bioethics* 9.9 (2009): 34–38.

21. Angell M. Drug companies and doctors: A story of corruption. *New York Rev Books*; January 15, 2009. http://www.nybooks.com/articles/ archives/2009/jan/15/drug-companies-doctorsa-story-of-corruption/?pa gination=false. Accessed December 17, 2013.

22. Feifel D. The use of placebo-controlled clinical trials for the approval of psychiatric drugs: Part I—Statistics and the case for the "greater good." *Psychiatry MMC* 6.3 (2009): 41–43.

23. Dunlop BW, Banja J. A renewed, ethical defense of placebo-controlled trials of new treatments for major depression and anxiety disorders. *Journal of Medical Ethics* 35 (2009): 384–389.

24. Laughren TP. The scientific and ethical basis for placebo-controlled trials in depression and schizophrenia: An FDA perspective. *European Psychiatry.* 2001;16(7): 418–423.

25. Steinbrook R. Protecting research subjects—the crisis at Johns Hopkins. *New England Journal of Medicine.* 2002; 346(9): 716–720.

Chapter 5

1. Steinbrook R. Protecting research subjects—the crisis at Johns Hopkins. *New England Journal of Medicine.* 346.9 (2002): 716–720.

2. Hexamethonium Chloride for Oral Use; Notice of Withdrawal of Approval of New-Drug Application. *Federal Register* 37.62 (1972): 6510.

3. Katz J. Informed consent—Must it remain a fairy tale? *Journal of Contemporary Health Law and Policy* 69 (1994): 69–91.

4. Albala I, Doyle M, Appelbaum PS. The evolution of consent forms for research: A quarter century of changes. *IRB: Ethics & Human Research* 32.3 (2010): 7–11.

5. US Department of Health and Human Services, 45 C.F.R. § 46 (2009). Available at: http://www.hhs.gov/ohrp/humansubjects/guidance/45cfr46.html. Accessed December 27, 2012.

6. Stark AR, Tyson JE, Hibberd PL. Variation among institutional review boards in evaluating the design of a multicenter randomized trial. *Journal of Perinatology* 30.3 (2009): 163–169.

7. Dziak K, Anderson R, Sevick MA, Weisman CS, Levine DW, Scholle SH. Variations among institutional review boards in a multisite health services research study. *Health Services Research* 40.1 (2005): 279–290.

8. Paasche-Orlow MK, Taylor HA, Brancati F. (2003). Readability standards for informed consent forms as compared with actual readability. *NEJM* 348: 721-726.

9. Baskin P. Academe hath no fury like a fellow professor deceived. *The Chronicle of Higher Education,* May 9, 2010. Available at http://chronicle.com/article/Academe-Hath-No-Fury-Like-a/65466/. Accessed April 18, 2013.

10. Cornell University Media Relations Office. Media statement on Cornell University's role in Facebook "emotional contagion" research. (2014, June 30). http://mediarelations.cornell.edu/2014/06/30/media-statement-on-cornell-universitys-role-in-facebook-emotional-contagion-research/. Accessed August 5, 2014.

11. Amber D. Case at VCU brings ethics to forefront. *The Scientist*, May 1, 2000. Available at http://www.the-scientist.com/?articles.view/articleNo/12810/title/Case-at-VCU-Brings-Ethics-To-Forefront/. Accessed May 1, 2013.

12. US Department of Health and Human Services, 45 C.F.R. § 46 (2009). Available at: http://www.hhs.gov/ohrp/humansubjects/guidance/45cfr46.html. Accessed December 27, 2012.

13. Department of Health and Human Services. Human subjects research protections: Enhancing protections for research subjects and reducing burden, delay, and ambiguity for investigators. *Federal Register* 76.143 (2011): 44512–44531.

14. Klitzman R. Views of the process and content of ethical reviews of HIV vaccine trials among members of US Institutional Review Boards and South African Research Ethics Committees. *Developing World Bioethics* 8.3 (2008) 207–218.

15. Appelbaum PS, Waldman CR, Fyer A, Klitzman R, Parens E, Martinez J, Price N, Chung WK. Informed consent for return of incidental findings in genomic research. *Genetics in Medicine* (2013): ePub.

16. ClinicalTrials.gov. A service of the U.S. National Institutes of Health (2012). Available at: http://www.clinicaltrials.gov/ct2/home.

Chapter 6

1. Olfson M, Marcus SC. Decline in placebo-controlled results suggests new directions for comparative effectiveness research. *Health Affairs* 32.6 (2013): 1116–1125.

2. Manzo AN, Burke JM. Increasing response rate in web-based/internet surveys. In L. Gideon (Ed.), *Handbook of Survey Methodology for the Social Sciences*. New York: Springer Science+Business Media, 2012: 327–343.

3. Melnyk, SA, Page TJ, Wu SJ, Burns LA. Would you mind completing this survey: Assessing the state of survey research in supply chain management. *Journal of Purchasing and Supply Management* 18.1 (2012): 35–45.

4. Kaur S. How IRBs make decisions: Should we worry if they disagree? *Journal of Medical Ethics* (Published online October 17, 2012): doi:10.1136/medethics-2012-100965.

5. McWilliams R, Hoover-Fong J, Hamosh A, et al. Problematic variation in local institutional review of a multicenter genetic epidemiology study. *JAMA* 290.3 (2003): 360–366.

6. Stair TO, Reed CR, Radeos MS, et al. Variation in institutional review board responses to a standard protocol for a multicenter clinical trial. *Academic Emergency Medicine* 8.6 (2001): 636–641.

7. Greene SM, Geiger AM. A review finds that multicenter studies face substantial challenges but strategies exist to achieve Institutional Review Board approval. *Journal of Clinical Epidemiology* 59.8 (2006): 784–790.

8. Jaeger JF. An ethnographic analysis of institutional review board decision-making. (January 1, 2006). Dissertations available from ProQuest. Paper AAI3246172. http://repository.upenn.edu/dissertations/AAI3246172.

9. Diekema DS. Examining the quest to eliminate discrepancies in IRB decisions. *AJOB Primary Research* 2.2 (2011): 34–36.

10. Pinker, S. My genome, myself. *The New York Times* (January 9, 2009). Available at: http://www.nytimes.com/2009/01/11/magazine/11Genome-t.html?pagewanted=all. Accessed August 13, 2012.

11. Bekelman JE, Li Y, Gross CP. Scope and impact of financial conflicts of interest in biomedical research: A systematic review. *JAMA* 289.4 (2003): 454–465.

12. Haidt, J. 2001. The emotional dog and its rational tail: A social intuitionist approach to moral judgment. *Psychological Review* 108: 814–834.

13. Catania JA, Lo B, Wolf LE, et al. Survey of US human research protection organizations: Workload and membership. *Journal of Empirical Research on Human Research Ethics* 3.4 (2008): 57–69.

14. Shah S, Whittle A, Wilfond B, et al. How do institutional review boards apply the federal risk and benefit standards for pediatric research? *JAMA* 291.4 (2004): 476–482.

15. Klitzman R. Views of the process and content of ethical reviews of HIV vaccine trials among members of US Institutional Review Boards and South African Research Ethics Committees. *Developing World Bioethics* 8.3 (2008): 207–218.

16. Rich W, Finer NN, Gantz MG, Newman NS, Hensman AM, Hale EC, Auten KJ, Schibler K, Faix RG, Laptook AR, Yoder BA, Das A, Shankaran S; SUPPORT and Generic Database Subcommittees of the Eunice Kennedy Shriver National Institute of Child Health and Human Development Neonatal Research Network. Enrollment of extremely low birth weight infants in a clinical research study may not be representative. *Pediatrics* 129.3 (2012): 480–484.

Chapter 7

1. Emirbayer M. Manifesto for a relational sociology. *American Journal of Sociology* 103.2 (1997): 281–317.

2. Von Bertalanffy L. An outline of general system theory. *The British Journal for the Philosophy of Science* 1.2 (1950): 134–165.

3. Begun JW, Zimmerman B, Dooley K. Health care organizations as complex adaptive systems. In: Mick SM, Wyttenbach M, Eds. *Advances in Health Care Organization Theory*. San Francisco: Jossey-Bass, 2003: 253–288.

4. Parsons T. *The Social System*. Glencoe, Illinois: Free Press, 1951.

5. Silbey SS. The sociological citizen: Pragmatic and relational regulation in law and organizations. *Regulation & Governance* 5.1 (2011): 1–13.

6. Endicott T. Law is necessarily vague. *Legal Theory* 7.4 (2001): 389–385.

7. Bellis MD. The illusion of clarity: A critique of "pure" clarity using examples drawn from judicial interpretations of the Constitution of the United States. In: Wagner A, Cacciaguidi-Fahy, S, Eds. *Obscurity and Clarity in the Law: Prospects and Challenges*. United Kingdom: Ashgate Publishing Ltd., 2008.

8. Klitzman R. Local IRBs *vs.* federal agencies: Shifting dynamics, systems, and relationships. *Journal of Empirical Research on Human Ethics* 7.3 (2012): 50–62.

9. US Department of Health & Human Services Office of Extramural Research. Frequently Asked Questions From Applicants: Human Subjects Research—Exemptions (2010). Available at http://grants.nih.gov/grants/policy/hs/faqs_aps_exempt.htm#635. Accessed December 27, 2012.

10. The Health Insurance Portability and Accountability Act (HIPAA) (1996). Available at http://www.hhs.gov/ocr/privacy/index.html. Accessed August 11, 2013.

11. Kevles DJ. *The Baltimore Case: A Trial of Politics, Science, and Character*. New York: W.W. Norton & Company, 1998.

12. Emanuel EJ, Menikoff J. Reforming the regulations governing research with human subjects. *NEJM* 365 (2011): 1145–1150.

13. Zern COH. Is the customer always right? Department of Health and Human Services' proposed regulations allow institutional review boards to place customer service ahead of the welfare of research participants. *Saint Louis University Public Law Review* 32 (2013): 411–446.

14. Resnik DB. Liability for institutional review boards: From regulation to litigation. *The Journal of Legal Medicine* 25 (2004): 131–184.

15. Hoffman S. Berg JW. The suitability of IRB liability. *University of Pittsburgh Law Review* 67 (2005-2006): 365–427.

16. Schrag ZM. *Ethical Imperialism: Institutional Review Boards and the Social Sciences, 1965-2009*. Baltimore: The Johns Hopkins University Press, 2010.

17. Heimer CA, Petty J. Bureaucratic ethics: IRBs and the legal regulation of human subjects research. *Annual Review of Law and Social Science* 6.1 (2010): 601–626.

18. Hamburger P. The new censorship: Institutional review boards. *Supreme Court Review* 1 (2004): 271–354.

19. Keith-Spiegel P, Koocher GP. The IRB paradox: Could the protectors also encourage deceit? *Ethics & Behavior* 15.4 (2005): 339–349.

20. US Department of Health and Human Services. Human subjects research protections: Enhancing protections for research subjects and reducing burden, delay, and ambiguity for investigators. *Federal Register* 76.143 (2011): 44512–44531.

Chapter 8

1. Steinbrook R. The Gelsinger case. In Emanuel EJ, Grady C, Crouch RA et al., eds. *The Oxford Textbook of Clinical Research Ethics*. New York: Oxford University Press, 2008.

2. Dorsey ER, de Roulet J, Thompson JP, Reminick JI, Thai A, White-Stellato Z, Beck CA, George BP, Moses H. Funding of US biomedical research, 2003-2008. *JAMA* 303.2 (2010): 137–143.

3. http://www.faseb.org/portals/2/PDFs/opa/5.16.13%20NIH%20 Funding%20Cuts%202-pager.pdf

4. http://www.researchamerica.org/uploads/healthdollar12.pdf

5. The Bayh-Dole Act. Pub. L. No. 96-517 (December 12, 1980). Available at http://www.gpo.gov/fdsys/pkg/CFR-2002-title37-vol1/content-detail. html. Accessed July 22, 2013.

6. Blumenthal D, Campbell EG, Causino N, Louis KS. Participation of life-science faculty in research relationships with industry. *NEJM* 335 (1996): 1734–1739.

7. Welsh R, Glenna L, Lacy W, Biscotti D. Close but not too far: Assessing the effects of the university–industry relationships and the rise of academic capitalism. *Research Policy* 37 (2008): 1854–1864.

8. Bourgeius FT, Murthy S, Mandl KD. Outcome reporting among drug trials registered in Clinicaltrials.gov. *Annals of Internal Medicine* 153.3 (2010): 158–166.

9. Editorial Board. In science we trust. *Nature Medicine* 7.8 (2001): 871.

10. Bekelman JE, Li Y, Gross CP. Scope and impact of financial conflicts of interest in biomedical research: A systematic review. *JAMA* 289 (2003): 454–465.

11. US Department of Health and Human Services, 45 C.F.R. § 46 (2009) Available at: http://www.hhs.gov/ohrp/humansubjects/ guidance/45cfr46.html. Accessed December 27, 2012.

12. Weinfurt KP, Hall MA, Hardy NC, et al. Oversight of financial conflicts of interest in commercially sponsored research in academic and nonacademic settings. *Journal of General Internal Medicine* 25.5 (2010): 460–464.

13. Hall MA, Weinfurt KP, Lawlor JS, et al. Community hospital oversight of clinical investigators' financial relationships. *IRB: Ethics & Human Research* 31.1 (2009): 7–13.

14. Vogeli C, Koski G, Campbell EG. Policies and management of conflicts of interest within medical research institutional review boards: Results of a national study. *Academic Medicine* 84.4 (2009): 488–494.

15. Markman M. "Conflict-of-interest" and participation in IRB deliberations: An alternative perspective. *Cancer Investigation* 26.2 (2008): 115–117.

16. Psaty BM, Burke SP. Protecting the Health of the Public—Institute of Medicine recommendations on drug safety. *NEJM 355.17* (2006): 1753–1755.

17. Sox HC, Rennie D. Seeding trials: just say "no." *Annals of Internal Medicine* 149.4 (2008): 279–281.

18. Hall MA, Friedman JY, King NMP, et al. Per capita payments in clinical trials: reasonable costs versus bounty hunting. *Academic Medicine* 85.10 (2010): 1554–1556.

19. Glasser SP, Salas M, Delzell E. Importance and challenges of studying marketed drugs: What is a Phase IV study? *Journal of Clinical Pharmacology* 47.9 (2007): 1074–1086.

20. Katz K. Time to nip "seeding trials" in the bud. *Archives of Dermatology* 144.3 (2008): 403–404.

21. Emanuel EJ, Wendler D, Grady C. What makes clinical research ethical? *JAMA.* 283.20 (2000): 2701–2711.

22. Wynia M, Boren D. Better regulation of industry-sponsored clinical trials is long overdue. *Journal of Law, Medicine and Ethics* 37.3 (2009): 410–419.

23. Cauchon D. FDA advisers tied to industry. *USA Today,* September 25, 2000. Available at http://www.commondreams.org/headlines/092500-01.htm. Accessed December 28, 2012.

24. Lurie P, Almeida CM, Stine N, et al. Financial conflict of interest disclosure and voting patterns and Food and Drug Administration Drug Advisory Committee meetings. *JAMA.* 295.16 (2006): 1921–1928.

25. Institute of Medicine (US) Committee on Assessing the System for Protecting Human Research Participants; Federman DD, Hanna KE, Rodriguez LL, Eds. *Responsible research: A systems approach to protecting research participants.* Washington DC: National Academies Press, 2002.

26. Responsibility of applicants for promoting objectivity in research for which public health service funding is sought and responsible prospective contractors; HHS Final Rule. 76 Fed. Reg. 53256 (August 25, 2011) (to be codified at 42 C.F.R 50, 45 C.F.R 94).

27. The Institute of Internal Auditors (IIA). Available at https://na.theiia.org/Pages/IIAHome.aspx.

28. Grant G, Guyton O, Forrester R. Creating effective research compliance programs in academic institutions. *Academic Medicine* 74.9 (1999): 951–971.

29. Iserson KV, Cerfolio RJ, Sade RM. Politely refuse the pen and note pad: Gifts from industry to physicians harm patients. *Annals of Thoracic Surgery*. 84.4 (2007): 1077–1084.

30. Licurse A, Barber E, Joffe S, Gross C. The impact of disclosing financial ties in research and clinical care: A systematic review. *Archives of Internal Medicine* 170.8 (2010): 675–682.

31. Grattini S, Bertele V. Non-inferiority trials are unethical because they disregard patients' interests. *The Lancet* 370 (2007): 1875–1877.

32. Chuang-Stein C, Beltangady M, Dunne M, et al. The ethics of non-inferiority trials. *The Lancet* 371 (2008): 895–896.

33. Piaggio G, Elbourne DR, Altman DG, et al. Reporting of non-inferiority and equivalence randomized trials: An extension of the CONSORT statement. *JAMA* 295.10 (2006): 1152–1160.

34. Wangge G, Klungel OH, Roes KCB, et al. Room for improvement in documenting and reporting non-inferiority randomized controlled trials on drugs: A systematic review. *PLoS ONE* 5.10 (2010).

35. Appelbaum P, Roth LH, Lidz CW, et al. False hopes and best data: Consent to research and the therapeutic misconception. *Hastings Center Reports* 17.2 (1987): 20–24.

36. Department of Health, Education, and Welfare, *The Belmont report: Ethical principles and guidelines for the protection of human subjects of research*, Washington, DC: OPRR Reports, 1979. Available at: http://ohsr.od.nih.gov/guidelines/belmont.html.

Chapter 9

1. Renwick RB. In a scandal's wake: An interview with Dr. Nancy Olivieri. *University of Toronto Medical Journal* 81.3 (2004): 196–199.

2. Emirbayer M. Manifesto for a relational sociology. *American Journal of Sociology* 103.2 (1997): 281–317.

3. Silbey SS. The sociological citizen: Pragmatic and relational regulation in law and organizations. *Regulation & Governance* 5.1 (2011): 1–13.

4. Speckman JL, Byrne MM, Gerson J, et al. Determining the costs of institutional review boards. *IRB: Ethics & Human Research* 29.2 (2007): 7–13.

5. Wagner TH, Bhandari A, Chadwick GL, Nelson DK. The cost of operating institutional review boards (IRBs). *Academic Medicine* 78.6 (2003): 638–644.

6. Woodward B. Challenges to human subject protections in US medical research. *JAMA* 282.20 (1999): 1947–1952.

7. Department of Health and Human Services. Human subjects research protections: Enhancing protections for research subjects and reducing burden, delay, and ambiguity for investigators. *Federal Register* 76.143 (2011): 44512–44531.

8. Emanuel EJ, Menikoff J. Reforming the regulations governing research with human subjects. *NEJM* 365 (2011): 1145–1150.

9. Vogeli C, Koski G, Campbell EG. Policies and management of conflicts of interest within medical research institutional review boards: Results of a national study. *Academic Medicine* 84.4 (2009): 488–494.

10. Horrobin DF. Non-financial conflicts of interest are more serious than financial conflicts. *BMJ* 318 (1999): 466.

11. Maj M. Non-financial conflicts of interests in psychiatric research and practice. *British Journal of Psychiatry* 193.2 (2008): 91–92.

12. Kesselheim AS, Maisel WH. Managing financial and nonfinancial conflicts of interest in healthcare delivery. *American Journal of Therapeutics*. 17.4 (2010): 440–443.

13. Levinsky NG. Nonfinancial conflicts of interest in research. *NEJM* 347.10 (2002): 759–761.

14. Sollitto S, Hoffman S, Mehlman M, et al. Intrinsic conflicts of interest in clinical research: A need for disclosure. *Kennedy Institute of Ethics Journal* 13.2 (2003): 83–91.

15. Emanuel EJ, Lemmens T, Elliot C. Should society allow research ethics boards to be run as for-profit enterprises? *PLoS Medicine* 3.7 (2006): e309.

Chapter 10

1. Gunsalus CK, Bruner EM, Burbules NC, et al. Mission creep in the IRB world. *Science* 312 (2006): 1441.

2. Burris S, Moss K. U.S. health researchers review their ethics review boards: A qualitative study. *Journal of Empirical Research on Human Research Ethics* 1.2 (2006): 39–58.

3. Bell J, Whiton J, Connelly S. *Final Report: Evaluation of NIH Implementation of Section 491 of the Public Health Service Act, Mandating a Program of Protection for Research Subjects.* Arlington, VA: James Bell Associates, 1998.

4. Klitzman R. The myth of community differences as the cause of discrepancies between IRBs. *American Journal of Bioethics* 2.2 (2011): 24–33.

5. Bass S. Policing space, policing race: Social control imperatives and police discretionary decisions. *Social Justice* 28.1 (2001): 156–176.

6. Tyler T, Kramer R. Whither trust? In R. Kramer and T. Tyler, Eds. *Trust in Organizations*. Thousand Oaks, CA: Sage, 1996.

7. Weber M. *Economy and Society* (Posthumously published 1920–1921). Berkeley, CA: University of Southern California Press, 1978.

8. Merton RK. *Social Theory and Social Structure*. Glencoe, IL: Free Press, 1957, pp. 195–206.

9. Hardin R. *Trust and Trustworthiness*. New York: Russell Sage Foundation, 2002.

10. Burris S. Regulatory innovation in the governance of human subjects research: A cautionary tale and some modest proposals. *Regulation & Governance* 2.1 (2008): 65–84.

11. Keith-Spiegel P, Koocher GP, Tabachnick B. What scientists want from their research ethics committees. *Journal of Empirical Research Human Research Ethics* 1.1 (2006): 67–82.

12. Koerner AF. Communication scholars' communication and relationship with their IRBs. *Journal of Applied Communication Research* 33.3 (2005): 231–241.

13. Burris S, Moss K. US health researchers review their ethics review boards: A qualitative study. *Journal of Empirical Research Human Research Ethics* 1.2 (2006): 39–58.

14. Aristotle (Saunders TJ, ed.). *The Politics* (350 B.C.). New York: Penguin Classics, 1981.

15. Hamilton A, Madison J, Jay J. *The Federalist Papers*. (1787-1788). Available at http://www.foundingfathers.info/federalistpapers/. Accessed January 3, 2013.

16. Emanuel EJ, Menikoff J. Reforming the regulations governing research with human subjects. *NEJM* 365 (2011): 1145–1150.

17. Ahmed AH, Nicholson KG. Delays and diversity in the practice of local research ethics committees. *Journal of Medical Ethics* 22.5 (1996): 263–266.

18. Millum J, Menikoff J. Streamlining ethical review. *Ann Intern Med.* 153.10 (2010): 655–657.

Chapter 11

1. Wakefield AJ, Murch SH, Anthony A et al. Ileal-lymphoid-nodular hyperplasia, non-specific colitis, and pervasive developmental disorder in children. *Lancet* 351 (1998): 637–641. (Retracted).

2. Ross O. Andrew Wakefield's fraudulent vaccine research. *The Star* (Toronto), January 7, 2011. Accessed September 4, 2012.

3. The Associated Press. Disgraced Korean cloning scientist indicted. *The New York Times*, May 12, 2006. http://www.nytimes.com/2006/05/12/world/asia/12korea.html. Accessed September 4, 2012.

4. Kennedy D. Responding to fraud. *Science* 314 (2006): 1353.

5. Heath E. The IRB's monitoring function: Four concepts of monitoring. *IRB: Ethics and Human Research* 1.5 (1979): 1-3+12.

6. Weijer C, Shapiro S, Fuks A, Glass KC, Skrutkowska M. Monitoring clinical research: An obligation unfulfilled. *Canadian Medical Association Journal* 152.12 (1995): 1973–1980.

7. Stevenson A, Siefring J, Brown L, Trumble WR, Eds. *Oxford English Dictionary*. Oxford: Oxford University Press, 2002.

8. Office of Research Integrity. US Department of Health and Human Services. Available at http://ori.hhs.gov/research/extra/index.shtml Accessed September 8, 2005.

9. Martinson B, Anderson M, de Vries R. Scientists behaving badly. *Nature* 435.9 (2005): 737–738.

10. Greene SM, Geiger AM. A review finds that multicenter studies face substantial challenges but strategies exist to achieve Institutional Review Board approval. *Journal of Clinical Epidemiology* 59.8 (2006): 784–790.

11. Jones J, White L, Pool L, Dougherty J. Structure and practice of institutional review boards in the United States. *Academic Emergency Medicine* 3.8 (1996): 804–809.

12. Parsons T. *The Social System*. Glencoe, Illinois: Free Press, 1951.

13. Korenman SG, Berk R, Wenger NS, Lew V. Evaluation of the research norms of scientists and administrators responsible for academic research integrity. *JAMA* 279.1 (1998): 41–47.

14. Koocher, GP. 2005. The IRB paradox: Could the protectors also encourage deceit? *Ethics & Behavior* 15.4 (2005): 339–349.

15. Mello M, Clarridge B, Studdert D. Academic medical centers' standards for clinical-trial agreements with industry. *NEJM* 352.21 (2005): 2202–2210.

16. Koocher G, Keith-Speigel P. *IRB Researcher Assessment Tool (IRB-RAT): A Users Guide*. Boston: Harvard Medical School, 2005.

17. Kifner J. Scholar sets off gastronomic false alarm. *The New York Times*, September 8, 2001. Available at http://www.nytimes.com/2001/09/08/nyregion/scholar-sets-off-gastronomic-false-alarm.html. Accessed April 16, 2013.

18. Burris S, Moss K. U.S. health researchers review their ethics review boards: A qualitative study. *Journal of Empirical Research on Human Research Ethics* 1.2 (2006): 39–58.

19. Leonard NH, Beauvais LL, Scholl RW. Work motivation: The incorporation of self-concept-based processes. *Human Relations* 52.8 (1999): 969–998.

20. Keith-Spiegel P, Koocher GP. The IRB paradox: Could the protectors also encourage deceit? *Ethics & Behavior* 15.4 (2005): 339–349.

21. Merton RK. Social structure and anomie. *American Sociological Review* 3.5 (1938): 672–682.

22. Institute of Medicine (US) Committee on Assessing the System for Protecting Human Research Participants; Federman DD, Hanna KE, Rodriguez LL, Eds. *Responsible research: A systems approach to protecting research participants.* Washington DC: National Academies Press, 2002.

23. Nagel T. Concealment and exposure. *Philosophy and Public Affairs* 27.1 (1998): 3–30.

24. Callahan ES, Dworkin TM. The state of state whistleblower protection. *American Business Law Journal* 38.1 (2000): 99–175.

25. Katz D, Kahn RL. *The Social Psychology of Organizations.* New York: Wiley, 1996.

Chapter 12

1. Stephens J. Cable: Pfizer hired investigators to press Nigeria to drop suit. *Washington Post.* December 12, 2010. Available at http://www.washingtonpost.com/wp-dyn/content/article/2010/12/11/AR2010121102884.html. Accessed October 14, 2013

2. Stephens J. Where profits and lives hang in the balance. *Washington Post.* December 17, 2000. Available at http://www.washingtonpost.com/wp-dyn/content/story/2008/10/01/ST2008100101390.html Accessed October 14, 2013.

3. Leaked Cable is reprinted in full at http://www.theguardian.com/world/us-embassy-cables-documents/203205?guni=Article:in%20body%20link.

4. Thomas K. Drug research in China falls under cloud. *The New York Times,* July 22, 2013. Available at http://www.nytimes.com/2013/07/23/business/global/drug-research-in-china-falls-under-a-cloud.html?pagewanted=all&_r=0.

5. Samson K. Glaxo under fire over MS clinical trial allegations at R&D center in China. *Neurology Today* 13.17 (2013): 42–43

6. Angell M. Investigators' responsibilities for human subjects in developing countries *NEJM* 342 (2000): 967–969.

7. Kass NE, Hyder AA, Ajuwon A, et al. The structure and function of research ethics committees in Africa: A case study. *PLoS Medicine* 4.1 (2007): e3.

8. Nyika A, Kilama W, Chilengi R, et al. Composition, training needs and independence of ethics review committees across Africa: Are the gate-keepers rising to the emerging challenges? *Journal of Medical Ethics* 35.3 2009: 189–193.

9. Bhan A, Desikan P, Swarnalakshmi S, Kalantri SP. Process, pitfalls and probity: Sharing experiences on setting up and running ethics committees in India. *Indian Journal of Medical Ethics* 7.1 (2010): 48–51.

10. Rivera R, Ezcurra E. Composition and operation of selected research ethics review committees in Latin America. *IRB: Ethics & Human Research* 23.5 (2001): 9–12.

11. Bartlett EE. International analysis of institutional review boards registered with the US Office for Human Research Protections. *Journal of Empirical Research Human Research Ethics* 3 (2008): 49–56.

12. Kirigia JM, Wambebe C, Baba-Moussa A. Status of national research bioethics committees in the WHO African region. *BMC Medical Ethics* 6 (2005): 10.

13. Ikingura JKB, Kruger M, Zeleke W. Health research ethics review and needs of institutional ethics committees in Tanzania. *Tanzania Health Research Bulletin* 9.3 (2007): 154–158.

14. Klitzman R. Views of the process and content of ethical reviews of HIV vaccine trials among members of US institutional review boards and South African research ethics committees. *Developing World Bioethics* 8.3 (2008): 207–218.

15. Sugarman J, Popkin B, Fortney J, Rivera R. Ethical and Policy Issues in International Research: Clinical Trials in Developing Countries. Bethesda, MD: Report and Recommendations of the National Bioethics Advisory Commission. *International perspectives on protecting human research subjects*, Commissioned paper (2001): E1–E11.

16. Klitzman R. The importance of social, cultural and economic contexts, and empirical research in examining "undue inducement." *The American Journal of Bioethics* 5.6 (2005): 56–58.

17. Mystakidou K, Panagiotou I, Katsaragakis S, Tsilika E, Parpa E. Ethical and practical challenges in implementing informed consent in HIV/AIDS clinical trials in developing or resource-limited countries. *Journal of Social Aspects of HIV/AIDS* 6.2 (2009): 46–57.

18. Krosin M, Klitzman R, Levin B, Cheng J, Ranney ML. Problems in comprehension of informed consent in rural and peri-urban Mali, West Africa. *Clinical Trials* 3.3 (2006): 306–313.

19. Klitzman R. US IRBs confronting research in the developing world. *Developing World Bioethics* 12.2 (2012): 63–73.

20. Wichman A, Smith J, Mills D, Sandler AL. Collaborative research involving human subjects: A survey of researchers using international single project assurances. *IRB* 19.1 (1997): 1–6.

21. Chin LJ, Rifai-Bashjawish H, Kleinert K, Saltman A, Leu C-S, Klitzman R. HIV/AIDS research conducted in the developing world and sponsored by the developed world: Reporting of research ethics committee review in two countries. *Journal of Empirical Research on Human Research Ethics* 6.3 (2011): 83–91.

22. Angell M. Ethical imperialism? Ethics in international collaborative clinical research. *New England Journal of Medicine* 319.16 (1988): 1081–1083.

23. Said EW. *Culture and Imperialism* (1993). New York: Alfred A. Knopf, 1994.

24. Connor EM, Sperling RS, Gelber R, Kiselev P, Scott G, O'Sullivan MJ, Balsley J. Reduction of maternal-infant transmission of human immunodeficiency virus type 1 with zidovudine treatment. *NEJM* 331.18 (1994): 1173–1180.

25. Bayer R. The debate over maternal-fetal HIV transmission prevention trials in Africa, Asia, and the Caribbean: Racist exploitation or exploitation of racism? *American Journal of Public Health* 88.4 (1998): 567–570.

26. Sawires SR., Dworkin SL, Fiamma AF, Peacock D, Szekeres G, Coates TJ. Male circumcision and HIV/AIDS: Challenges and opportunities. *Lancet* 369 (2007): 708–713.

27. Fogarty International Center. Available at: http://www.fic.nih.gov/Pages/Default.aspx.

28. Gazzinelli MF, Lobato L, Matoso L, et al. Health education through analogies: Preparation of a community for clinical trials of a vaccine against hookworm in an endemic area of Brazil. *PLoS Neglected Tropical Diseases* 4.7 (2010): 1–12.

29. Sarkar R, Sowmyanarayanan TV, Samuel P, et al. Comparison of group counseling with individual counseling in the comprehension of informed consent: A randomized controlled trial. *BMC Medical Ethics* 11.8 (2010).

30. Sexton P, Hui K, Hanrahan D, Barnes M, Sugarman J, London AJ, Klitzman R. The roles of governmental agencies in emerging economies in reviewing HIV related research. *Developing World Bioethics*, (Published online 10 November 2014): DOI: 10.1111/dewb.12072.

31. Hanrahan D, Sexton P, Hui K, Teitcher J, Klitzman R. Linguistic and cultural challenges in translating informed consent in US-sponsored HIV prevention research in emerging economies. (Submitted for publication).

Chapter 13

1. Office for Human Research Protections (OHRP). Available at http://www.hhs.gov/ohrp/. Accessed March 12, 2014.

2. Greene SM, Geiger AM. A review finds that multicenter studies face substantial challenges but strategies exist to achieve Institutional Review Board approval. *Journal of Clinical Epidemiology* 59.8 (2006): 784–790.

3. Hedgecoe A, Carvalho F, Lobmayer P, Raka F. Research ethics committees in Europe: Implementing the directive, respecting diversity. *Journal of Medical Ethics* 32.8 (2006): 483–486.

4. Christey S. Impact of EU clinical trial directive. *European Journal of Cancer* 37.15 (2001): 1805.

5. Porcu L, Poli D, Torri V, et al. Impact of recent legislative bills regarding clinical research on Italian ethics committee activity. *Journal of Medical Ethics* 34.10 (2008): 747–750.

6. Simek J, Zamykalova L, Mesanyova M. Ethics committee or community? Examining the identity of Czech Ethics Committees in the period of transition. *Journal of Medical Ethics* 36.9 (2010): 548–552.

7. European Parliament. Directive 2001/20/EC of the European Parliament and of the Council of 4 April 2001 on the approximation of the laws, regulations and administrative provisions of the Member States relating to the implementation of good clinical practice in the conduct of clinical trials on medicinal products for human use. *Official Journal of the European Communities* L121 (2001): 34–44.

8. Menikoff J. The paradoxical problem with multiple-IRB review. *New England Journal of Medicine* 363.17 (2010): 1591–1593.

9. Ahmed AH, Nicholson KG. Delays and diversity in the practice of local research ethics committees. *Journal of Medical Ethics* 22.5 (1996): 263–266.

10. Christian MC, Goldberg JL, Killen J, et al. A central institutional review board for multi-institutional trials. *New England Journal of Medicine* 346.18 (2002): 1405–1408.

11. The National Cancer Institute. Current status of the CIRBs. Available at https://ncicirb.org/cirb/project.action. Accessed March 11, 2014.

12. Wagner TH, Murray C, Goldberg J, Adler JM, Abrams J. Costs and benefits of the National Cancer Institute Central Institutional Review Board. *Journal of Clinical Oncology* 28.4 (2010): 662–666.

13. Loh ED, Meyer RE. Medical schools' attitudes and perceptions regarding the use of central institutional review boards. *Academic Medicine* 79.7 (2004): 644–651.

14. Iserson KV, Cerfolio RJ, Sade RM. Politely refuse the pen and note pad: Gifts from industry to physicians harm patients. *The Annals of Thoracic Surgery* 4.4 (2007): 1077–1084.

15. Department of Health and Human Services. Human subjects research protections: Enhancing protections for research subjects and reducing burden, delay, and ambiguity for investigators. *Federal Register* 76.143 (2011): 44512–44531.

16. Klitzman R, Appelbaum PS. To protect human subjects, review what was done, not proposed. *Science* 335 (2012):1576–1577.

17. IRB Forum. Available at http://www.irbforum.org/. Accessed March 11, 2014.

18. Lantos J. It is time to professionalize Institutional Review Boards. *Archives of Pediatrics & Adolescent Medicine* 163.12 (2009): 1163–1164.

Chapter 14

1. Beecher HK. Ethics and clinical research. *New England Journal of Medicine* 274.4 (1966): 1354–1360.

2. Diekema DS. Examining the quest to eliminate discrepancies in IRB decisions. *AJOB Primary Research* 2.2 (2011): 34–36.

3. Dziak K, Anderson R, Sevick MA, Weisman CS, Levine DW, Scholle SH. Variations among institutional review boards in a multisite health services research study. *Health Services Research* 40.1 (2005): 279–290.

4. Fox RC, Swazey JP. *Observing Bioethics*. New York: Oxford University Press, 2008.

5. Charon R. *Narrative Medicine*. New York, Oxford University Press, 2006.

6. Churchill WS. Speech in the House of Commons. November 11, 1947. *Winston S. Churchill: His Complete Speeches, 1897–1963*, Ed. Robert Rhodes James, vol. 7. New York: Chelsea House, 1974: 7566.

Appendix A

1. Geertz C. *Interpretation of Cultures*. New York: Basic Books, 1973.

2. Strauss A. Corbin J. *Basics of qualitative research-techniques and procedures for developing grounded theory*. Sage Publications; Newbury Park, CA: 1990.

INDEX